PSYCHOLOGICAL FACTORS AND CARDIOVASCULAR DISORDERS: THE ROLE OF PSYCHIATRIC PATHOLOGY AND MALADAPTIVE PERSONALITY FEATURES

Psychological Factors and Cardiovascular Disorders: The Role of Psychiatric Pathology and Maladaptive Personality Features

Leo Sher
Editor

2008

Nova Biomedical Books
New York

For permission to use material from this book please contact us:
Telephone 631-231-7269; Fax 631-231-8175
Web Site: http://www.novapublishers.com

NOTICE TO THE READER

LIBRARY OF CONGRESS CATALOGING-IN-PUBLICATION DATA

Psychological factors and cardiovascular disorders : the role of psychiatric pathology and maladaptive personality features / Leo Sher, editor.   p. ; cm.
Includes bibliographical references and index.
ISBN 978-1-60456-871-4 (hardcover)
1. Cardiovascular system--Diseases--Psychosomatic aspects. I. Sher, Leo.
[DNLM: 1. Cardiovascular Diseases--etiology. 2. Cardiovascular Diseases--complications. 3. Cardiovascular Diseases--psychology. 4. Mental Disorders--complications. 5. Mental Disorders--psychology. WG 120 P974 2008]
RC669.P76 2008
616.1001'9--dc22   2008023216

Published by Nova Science Publishers, Inc. ✦ New York

CONTENTS

PREFACE

Psychiatric disorders and certain personality features are frequently associated with cardiovascular disorders. For the past several decades attention to the psychosocial and behavioral factors in cardiovascular disease has increased significantly. Understanding the integration of the interactions among multiple psychological and biological factors in the regulation of the cardiovascular system and the development of cardiovascular disorders is an important challenge for future research. I hope that this book will contribute to this goal. The contributors to this book are the leading international experts in the field of the relation between psychological processes and cardiovascular disorders. I would like to acknowledge and thank all the contributors. My task as the editor was greatly facilitated by their swift and positive response to my initial inquiry, and thereafter by producing their manuscripts diligently. I believe that this book will be of interest to clinicians, researchers, and the general public. This book is dedicated to the Memory of my Parents, Ivetta Sher (1927-2007) and Aleksandr Sher (1926-2008).

Leo Sher
April 2008

In: Psychological Factors and Cardiovascular Disorders   ISBN: 978-1-60456-871-4

Editor: Leo Sher   © 2008 Nova Science Publishers, Inc.

Chapter I

ROLE OF PSYCHOLOGICAL RISK FACTORS IN PATHOGENESIS OF CORONARY ARTERY DISEASE

Rajesh Vijayvergiya

Department of Cardiology, Post Graduate Institute of Medical Education and Research, Chandigarh, India.

ABSTRACT

Chronic psychosocial factors like depression, anxiety and cognitive disorders play an important role in pathogenesis of atherosclerotic coronary artery disease (CAD). These factors are frequently observed in CAD patients and in healthy individuals who are prone to develop CAD. The evidences based on observational, case control and epidemiological studies are sufficient to establish their significant contribution in atherosclerotic cardiovascular diseases. The common patho-physiological mechanism of adverse cardiovascular outcome is related with hypothalamic-adrenocortical and sympatho-adrenal system stimulation, which resulted in acute coronary syndrome, arrhythmias and sudden cardiac death. For management of these patients, there is a need for integrated psychosocial intervention including individual or group psychotherapy, support and stress reduction in cardiac patients and healthy individuals. As psychosocial interventions needs persistent perusal, chronic & regular follow-up session with the patients, patient specific treatment strategy, antidepressant pharmacotherapy and integration with de-addiction, physiotherapy department and various social organizations; there should be combined approach of clinical psychiatrist and primary physician in management of these patients. Behavioral risk factors for CAD such as smoking, overweight, physical inactivity, overeating, and non–compliance to drug treatment for CAD and its risk factors like hypertension, diabetes mellitus, dyslipidemia needs the active and coordinated interdisciplinary approach for prevention of adverse cardiac outcome in these patients.

INTRODUCTION

Psychosocial factors play an important role in onset and progression of coronary artery disease (CAD). There is enough literature evidence to establish their significant contribution in pathogenesis of CAD. Depression, anxiety and cognitive disorders are few of the psychiatric problems which frequently occur as the complications or association with cardiovascular diseases. These factors have the multi-organ effects; hence their strength of association with cardiovascular diseases might be under estimated in various epidemiological studies. In the present chapter, the role of chronic and acute psychological factors in pathogenesis of cardiovascular diseases especially of CAD will be discussed.

CHRONIC PSYCHOLOGICAL FACTORS

1. Depression and Related Syndromes

Depression is an important psychosocial predictor of CAD onset and progression [1]. The major depression in CAD patients is about 3 fold higher than its prevalence in the general community [2]. Recent epidemiological studies evaluating the relationship between depression and CAD among healthy [3-6] and CAD [7-10] populations consistently demonstrate a significant prospective relationship between the occurrence of major depression episodes and the incidence of cardiac events. There is a continuous, linear relationship between the severity of depression and the risk of subsequent cardiac events [11]. Even the minor depressive symptoms not enough to be defined as major depression, is associated with increased cardiac events [7]. Clinically significant depression is present in 40 to 65% of patients following myocardial infarction, and major depression is found in 15-25% of such patients [12,13]. In one study, 31.5% patients experienced major depression during 1 year following myocardial infarction [14]. It is twice high in women with CAD than in men. It increases the risk of reinfarction, cardiac arrest and death following myocardial infarction [11,12,14]. Depressed individual also have exaggerated cardiac symptoms, decreased exercise capacity, poor compliance to drugs & cardiac rehabilitation therapy [15]. In conclusion, depression is a negative prognostic marker for CAD patients and a risk factor for development of CAD in healthy individuals. It is associated with increased morbidity, mortality, disability and impaired quality of life. The degree of risk associated with major depression is equivalent to conventional risk factor for development of CAD. In a recent meta-analysis, major depression is also prevalent in at least 1 out of 5 heart failure patients; the incidence of mortality, clinical events, rehospitalization, and general health care was markedly higher in patients with more sever depression [16]. There is also a relationship between hopelessness- one of the manifestations of depression, with development of CAD [17] and sudden cardiac death [18]. It also contributes to accelerated progression of carotid atherosclerosis, particularly among men with early evidence of atherosclerosis [19]. Among the various depressive symptoms, hopelessness is the most cardiotoxic and associated with a more than three-fold risk of clinical events 2 years following coronary angioplasty [20]. Another related phenomenon of "vital exhaustion" characterized by triad of fatigue, irritability, and demoralized feelings is also being reported to predict cardiac events in healthy and CAD populations [21,22]. It is also observed that individuals who are hostile or of type A behavior are more prone to have vital exhaustion following exposure to prolonged and uncontrolled psychological stress.

The patho-physiological mechanism of depression's association with CAD is explained by hyperactivity of hypothalamic-adrenocortical and sympatho-adrenal system. There is hypercortisolemia, attenuation of adrenocorticotropin hormone response to corticotropin-releasing factor, and nonsuppression of cortisol secretion after dexamethosone administration [23]. Hypercortisolemia is atherogenic and causes high blood pressure, increases cholesterol and free fatty acids [23]. It also causes endothelial dysfunction [24]. In addition, there is increase level of catecholamines which causes tachycardia, high blood pressure and increase cardiac workload [25]. There is imbalance between vagal and sympathetic tone, reduced heart rate variability, which can explain the enhanced arrhythmogenic potential and sudden cardiac death in these individuals [26]. They also have significant impairments in platelet function, including enhanced platelet reactivity/aggregation and release of platelet factor 4 and ß-thromboglobulin [27]. The combination of endothelial dysfunction and increased platelet activation results into impaired coronary autoregulatory circulation and clinically manifested as acute coronary syndrome.

2. Anxiety Syndromes

Along with the depression, the chronic anxiety state is another important psychological risk factor associated with the development of CAD [28,29] and a negative prognostic factor for established CAD [30]. There is enough literature evidence of anxiety disorder's association with development of arteriosclerotic plaques, carotid artery intimal thickness, non-fatal myocardial infarction and cardiac death in initially healthy men and women [28,30,31]. The anxious individuals have significantly more ischemic and arrhythmic complications like reinfarction, new onset ischemia, ventricular fibrillation, sustained ventricular tachycardia, or in-hospital death, within 48 hours of myocardial infarction [32]. In a recent study of 516 stable CAD patients who were followed up for 3.4 years, the high cumulative anxiety score was associated with increased risk for non-fatal myocardial infarction and total mortality [33]. There is a dose dependant relationship between anxiety levels and arrhythmic cardiac death. In an another study, the major depression and generalized anxiety disorder in stable CAD patients revealed more than 2 fold increase risk of major adverse cardiac events at 2 years of follow-up [30]. Similar to the pathophysiological mechanism of depression, the chronic anxiety state is also associated with altered autonomic tone including increased sympathetic activity, impaired vagal tone, and impaired heart rate variability [34,35].

3. Personality and Character Traits

Initial reports observed that type A personality is associated with increased risk for CAD and myocardial infarction [36]; however the finding was not consistent in later studies because of potential confounding variable of social support [37-39]. The various components of type A personality being investigated to know the exact association with cardiac events. Hostility, a major aspect of type A behavior, is a broad psychological construct, encompassing negative orientations toward interpersonal relationships, and includes anger, cynicism, and mistrust. Anger and cynical mistrust are noted to be associated with future cardiac events [40]. Even CAD patients with high hostility have a greater restenosis following coronary angioplasty [41], experience more rapid atherosclerosis progression during serial carotid ultrasonography [42], and manifest more ischemia during stress testing than other CAD patients [43]. Unhealthy lifestyle behaviors like smoking, poor diet and obesity, and psychological factors like social isolation and lack of social support, which is common with hostile individuals predisposes them for CAD [44]. They also have high cortisols and cathecholamines levels, manifest higher heart rate and blood pressure to routine activities, which predispose them for adverse cardiac events [45]. An another type of personality known as type D (distressed), which is characterized by a combination of pessimistic emotions and introversion has also received the attention as a possible cause of cardiovascular risk [46].

4. Social Isolation, Lack of Social Support and Social Disruption

Social factors like living alone, marital status, and/or marital disruption, and substantial social support by the community plays an important role in prevention of future cardiac events in healthy individuals [47] or patients with preexisting CAD [48,49]. There is about 2-3 fold increase in future cardiac events in healthy population with adverse social factors. A low level of perceived emotional support confers even a greater increase risk for future cardiac events. In preexisting CAD, there is 3 fold increase in subsequent cardiac events in post MI patients reported to have low emotional support [50]; and 3 fold increases in 5 year mortality in unmarried or low confidence individuals [51]. Social support and depression counteract in the sense that high level of social support blunt the impact of depression on cardiac mortality [52]. A favorable and emotionally encouraging social support helps in healthy lifestyle, adherence to medical regimen and improvement in depression & stress. Lower socioeconomic status whether it is education, income or occupation based, prospectively predispose healthy people to an increase risk of CAD and CAD patients to poorer prognosis. The possible mechanism of adverse cardiac outcome is secondary to unhealthy lifestyle behaviors like smoking, alcoholism, poor weight control, non-compliance to medical treatment, and other associated clustering of psychosocial risk factors like lack of social support, social isolation, depression, job strain, hostility etc [53].

5. Life stress and Job strain

The life stress can be secondary to either a major life event like getting divorced, encountering financial loss, being involved in lawsuit etc; or a minor, recurrent irritation, tension or frustration. Both are associated with increased risk for CAD and sudden cardiac death. When considering the recurrent, daily stresses, job strain and work related pressures have received the considerable attention. It is observed that job strain with high demand and low ability for decision making or low reward is more harmful than isolated high demand job strain with affirmative working atmosphere [54]. Both cross sectional and longitudinal studies have supported the relationship of job strain with increase risk of CAD and cardiac death in healthy population. In a longitudinal study of 12,517 Swedish men over a 14 year period, low level of control over one's work conditions were an independent risk factor for cardiac mortality with the relative risk of 1.83 [55]. A review of 36 cross-sectional, case control and cohort studies concluded a positive link between job strain and development of CAD in both men and women [56]. It tends to be more in individuals with lower socioeconomic group, and is associated with poor social support, high incidence of conventional CAD risk factors, less education and certain psychological traits [57]. An another type of chronic life stress is marital and domestic stress, which is common in women, and predicts the depressive symptoms and also CAD [58]. It is observed that women with job strain or marital stress have the progression of angiographically proven coronary atherosclerosis during the period of 3 years [59]. The effect of domestic stress is more pronounced in women with low socioeconomic status, poor social support and depression [60]. Another form of domestic stress is caring responsibilities of disabled or ill spouse. An analysis from the Nurses' Health Study has shown that women who looked after a disabled or ill spouse for 9 or more hours per week had a significant increase risk of cardiovascular death and non-fatal myocardial infarction [61].

ACUTE LIFE STRESS

Acute life stress has negative cardiovascular outcomes as evident by increased mortality in the month following a bereavement event or immediately following natural disaster or military/terrorist attack. The risk of mortality is >2 fold for men and >3 fold for women following such events [62]. An episode of intense anger or frustration also results in myocardial ischemia, arrhythmias and sudden cardiac death [63]. An acute stress of high work load entailed a six fold increase in risk of acute myocardial infarction during 24 hours [64]. The myocardial ischemia following acute mental stress has been documented by various laboratory methods like radionuclide ventriculography, echocardiography, positron emission tomography and ^{99m}Tc-sestamibi myocardial perfusion tomography [65]. Approximately half of CAD patients with exercise-induced myocardial ischemia also demonstrate inducible ischemia during mental stress testing. Mental stress–induced ischemia generally occurs at relatively low heart rate elevations compared with exercise testing. The mental stress with emotional component or matter related with personal faults/problems leads to greater frequency and magnitude of ischemia than the simple laboratory based mental arithmetic exercise [65]. CAD patients who exhibit mental stress induced ischemia have increase risk of subsequent fatal and non-fatal cardiac events [66].

An episode of anger can trigger the intense sympathetic stimulation resulting into coronary spasm, atherosclerotic plaque rupture and platelet activation in addition to onset of ventricular arrhythmias. The mechanism of mental stress related myocardial ischemia constitutes increase cardiac workload following increase in heart rate and blood pressure, coronary vasoconstriction and spasm secondary to neuroharmonal and platelet activation [67]. Arrhythmias and sudden cardiac death following acute mental stress is mediated via neuroharmonal activation and autonomic imbalance [68]. Hypercortisolemia mediated endothelial dysfunction also contribute to adverse cardiac events in such situations [69]. Some individuals have sympathetic nervous system hyperreactivity, also known as "hot reactors" who have disproportional increase in blood pressure and heart rate, more vasoconstriction and catecholamine release and have prolonged recovery phase following a stressful situation. These individuals are subsequently prone to develop hypertension and atherosclerosis [70,71].

THERAPEUTIC IMPLICATIONS

As both acute and chronic stress contribute in pathogenesis of atherosclerosis, it is important to have psychosocial intervention including individual or group psychotherapy, support and stress reduction in cardiac patients and healthy individuals. As acute stress is mostly unavoidable, the best way of management of untoward cardiac events is to prevent and treat underlying CAD. The chronic psycho-social stress which can be intervened and modified alter the adverse cardiac outcomes. There is a need for studying and integrating psychosocial interventions into routine clinical practice for the management of CAD patients. Physician should take the active participation in modification of lifestyle and psychosocial factors adversely affecting the health of individuals. There is a need for educating the general practitioners about strength of association between psychosocial factors and CAD, and integration of various behavioral modification techniques in routine practice. As psychosocial interventions needs persistent perusal, chronic & regular follow-up session with the patients, patient specific treatment strategy, antidepressant pharmacotherapy and integration with de-addiction, physiotherapy department and various social organizations; there should be a combined approach of clinical psychiatrist and primary physician in management of these patients. Behavioral risk factors for CAD such as smoking, overweight, physical inactivity, overeating, and non–compliance to drug treatment for CAD and its risk factors like hypertension, diabetes mellitus, dyslipidemia needs the active and coordinated interdisciplinary approach for prevention of adverse cardiac outcome. There is also a need for future research into common genetic, environmental and pathophysiological pathways and treatment of both psychological stress and CAD.

REFERENCES

[1]   Musselman DL, Evans DL, Nemeroff CB. The relationship of depression to cardiovascular disease: epidemiology, biology, and treatment. *Arch Gen Psychiatry* 1998; 55: 580–92.

[2]   Hans M, Carney RM, Freedland KE, Skala J. Depression in patients with coronary heart disease: a 12-month follow-up. *Gen Hosp Psychiatry.* 1996;18:61–65.

[3]   Ford DE, Mead LA, Chang PF, Cooper-Patrick L, Wang N, Klag MJ. Depression is a risk factor for coronary artery disease in men. *Arch Intern Med.* 1998;158:1422–1426.

[4]   Pratt LA, Ford DE, Crum RM, Armenian HK, Gallo JJ, Eaton WW. Depression, psychotropic medication, and risk of myocardial infarction: prospective data from the Baltimore ECA follow-up. *Circulation.* 1996;94:3123–3129.

[5]   Vogt T, Pope C, Mullooly J, Hollis J. Mental health status as a predictor of morbidity and mortality: a 15-year follow-up of members of a health maintenance organization. *Am J Public Health.* 1994;84:227–231.

[6]   Anda R, Williamson D, Jones D, Macera C, Eaker E, Glasman A, Marks J. Depressed affect, hopelessness, and the risk of ischemic heart disease in a cohort of U. S. adults. *Epidemiology.* 1993;4:285–294.

[7]   Frasure-Smith N, Lesperance F, Talajic M. Depression and 18-month prognosis after myocardial infarction. *Circulation.* 1995;91:999–1005.

[8]   Barefoot JC, Helms MJ, Mark DB. Depression and long-term mortality risk in patients with coronary artery disease. *Am J Cardiol.* 1996;78:613–617.

[9]   Denoillet J, Brutsaert DL. Personality, disease severity, and the risk of long term cardiac events in patients with a decreased ejection fraction after myocardial infarction. *Circulation.* 1998;97:167–173.

[10]   Frasure-Smith N, Lesperance F, Juneau M, Talajic M, Bourassa MG. Gender, depression, and one-year prognosis after myocardial infarction. *Psychosom Med.* 1999;61:26–37.

[11]   Lesperance, F.; Frasure-Smith, N.; Talajic, M., and Bourassa, M. G. Five-year risk of cardiac mortality in relation to initial severity and one-year changes in depression symptoms after myocardial infarction. *Circulation.* 2002; 105:1049-53.

[12]   Frasure-Smith N, Lesperance F, Talajic M. Depression following myocardial infarction. Impact on 6-month survival. *JAMA.* 1993; 270:1819-25.

[13]   Glassman AH, O'Connor CM, Califf RM, Swedberg K, Schwartz P, Bigger JT Jr, Krishnan KR, van Zyl LT, Swenson JR, Finkel MS, et al. Sertraline treatment of major depression in patients with acute MI or unstable angina. *JAMA* 2002; 288:701-9.

[14]   Lesperance F, Frasure-Smith N, Talajic M. Major depression before and after myocardial infarction: its nature and consequences. *Psychosom Med* 1996; 58:99-110.

[15]   Sullivan MD, LaCroix AZ, Baum C, Grothaus LC, Katon WJ. Functional status in coronary artery disease: a one-year prospective study of the role of anxiety and depression. *Am J Med* 1997; 103:348-56.

[16]   Rutledge T, Reis VA, Linke SE, Greenberg BH, Mills PJ. Depression in heart failure a meta-analytic review of prevalence, intervention effects, and associations with clinical outcomes. *J Am Coll Cardiol.* 2006; 48:1527-37.

[17] Kubzansky LD, Davidson KW, Rozanski A. The clinical impact of negative psychological states: expanding the spectrum of risk for coronary artery disease. *Psychosom Med* 2005; 67 (Suppl 1):S10-4.

[18] Davidson PM, Dracup K, Phillips J, Daly J, Padilla G. Preparing for the worst while hoping for the best: the relevance of hope in the heart failure illness trajectory. *J Cardiovasc Nurs* 2007;22:159-65.

[19] Everson SA, Kaplan GA, Goldberg DE, Salonen R, Salonen JT. Hopelessness and 4-year progression of carotid atherosclerosis. The Kuopio Ischemic Heart Disease Risk Factor Study. *Arterioscler Thromb Vasc Biol* 1997; 17:1490-5.

[20] Pedersen SS, Denollet J, Daemen J, van de Sande M, de Jaegere PT, Serruys PW, Erdman RA, van Domburg RT. Fatigue, depressive symptoms, and hopelessness as predictors of adverse clinical events following percutaneous coronary intervention with paclitaxel-eluting stents. *J Psychosom Res* 2007; 62:455-61.

[21] Kopp MS, Falger PR, Appels A, Szedmak S. Depressive symptomatology and vital exhaustion are differentially related to behavioral risk factors for coronary artery disease. *Psychosom Med* 1998; 60:752-8.

[22] Appels A. Exhaustion and coronary heart disease: the history of a scientific quest. *Patient Educ Couns* 2004; 55:223-9.

[23] Carroll BJ, Cassidy F, Naftolowitz D, Tatham NE, Wilson WH, Iranmanesh A, Liu PY, Veldhuis JD. Pathophysiology of hypercortisolism in depression. *Acta Psychiatr Scand Suppl.* 2007; (433): 90-103.

[24] Tomfohr LM, Martin TM, Miller GE. Symptoms of depression and impaired endothelial function in healthy adolescent women. *J Behav Med* 2007 Dec 29. [Epub ahead of print]

[25] Barton DA, Dawood T, Lambert EA, Esler MD, Haikerwal D, Brenchley C, Socratous F, Kaye DM, Schlaich MP, Hickie I, et al. Sympathetic activity in major depressive disorder: identifying those at increased cardiac risk? *J Hypertens* 2007; 25:2117-24.

[26] Kamphuis MH, Geerlings MI, Dekker JM, Giampaoli S, Nissinen A, Grobbee DE, Kromhout D. Autonomic dysfunction: a link between depression and cardiovascular mortality? The FINE Study. *Eur J Cardiovasc Prev Rehabil* 2007; 14:796-802.

[27] Bruce EC, Musselman DL. Depression, alterations in platelet function, and ischemic heart disease. *Psychosom Med* 2005; 67 (Suppl 1):S34-6.

[28] Kawachi I, Colditz GA, Ascherio A, Rimm EB, Giovannucci E, Stampfer MJ, Willert WC. Prospective study of phobic anxiety and risk of coronary heart disease in men. *Circulation.* 1994; 89:1992–1997.

[29] Shen BJ, Avivi YE, Todaro JF, Spiro A 3rd, Laurenceau JP, Ward KD, Niaura R. Anxiety characteristics independently and prospectively predict myocardial infarction in men the unique contribution of anxiety among psychologic factors. *J Am Coll Cardiol.* 2008; 51:113-9.

[30] Frasure-Smith N, Lesperance F. Depression and anxiety as predictors of 2-year cardiac events in patients with stable coronary artery disease. *Arch Gen Psychiatry* 2008; 65:62-71.

[31] Paterniti S, Zureik M, Ducimetiere P, Touboul PJ, Feve JM, Alperovitch A. Sustained anxiety and 4-year progression of carotid atherosclerosis. *Arterioscler Thromb Vasc Biol* 2001; 21:136-41.

[32] Moser DK, Dracup K. Is anxiety early after myocardial infarction associated with subsequent ischemic and arrhythmic events? *Psychosom Med* 1996; 58:395-401.

[33] Shibeshi WA, Young-Xu Y, Blatt CM. Anxiety worsens prognosis in patients with coronary artery disease. *J Am Coll Cardiol* 2007; 49:2021-7.

[34] Martens EJ, Nyklicek I, Szabo BM, Kupper N. Depression and anxiety as predictors of heart rate variability after myocardial infarction. *Psychol Med* 2008; 38:375-83.

[35] Friedman BH. An autonomic flexibility-neurovisceral integration model of anxiety and cardiac vagal tone. *Biol Psychol* 2007; 74:185-99.

[36] Rosenman RH, Brand RJ, Jenkins CD, Friedman M, Straus R, Wurm M. Coronary heart disease in the Western Collaborative Group Study: final follow-up experience of 8 1/2 years. *JAMA.* 1975; 233:872–877.

[37] Kawachi I, Sparrow D, Kubzansky LD, Spiro A 3rd, Vokonas PS, Weiss ST. Prospective study of a self-report type A scale and risk of coronary heart disease: test of the MMPI-2 type A scale. *Circulation* 1998; 98: 405–12.

[38] Ragland DR, Brand RJ. Type A behavior and mortality from coronary heart Disease. *N Engl J Med* 1988; 318: 65–69.

[39] Schroeder KE, Narkiewicz K, Kato M, Pesek C, Phillips B, Davison D, Somers VK. Personality type and neural circulatory control. *Hypertension* 2000; 36:830-3.

[40] Wielgosz AT, Nolan RP. Biobehavioral factors in the context of ischemic cardiovascular diseases. *J Psychosom Res.* 2000; 48:339-45.

[41] Goodman M, Quigley J, Moran G, Meilman H, Sherman M. Hostility predicts restenosis after percutaneous transluminal coronary angioplasty. *Mayo Clin Proc* 1996; 71:729-34.

[42] Julkunen J, Salonen R, Kaplan GA, Chesney MA, Salonen JT. Hostility and the progression of carotid atherosclerosis. *Psychosom Med.* 1994; 56:519–525.

[43] Helmers KF, Krantz DS, Howell RH, Klein J, Bairey N, Rozanski A. Hostility and myocardial ischemia in coronary artery disease patients: evaluation by gender and ischemic index. *Psychosom Medicine.* 1993; 55:29–36.

[44] Lavie CJ, Milani RV. Adverse psychological and coronary risk profiles in young patients with coronary artery disease and benefits of formal cardiac rehabilitation. *Arch Intern Med* 2006; 166:1878-83.

[45] Januzzi JL, Pasternak RC. Depression, Hostility, and Social Isolation in Patients with Coronary Artery Disease. *Curr Treat Options Cardiovasc Med* 2002; 4:77-85.

[46] Denollet J, Pedersen SS, Vrints CJ, Conraads VM. Usefulness of type D personality in predicting five-year cardiac events above and beyond concurrent symptoms of stress in patients with coronary heart disease. *Am J Cardiol* 2006; 97:970-3.

[47] Orth-Gomer K, Rosengren A, Wilhelmsen L. Lack of social support and incidence of coronary heart disease in middle-aged Swedish men. *Psychosom Med.* 1993; 55:37–43.

[48] Jenkinson CM, Madeley RJ, Mitchell JRA, Turner ID. The influence of psychosocial faction on survival after myocardial infarction. *Public Health.* 1993; 107:305–317.

[49]   Wang HX, Mittleman MA, Leineweber C, Orth-Gomer K. Depressive symptoms, social isolation, and progression of coronary artery atherosclerosis: the Stockholm Female Coronary Angiography Study. *Psychother Psychosom* 2006; 75:96-102.

[50]   Berkman LF, Leo-Summers L, Horwitz RI. Emotional support and survival after myocardial infarction: a prospective, population-based study of the elderly. *Ann Intern Med.* 1992; 117:1003–1009.

[51]   Williams RB, Barefoot JC, Califf RM, Haney TL, Saunders WB, Pryor DB, Hlatky MA, Siegler IC, Mark DB. Prognostic importance of social and economic resources among medically treated patients with angiographically documented coronary artery disease. *JAMA.* 1992; 267:520–524.

[52]   Frasure-Smith N, Lesperance F, Gravel G, Masson A, Juneau M, Talajic M, Bourassa MG. Social support, depression, and mortality during the first year after myocardial infarction. *Circulation* 2000; 101:1919-24.

[53]   Pollitt RA, Rose KM, Kaufman JS. Evaluating the evidence for models of life course socioeconomic factors and cardiovascular outcomes: a systematic review. *BMC Public Health.* 2005; 5:7.

[54]   Greenlund KJ, Liu K, Knox S, McCreath H, Dyer AR, Gardin J. Psychosocial work characteristics and cardiovascular disease risk factors in young adults: the CARDIA study. Coronary Artery Risk Disease in Young Adults. *Soc Sci Med* 1995; 41:717-23.

[55]   Johnson JV, Stewart W, Hall EM, Fredlund P, Theorell T. Long-term psychosocial work environment and cardiovascular mortality among Swedish men. *Am J Public Health* 1996; 86:324-31.

[56]   Schnall PL, Landsbergis PA, Baker D. Job strain and cardiovascular disease. *Annu Rev Public Health* 1994; 15:381-411.

[57]   Strike PC, Steptoe A. Psychosocial factors in the development of coronary artery disease. *Prog Cardiovasc Dis* 2004; 46:337-47.

[58]   Balog P, Janszky I, Leineweber C, Blom M, Wamala SP, Orth-Gomer K. Depressive symptoms in relation to marital and work stress in women with and without coronary heart disease. The Stockholm Female Coronary Risk Study. *J Psychosom Res* 2003; 54:113-9.

[59]   Wang HX, Leineweber C, Kirkeeide R, Svane B, Schenck-Gustafsson K, Theorell T, Orth-Gomer K. Psychosocial stress and atherosclerosis: family and work stress accelerate progression of coronary disease in women. The Stockholm Female Coronary Angiography Study. *J Intern Med* 2007; 261:245-54.

[60]   Blom M, Georgiades A, Laszlo KD, Alinaghizadeh H, Janszky I, Ahnve S. Work and marital status in relation to depressive symptoms and social support among women with coronary artery disease. *J Womens Health (Larchmt)* 2007; 16:1305-16.

[61]   Lee S, Colditz GA, Berkman LF, Kawachi I. Caregiving and risk of coronary heart disease in U.S. women: a prospective study. *Am J Prev Med.* 2003; 24:113-9.

[62]   Kaprio J, Koskenvuo M, Rita H. Mortality after bereavement: a prospective study of 95,647 persons. *Am J Public Health.* 1987; 77:283–287.

[63]   Krantz DS, Kop WJ, Santiago HT, Gottdiener JS. Mental stress as a trigger of myocardial ischemia and infarction. *Cardiol Clin* 1996; 14:271-87.

[64] Moller J, Theorell T, de Faire U, Ahlbom A, Hallqvist J. Work related stressful life events and the risk of myocardial infarction. Case-control and case-crossover analyses within the Stockholm heart epidemiology programme (SHEEP). *J Epidemiol Community Health* 2005; 59:23-30.

[65] Rozanski A, Blumenthal JA, Kaplan J. Impact of psychological factors on the pathogenesis of cardiovascular disease and implications for therapy. *Circulation* 1999; 99:2192-217.

[66] Jiang W, Babyak M, Krantz DS, Waugh RA, Coleman RE, Hanson MM, Frid DJ, McNulty S, Morris JJ, O'Connor CM, et al. Mental stress--induced myocardial ischemia and cardiac events. *JAMA* 1996; 275:1651-6.

[67] Goldberg AD, Becker LC, Bonsall R, Cohen JD, Ketterer MW, Kaufman PG, Krantz DS, Light KC, McMahon RP, Noreuil T, et al. Ischemic, hemodynamic, and neurohormonal responses to mental and exercise stress. Experience from the Psychophysiological Investigations of Myocardial Ischemia Study (PIMI). *Circulation* 1996; 94:2402-9.

[68] Pellizzon OA, Beloscar JS, Mariani E. Adrenergic nervous system influences on the induction of ventricular tachycardia. *Ann Noninvasive Electrocardiol* 2002; 7:281-8.

[69] Broadley AJ, Korszun A, Abdelaal E, Moskvina V, Jones CJ, Nash GB, Ray C, Deanfield J, Frenneaux MP. Inhibition of cortisol production with metyrapone prevents mental stress-induced endothelial dysfunction and baroreflex impairment. *J Am Coll Cardiol* 2005; 46:344-50.

[70] McKinney ME, McIlvain HE, Hofschire PJ, Collins RE, Somers JA, Ruddel H, Buell JC, Eliot RS. Cardiovascular changes during mental stress: correlations with presence of coronary risk factors and cardiovascular disease in physicians and dentists. *J Hum Hypertens* 1987; 1:137-45.

[71] Weidner G, Kohlmann CW, Horsten M, Wamala SP, Schenck-Gustafsson K, Hogbom M, Orth-Gomer K. Cardiovascular reactivity to mental stress in the Stockholm Female Coronary Risk Study. *Psychosom Med* 2001; 63:917-24.

In: Psychological Factors and Cardiovascular Disorders   ISBN: 978-1-60456-871-4
Editor: Leo Sher   © 2008 Nova Science Publishers, Inc.

Chapter II

RISK FACTORS IN CORONARY ARTERY DISEASE: GENDER MATTERS

Anne Maria Möller-Leimkühler

Department of Psychiatry, Ludwig-Maximilians-University of Munich, Munich, Germany.

ABSTRACT

Since recently, coronary artery disease (CAD) has been held to be a "male" disease due to men´s higher absolute risk compared to women, but the relative risk of women for CAD morbidity and mortality is actually higher. Current knowedge points to important gender differences in age of onset, symptom presentation, management, outcome as well as traditional and psychosocial risk factors. Compared to men, CAD risk in women is more strongly increased by some traditional factors, and socioeconomic and psychosocial factors seem to have a higher impact on CAD in women as well. With respect to differences in CAD management, a gender-bias in favour of men has to be taken into account in spite of older age and higher comorbidity in women, possibly contributing to a poorer outcome. With regard to depression which has been shown to be an independent risk factor and consequence of CAD, current evidence suggests that depression causes a greater increase in CAD incidence in women, and that female CAD patients experience higher levels of depression than men. Gender aspects should be more intensively considered in further cardiac research as well as in treatment and rehabilitation.

WHY IS GENDER SO IMPORTANT?

One of the more robust factors in explaining differences in morbidity and mortality is gender. In contrast to the term sex, gender is a multidimensional construct including biological/ genetic, psychological and social differences between men and women. Although gender is based on biology, and biological factors in men and women may predispose behaviour and vulnerability differently, these factors do not determine the entire scope of gender-related behaviour, emotions and attitudes. Beyond genetic and biological differences, gender refers to the socially constructed roles for men and women implicating different social norms and cultural expectations for both sexes. Normative expectations even result in classifying disorders as male and female, such as `male´ heart disease and ´female` depression which can have serious consequences for the health outcomes of both men and women [1].

Although traditional gender norms have changed during the last three decades and concepts of being male and female have become more individualistic, stereotypes of typical male and female attributes still remain influential in social perception and evaluation [2], including health care (gender bias).

Beyond biological sex, gender is a basic principle of societal organization structuring social roles and the access to personal, social and economic resources differently for men and women. It has been found that social structural and psychosocial determinants of health generally tend to be more important for women´s health, whereas behavioural determinants tend to be more important for men´s health [3]. Sociological stress research has become one of the most commonly used explanations of gender differences in health assuming that suspectibility to psychological or physical breakdown is shaped largely by inequalities in life chances emerging from the organization of gender, class, race and age. Women are mainly underprivilegded in these concerns, and generally experience poorer health and distress than men including psychiatric disorders and a variety of chronic disorders. This is explained by their reduced access to the material and social conditions of life that foster health and from the greater stress associated with their gender and marital roles. Additionally, there is evidence that women respond to life events and ongoing strain more sensitively than men [3,4].

CONORARY ARTERY DISEASE: A "MALE" DISEASE?

Coronary artery disease (CAD) is the leading cause of morbidity and mortality in economically more developed areas of the world being two to five times more common in men than in women in younger age groups [5]. CAD risk increases with age in both men and women, but with a more prominent increase in women older than 50 years. Despite better medical treatment of CAD, it remains the leading killer of women, too [6]. In Europe, about 55% of all females´ deaths are caused by CAD, especially coronary heart disease and stroke compared to 44% of all males´ deaths [7]. Age-adjusted mortality for CAD has continously declined in the last four decades, but to a lesser extent in women than in men. In fact, the temporal trend of the incidence of CAD even shows a rise in women (Figure 1) [8,9]. This has been mainly attributed to a decrease in myocardial infarction incidence in younger men with a concomitant increase in older women [8]. Recent data even suggest an increased incidence of women under the age of 54 [10].

The older age at onset of CAD in women (70 years) compared to men (60 years), probably related to estrogen deficiency in post-menopause, correlates with an increase in comorbid diseases and consequently increased mortality; 38% of women will die within one year of an initial unrecognized myocardial infarction compared to 25% of men [11].

Until the last decade, CAD in women had been underestimated because of their lower prevalence rate in younger age, and due to the image of CAD as a male disorder with the consequence that women had been largely underdiagnosed, undertreated and neglected in cardiological research. With regard to research, either the study populations exclusively consisted of male cohorts, the gender distribution was not specified or the number of females included in studies was too small to enable conclusions to be drawn about gender differences in risk factors. It was simply assumed that the knowledge derived from studies on men was similarly applicable to women, whether it concerned biological or psychosocial risk factors. Gender bias in constructing hypotheses on risk factors led to numerous methodological pitfalls and false conclusions; for example, it was assumed that men were harmed by work stress, while women were protected by being at home [12]. Now, the situation has changed, and several recent controlled cohort studies in men and women are available, which indicate important gender differences in clinical presentation, disease management, and outcome, as well as biological and psychosocial risk factors.

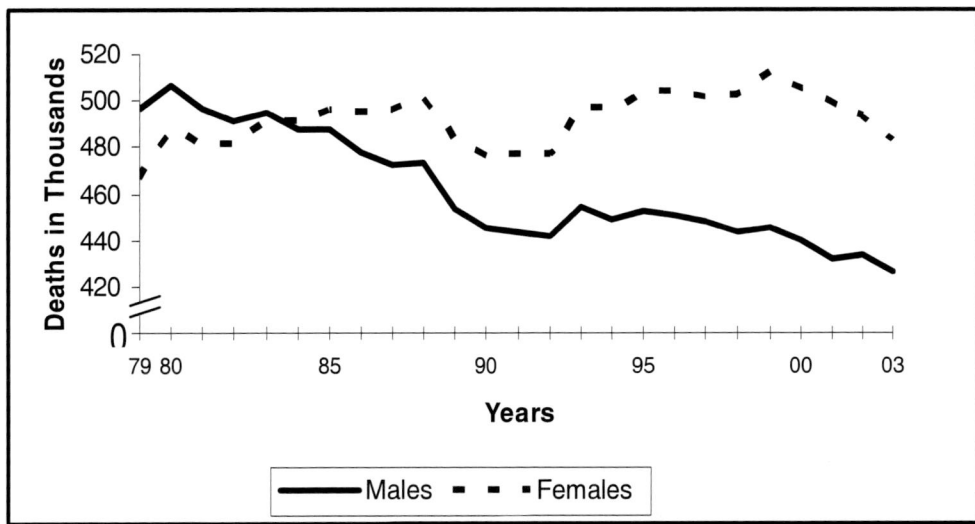

Figure 1. Cardiovascular disease mortality trends for males and females United States: 1979-2003 [9].

CAD MANAGEMENT AND OUTCOME: EVIDENCE FOR A GENDER-BIAS

Women with acute myocardial infarction (MI) tend to present with more atypical symptoms such as abdominal pain, dyspneoa, nausea, back and neck pain, indigestion, palpitations, and unexpected fatigue instead of clearly defined chest pain, which is the typical male complaint and probably better recognized by physicians [13,14]. Regarding the delay in help-seeking, it has been noted that women underestimate their risk for CAD because the general public still perceives CAD as primarily a health problem for men [15]. Misperception of risk and symptoms, as well as lack of immediate informal help to older women living alone, may result in late arrival in the emergency room. This might be the explanation for earlier reports noting that women were less likely to be referred for diagnostic and therapeutic procedures, and that younger women have higher rates of death during hospitalization after acute MI compared to men of the same age (< 50 years: 6.1% vs. 2.9%) [16]. Moreover, serious comorbidities are more common in older women, and may limit treatment options. Indeed, lower rates of specific treatments for women have been reported, but some authors suggest, that it is not clear whether gender differences in treatment would have consequences for outcome. However, despite an increasing awareness for CAD in women, outcome in women remains worser compared to men; e g, hospital mortality rates for acute MI are 16% for women and 11% for men [17]. The mortality for bypass surgery in women is twice that for men, they experience more heart failure and are more likely to require reoperation within 5 years [13]. Although the poor prognosis for women after MI is mostly attributed to their worse baseline characteristics, these differences do not account for the total gender differential in clinical outcome [18]. Poor clinical outcome in women has to be attributed as well to the psychosocial adjustment which has shown to be worse in women than in men in terms of quality of life, anxiety and depression, probably explaining their increased mortality risk [19].

In sum, management of CAD in men and women is obviously different, and these differences are partially due to a gender bias in favour of men. While some studies did not find a gender bias in the management and outcome of patients with acute CAD [20], unstable angina [21], and in selection for coronary angiography and revascularization early after MI [22], others did [23,24]. For example, in the Euro Heart Survey of Stable Angina [24], significant gender bias has been identified at multiple levels in the investigation and management of stable angina. Female patients were referred significantly less often for either noninvasive or invasive investigation than male patients and less likely to receive revascularization or optimal secondary preventive medication even in the presence of confirmed coronary disease. They were twice as likely to suffer death or nonfatal MI within a 1-year follow-up period.

In an Irish population of 15,590 patients with ischaemic heart disease, compared with male patients, female patients were less likely to receive a secondary preventive medication. However, they were more likely to receive anxiolytics [25]. A similar gender bias has been detected by a Scottish study [26], where the gender difference was independent of age, deprivation, and comorbidities, and even increased over time.

Gender-bias has also been reported with respect to cardiac rehabilitation. Most studies report poorer programme uptake, poorer adherence and higher drop-out rates for women than for men, although data indicate that women show improvements the same or greater than those of men [18]. This seems not only due to psychosocial barriers in women themselves (low self-esteem, multiple care-giving roles, economic concerns), but also to less strong recommendations for rehabilitation. Gender stereotypes in medicine may have fatal consequences as in the case of CAD, and the lack of secondary preventive medication in women may additionally expose them to a higher risk of MI and death, and may be one reason for the slower decline in female mortality rates.

TRADITIONAL CARDIAC RISK FACTORS: WOMEN HAVE A HIGHER RELATIVE RISK

Traditional cardiac risk factors are assumed to be essentially the same for men and women, although important quantitative differences have been observed. Women have smaller artery dimension, different electrical properties, and different plaque composition and development [27]. Men have generally less favorable cardiac risk factors than women; on the other hand, diabetes mellitus, hypertension, smoking, hypercholesterolemia, and obesity have been shown to contribute more to women´s than men´s CAD risk.

Most significant is *diabetes* which results in a 3- to7-fold increased CAD risk in women compared to a 2- to 3-fold elevation of risk in men. Diabetes negates the presumed gender-protective effect of estrogen in premenopausal women [13]. It is estimated, that two thirds of all diabetic deaths are due to CAD [11].

Hypertension, a major CAD risk factor for both sexes, is more prevalent in women than in men after the age of 65. Contrary to earlier belief, women do not tolerate effects of hypertension on cardiovasular and renal system better than men do [16].

In women younger than 50 years, *smoking* is the leading cause of CAD. Although the prevalence of smokers is still slightly higher in men than in women, the decline in tabacco use among women is less evident than in men [28]. In fact, in younger women there may even be an increase rather than a decrease, and this may explain the increased incidence rates of CAD [28,29,30]. The risk in young female smokers is additionally elevated by the use of oral contraceptives [31].

Hypercholesterolemia plays a central role in the development of CAD in men and women, with a linear relationship between low-density lipoprotein (LDL) levels and risk for CAD particularly in women less than 65 years. Additionally, low high-density lipoprotein (HDL) levels in women over 65 years convey a greater risk than in men [32,11].

Obesity, and particularly central obesity, more prevalent in men until 45 years and in women over 45 years, increases the CAD risk specifically in women [33] and is associated with diabetes, hypertension and dyslipidemia as well as other lifestyle-related risk factors such as physical inactivity and bad diet.

The above-mentioned risk factors account for only approximately 40% of the variance of CAD.

PSYCHOSOCIAL CARDIAC RISK FACTORS: GREATER IMPACT ON WOMEN

Since the late 1950´s, the role of potential psychosocial risk factors in the development and outcomes of CAD had been extensively studied. Type A personality (excesses of aggression, hurry and competitiveness) and more recently type D personality (inhibition of negative emotions in social situations), depression and anxiety, low socioeconomic status, lack of social support, social isolation and chronic work stress have all been evoked. While these factors were initially believed to indirectly increase CAD by affecting the traditional risk factors (strengthening unhealthy life-style behaviours), numerous prospective cohort studies have demonstrated also direct effects via mechanisms such as disturbed autonomic and neuroendocrine regulation [34,35]. In a critical evaluation of a number of systematical reviews on the association between psychosocial risk factors and CHD, Bunker et al. [36] found strong and consistent evidence of an independent causal association between depression, social isolation and lack of social support and the occurrence and prognosis of CHD, whereas a causal association with regard to Type A behaviour, hostiliy, anxiety disorders, chronic life events and work-related stressors was less evident. When psychosocial risk factors occur in combination, and they tend to cluster together (for example, high levels of chronic stress and social isolation), the rate of subsequent cardiac events is 4-fold higher, independently of preexisting CAD [34]. The above findings come predominantly from studies in men; knowledge of gender specific risk factor profiles remains limited, although some population-based prospective studies such as the Framingham Study [37], the WHO MONICA study (Monitoring trends and determinants in cardiovascular disease) [38], the Stockholm Heart Epidmiology Program [39] and the Whitehall II study [40] have included women.

With regard to gender differences in CAD incidence and mortality, there is consistent evidence, that *low socioeconomic status* as defined by occupational position, income, or education is not only a major psychosocial risk factor in men, but also in women. In women, the social gradient seems to be even stronger than in men [41,18,42]. For example, less than 8 years of education contributed to a 4-fold risk of women (compared with women with 12 and more years of education) of developing CAD over a 14-year follow-up period; even after adjustment for other coronary risk factors, level of education remained a significant predictor [43]. A strong gradient in CAD by years of education was also confirmed by the Swedish Women's Lifestyle and Health Cohort Study in a 10 years follow-up period [44]. Several studies focussing on a life course approach to socioeconomic position found that socioeconomic disadvantage in childhood and in later life both were associated with increased CAD risk in women (4-fold) [45,46], and a twofold risk for dying from CAD in men [47]. The fact that unhealthy lifestyles are more prevalent in men and women with low socioeconomic status, did not explain the different effects of social status on CAD risk and outcome: traditional CAD risk factors explain about 33% to 50% of the risk associated with the social CAD gradient (higher rates in lower employment grades) [48,49].

The risk gradient in CAD has been ascribed to *psychosocial stressors of the work environment*, mainly refering to Karasek's job strain model (high demands - low control) and Siegrist's effort-reward imbalance model [50,51]. Findings indicate odds ratios (OR) from 1.2 to 5.0 with respect to job strain, and from 1.5 to 6.1 with respect to effort-reward imbalance, These OR seem higher for men than for women, but whether this is due to scarce data in women or to other reasons remains unresolved. While low job control in the Whitehall II study was related to a higher risk of newly reported CAD during 5 year follow-up for males and females [52], other studies revealed only weak associations between psychosocial work characteristics and risk of CAD in women [44,53,54]. For example, the Framingham Offspring Study [55] did not find any support for high job strain as a significant risk factor for CAD or death in women or in men within a 10 year follow-up period. Contrary to expectation, and unlike men, women with 'active' job strain (high demands – high control) had a 2.8-fold risk of CAD compared with women with high job strain (high demands – low control). This may be due to more difficulties in adopting new social roles for women when traditional expectations remain normative as well. Recent evidence suggests that women who are occupied in male-dominated jobs have a 2-fold risk of myocardial infarction compared to those in women-dominated jobs [56].

With regard to *employment*, employed men as well as women are healthier than their unemployed counterparts, even after adjustment for low income and low level of education. The relationship between employment and CAD risk is more complex in women. Findings indicate that, although women of all occupational levels were protected against CAD relative to those performing home duties, the protective effect of employment seems to be more pronounced in women in professional and managerial occupations than those in blue-collar occupations [18]. However, there is evidence, that employed women with children have an increased risk of CAD, perhaps because of the double load of work and family, which can result in anger and frustration due to low control over their lives [57,58,59]. Other predictors of CAD risk in women are marital stress [60] and caring for a disabled or ill spouse. As the findings from the Nurses´ Health Study [61] show, women carers (> 9 hours per week) had a significantly increased risk of fatal CAD or nonfatal MI infarction that was independent of age, smoking, exercise, alcohol intake, body mass index, history of hypertension, diabetes, and other covariates.

Other gender differences in psychosocial risk factors had been demonstrated concerning *life events*. While events occuring at work and at home affect risk increase in women, work-related events seem to influence men to a greater extent [62,63], a finding which is due to the fact that men consider their role at work as central, thus making them more vulnerable to job stressors. In the case of bereavement, most of the studies report a brief increase in CAD mortality during the first months after bereavement for men and women, and then a later slight increase in mortality in men [18]. Loss of a spouse might be more disruptive for men, because they loose their only confident and seem to be more affected by a decrease in social network and social support than women, who usually have larger social networks.

Lack of *social support* and *social isolation* has proven to be major long-term predictors of mortality from all causes, including CAD. Although social support has been examined by a variety of methods, the results have been remarkably consistent [64]. The relative risk (RR) of CAD incidence owing to lack of social support is 2- to 3-fold, independent of conventional and sociodemographic CAD predictors [34]. Social support can have direct effects on CAD risk and can also act as a buffer by moderating the effect of adverse life events, job strain, anger and depression on CAD incidence. Lack of social support at work is particularly associated with increased risk of CAD [65]. Again, empirical evidence is more consistent for men than for women in this respect. Independent of work, the risk of fatal CAD was up to 3.7 times higher among women lacking social ties than those who did not [66], whereas no consistent association was found for women in a Finish study [37]. Single mothers in particular, as they are exposed to a combination of several psychosocial stressors and behavioural risk factors, have been shown to be at higher risk for CAD than mothers with partners [68]. Being lonely during the day was associated with higher MI or CAD mortality in housewives at 20-year follow-up, as reported from the Framingham Study [37]. For both men and women, social support (measured as being married) has been shown to be an independent predictor for survival rates and recurrent infarction in CAD patients [69,70]. However, women with CAD tended to report lesser informational, instrumental and emotional support than men [71,72].

Personality characteristics such as *Type A behaviour* have been investigated as psychosocial stressors in CAD research. Overall, data on Type A behaviour have not been conclusive, and the attention has more recently focused on hostility and anger, resulting again in mixed findings [73]. However, the literature shows a relationship between anger and CAD. One of the first prospective studies in this respect, the Framingham Offspring Study [55], found that trait anger, hostility, and symptoms of anger were independent risk factors for incident CAD in men, but not in women. This was supported by a population-based study of Haas et al. [74]. In contrast, other studies indicate that hostility is an independent of other CAD risk factor for nonfatal myocardial infarction and recurrent events in postmenopausal women with CAD [75,76].

GENDER DIFFERENCES IN COMORBID DEPRESSION

Like CAD, depression is a major public health problem with a lifetime prevalence of approximately 15% [77]. By the year 2020, it is estimated that disability worldwide will be determined largely by depression and heart disease [78]. It is well known that major depression is twice as common in women than in men [79,80]. The female predominance in depression begins in adolescence and persists into middle and early old age [81,82]. The reasons for this gender difference are not fully understood. A substantial part can be attributed to gender role related stressors to which women are more exposed than men such as low socioeconomic status, lack of power, role overload and sexual abuse, and associated psychological attributes such as interpersonal orientation and a respective vulnerability, anxiety, lowered self-esteem and emotion-focused coping styles. The differences between men and women reflect differences in endocrine stress reactions, and might influence processes leading to depression [82].

With respect to comorbidity, etiologic and prognostic studies indicate that depression may be a cause or a consequence of CAD, thus supporting a bidirectional relationship. Major depression has been identified as a prominent psychosocial risk factor in CAD incidence for initially healthy men and women with a relative risk of 1.5 to 2.0, independent of traditional risk factors [83,84,64]. However, as Rugulies [83] concluded from his meta-analysis, clinical depression has a stronger effect size in predicting CAD than depressive mood. The association between depression and CAD may have several mechanisms, including coronary prone behaviour and noncompliance, hypercortisolism and autonomic dysregulation. Among patients already suffering from CAD, 17% to 27% have major depression when diagnosed according to DSM criteria during the first year after MI, and a significantly larger percentage has subsyndromal symptoms of depression. In patients with MI or unstable angina pectoris, those who had been diagnosed as depressed had a 3-fold risk of dying compared to nondepressed patients, indicating that depression is an independent predictor of mortality as well [85]. Although the importance of depression in CAD is well documented, it remains largely underdiagnosed. According to recent data from a survey of cardiovascular physicians,

50% of the respondents were unaware of depression as an independent cardiac risk factor, 71% asked less than half their patients with CAD about depression, and 79% used no standard screening method to diagnose depression [86].

DEPRESSION AS A RISK FACTOR OF CAD: GENDER-RELATED FINDINGS ARE INCONSISTENT

There are very few studies which address depression as a primary risk factor in the development of CAD in gender-balanced samples through the lenses of gender. Wassertheil-Smoller et al. [87] did not find an association between baseline depression score and MI, but reported a significantly (25%) increased mortality risk for women who had a 5-unit increase in depression score (measured with the Center for Epidemiological Studies Depression Scale, CES-D) during a 4.5-year follow-up period. In the National Health and Nutrition Examination Survey [88], CAD mortality was only related to depressed men with a RR of 2.34 compared to nondepressed men, while depression had no effect on CAD mortality in women. However, it was associated with an increased risk of CAD incidence in women as well. In contrast, another study found an effect of depressive symptoms and CAD death only in women [89]. Brenda et al. [90] investigated the effects of recent-onset and chronic depression on CAD events in a prospective cohort study with men and women >=65 years during 5 years. Newly depressed older men (depressed at baseline, not earlier, CES-D), but not women, were twice as likely to have a CAD event as those who were never depressed. This association remained significant after adjusting for CAD risks. In men, recent onset of depression was a better predictor of CAD than chronic depression. In a similar designed study on the effects of depression (CES-D) on heart failure [91], findings indicate depression as an independent risk factor for heart failure only in elderly women, but not elderly men. Whether the under-representation of men was due to death before inception of the study, to a different help-seeking behaviour of depressed men and women or to different pathophysiological processes, remains unclear.

Diabetes and childhood maltreatment have been investigated with regard to factors affecting the relationship between gender, depression and CAD differently for men and women. Depression is common in diabetic patients, particularly in women with a prevalence of 28% (vs. 18% in men) [92]. Depression rates double in the presence of diabetes, and depressed diabetic women have more rapid development of CAD than nondepressed diabetic women [93]. Whether this association also holds true for men remain unclear. Concerning childhood maltreatment, a larger impact of traumatic experiences on the development of depression in women and a larger impact on CAD in men was postulated, but could not be confirmed in a representative sample over 5000 adults [94].

Childhood maltreatment was associated with an almost 9-fold increase in CAD in women only, and with a significant increase in lifetime depression for both men and women. Although depression and CAD were correlated, depression did not contribute to the prediction of CAD in women.

DEPRESSION AS A PROGNOSTIC FACTOR IN CAD: WOMEN HAVE A HIGHER RISK

Women have a rate of depression 2 times that of men in cardiac patient population, as well as in the general population [95]. Several studies have shown that woman after MI and coronary artery bypass surgery had more severe depressive symptoms than men, symptoms persisted longer [96] and affected women´s prognosis more detrimentally [97]. Studies agree that the occurrence of post-MI depression is unrelated to the severity of MI and other medical factors [98]. Younger women in particular (60 years or under) had a depression risk that was 3.1 times higher than that of the reference group of men older than 60 [99]. According to a large 5-year follow-up Norwegian study with 23 693 participants [98], men and women also differ in their long-term outcome after MI: women showed a higher risk for anxiety and depression (measured with the Hospital Anxiety and Depression Rating Scale) in the first 2 years after MI than men, which is followed by a significant symptom reduction. In men, the risk for depression increased after 2 years post-MI. These data lend support to the impact of gender specific coping as a significant factor mediating MI-outcome differently for men and women, what has been scarcely investigated.

Marital status and social network have also been explored as potential mediators of the link between CAD and depression. Being single has been found to increase the risk of post-MI depession in men, whereas unmarried women or those living alone were less likely to be depressed [100,85,101]. These findings are consistent with the fact that protective health effects of marriage are notably less strong for women than for men [102].

Social networks, in relation to recurrent CAD events were investigated in the Stockholm Female Coronary Risk Study [103]. It was demonstrated that two or more depressive symtoms (BDI) and lack of social integration (number and function of social contacts) contributed independently to a relapse of their CAD (cardiovascular death, MI or revascularization) within 5 years.

CONCLUSIONS

Due to the lack of studies on gender-balanced populations and randomised clinical studies including a larger amount of women, the current knowledge of gender-related risk profiles in CAD and comorbid depression is limited. Nevertheless, there is evidence for significant gender differences in some aspects, which points to several disadvantages for women. Men and women differ in their cardiac physiology and pathophysiology, CAD risks and symptoms, vulnerability to traditional and psychosocial CAD risk factors, medical management and outcome. Also, a gender-bias in symptoms evaluation and referral to CAD investigation, treatment and rehabilitation in favour of men has been demonstrated. Women tend to have a poorer prognosis after MI and bypass surgery, and psychosocial adjustment seems to be worse in women than in men. Socioeconomic and psychosocial factors seem to influence CAD in women to a greater extent than men; groups with a particularly high risk of CAD are single mothers with low socioeconomic status, working mothers in low employment grades, and older women who live alone and have little social support. At the same time, these groups are more vulnerable to depression. Depression in otherwise healthy subjects seems to increase the risk of CAD more strongly in women, and women with CAD possibly experience higher levels of depression and lower levels of social support than men. However, single male patients also seem to be prone to a poorer outcome of CAD.

While in general, depression has shown to be an independent risk factor and consequence of CAD, the question as to whether the impact of depression on the development and progression of CAD differs as a function of gender is still unresolved.

There is a need for more systematic gender studies in CAD and comorbid depression, and for the development of gender-related biopsychosocial explanatory models. Prospective studies are needed, because gender bias is of high clinical and public health importance. There is also a need for improving the detection of depression in CAD patients, and for paying more attention to the suspectability to CAD in patients with major depression. Consequently, gender-related issues have to be taken into account, not only in detecting CAD and depression, but also in treatment and rehabilitation programs with the goal of better meeting the specific needs of men and women, improving the prevention of CAD.

REFERENCES

[1]   Curry P, O´Brian M: The male heart and the female mind: A study in the gendering of antidepressants and cardiovascular drugs in advertisements in Irish medical publication. *Social Science and Medicine* 2006; 62:1970-1977

[2]   Glick P, Lameiras M, Fiske ST, Eckes T, Masser B, Volpato C et al: Bad but bold: Ambivalent attitudes toward men predict gender inequality in 16 nations. *J Pers Soc Psychol.* 2004; 86:713-728

[3]   Denton M, Prus S, Walters V: Gender differences in health: a Canadian study of the psychosocial, structural and behavioural determinants of health. *Social Science and Medicine* 2004; 58:2585-2600

[4]   McDonough P, Walters V: Gender and health: reassessing patterns and explanations. *Social Science and Medicine* 2001; 52:547-559

[5]   Jackson R, Chambless L, Higgins M, et al: Sex difference in ischemic heart disease mortality and risk factors in 46 communities: an ecologic analysis. WHO MONICA Project, and ARIC Study. *Cardiovasc Risk Factors* 1997; 7:43-54

[6]   Mosca L, Appel LJ, Benjamin EJ, Berra K, Chandra-Strobos N et al.: Evidence-based guidelines for cardiovascular disease prevention in women. *Circulation* 2004; 109:672-693.

[7]   European Cardiovascular Disease Statistics 2005. www.heartstats.org/1570

[8]   Tunstall-Pedoe H, Kuulasma K, Mahonen M, Tolonen H, Ruokokoski E, Amouyel P: Contribution of trends in survival and coronary-event rates to changes in coronary heart disease mortality: 10-year results from 37 WHO MONICA project populations. Monitoring trends and determinants in cardiovascular disease. *Lancet* 1999; 353:1547-1557

[9]   American Heart Association. Heart and Stroke Statistics 2003. www.americanheart.org/

[10]   Löwel H, Meisinger C, Heier M et al. Geschlechtsspezifische Trends on plötzlichem Herztod und akutem Herzinfarkt. Ergebnisse des bevölkerungsbasierten KORA/MONICA-Augsburg Herzinfarktregisters 1985-1998. *Dtsch Med Wochenschr.* 2002; 44:2311-2316

[11]   Bello N, Mosca L: Epidemiology of coronary heart disease in women. *Progress in Cardiovascular Diseases* 2004; 46:287-295

[12]   Barrett-Connor E: Sex differences in coronary heart disease. Why are women so superior? The 1995 Ancel Keys Lecture. *Circulation* 1997; 95:252-264

[13]   Eastwood JA, Doering LV: Gender differences in coronary artery disease. *Journal of Cardiovascular Nursing* 2005; 20:430-351

[14]   Gold LD, Krumholz HM: Gender differences in treatment of heart failure and acute myocardial infarction. A question of quality or epidemiology? *Cardiology in Review* 2006; 14:180-186

[15]   Hart PL: Women´s perceptions of coronary heart disease: an integrative review. *J Cardiovasc Nurs* 2005; 20:170-176

[16]   Vaccarino V, Parsons L, Every NR, Barron HV, Krumholz HM: Sex-based differences in early mortality after myocardial infarction. *The New England Journal of Medicine* 1999; 341:217-225

[17]   Wenger N: Coronary heart disease: the female heart is vulnerable. *Progress in Cardiovascular Diseases* 2003, 46: 199-229

[18]   Brezinka V, Kittel F: Psychosocial factors of coronary heart disease in women: a review. *Social Science and Medicine* 1995; 10:1351-1365

[19]   Carney RM, Freedland KE, Smith L, Lustman PJ, Jaffe AS: Relation of depression and mortality after myocardial infarction in women. *Circulation* 1991; 84:1876-1877

[20]   Raine RA, Black, NA Bowker TJ, Wood DA: Gender differences in the management and outcome of patients with actue coronary artery disease. *J Epidemiol Community Health* 2002; 56:791-797

[21]   Ben-Ami T, Gilutz H, Porath A, Sosna G, Liel-Cohen N: No gender difference in the clinical management and outcome of unstable angina. *Isr Med Assoc J* 2005; 7:228-232

[22]   Krumholz HM, Douglas PS, Lauer MS, Paternak RC: Selection of patients for coronary angiography and coronary revascularization early after myocardial infarction: is there evidence for a gender bias? *Ann Intern Med* 1992; 116:875-790

[23]   Shaw LJ, Miller DD, Romeis JC, Kargl D, Younis LT, Chaitman BR: Gender differences in the noninvasive evaluation and management of patients with suspected coronary artery disease. *Ann Intern Med* 1994;20:559.566

[24]   Daley C, Clemens F, Lopez Sendon JL, Tavazzi L, Boersma E, Danchin N et al: Gender differences in the management and clinical outcome of stable angina. *Circulation* 2006; 113:490-498

[25]   Williams D, Bennett K, Feely J: Evidence for an age and gender bias in the secondary prevention of ischaemic heart disease in primary care. *Br J Clin Pharmacol* 2002; 55:604-608

[26] Simpson CR, Hannaford PC, Williams D: Evidence for inequalities in the management of coronary heart disease in Scotland. *Heart*. 2005; 91:630-634

[27] Legato MJ. Gender-specific physiology: how real is it? How important is it? *Int J Fertil* 1997; 42:19-29

[28] Executive summary. Women and smoking: A report of the surgeon general. *MMRW* 2002; 51:1-30

[29] Ulmer H, Diem G, Bischof HP, Ruttmann E, Concin H: Recent trends and sociodemographic distribution of cardiovascular risk factors: results from two population surveys in the Austrian WHO CONDO demonstration area. *Wien Klin Wochenschr* 2001; 113:573-579

[30] Mähönen MS, McElduff P, Dobson AJ, Kuulasmaa KA, Evans AE: Current smoking and the risk of non-fatal myocardial infaction in the WHO MONICA Project populations. *Tabacco Control* 2004; 13:244-250

[31] Castelli WP: Cardiovascular disease: pathogenesis, epidemiology, and risk among users of oral contraceptives who smoke. *Am J Obstet Gynecol* 1999; 180:349-356

[32] Polk ND, Naqvi TZ: Cariovascular disease in women: sex differences in presentation, risk factors, and evaluation. *Curr Cardiol Pre* 2005; 7:166-172

[33] Kenachaiah S, Gaziano JM, Vasan RS: Impact of obesity on the risk of heart failure and survival after the onset of heart failure. *Med Clin North Am* 2004; 88:1273-1294

[34] Rozanski A, Blumenthal JA, Kaplan J: Impact of psychological factors on the pathogenesis of cardiovascular disease and implications for therapy. *Circulation* 1999; 99:2192-2217

[35] Hemingway H, Marmot M: Psychosocial factors in the aetiology and prognosis of coronary heart disease: systematic review of prospective cohort studies. *BMJ* 1999; 318:1460-1467

[36] Bunker SJ, Colquhoun DM, Esler MS, Hickie IB, Hunt D, Jelinek M et al: „Stress" and coronary heart disease: psychosocial risk factors. *MJA* 2003; 178:272-276

[37] Eaker ED, Pinky J, Castelli WP: Myocardial infarction and coronary death among women: pychosocial predictors from a 20-year follow-up of women in the Framingham Study. *Am J Epidemio* 1992; 135:854-864

[38] Tunstall-Pedoe H, Kuulasmaa K, Amouyel P, Arveiler D, Rajakangas AM, Pajak A: Myocardial infarction and coronary deaths in the World Health Organization MONICA Project. Registration procedures, event rates, and case-fatality rates in 38 populations from 21 countries in four continents. *Circulation* 1994; 90:583-612

[39] Reuterwall C, Hallqvist J, Ahlbom A, de Faire U, Didrichsen F, Hogstedt C et al: Higher relative, but lower absolute risks of myocardial infarction in women than in men: analysis of some major risk factors in the SHEEP study. *Journal of Internal Medicine* 1999; 246:161-174

[40] Kuper H, Marmot M, Hemingway H: Systematic review of prospective cohort studies of psychosocial risk factors in the etiology and prognosis of coronary heart disease. *Semin Vas Med* 2002; 2:267-314

[41] Morrison C, Woodward M, Leslie W, Tunstall-Pedoe H: Effect of socioeconomic group on incidence of, management of, and survival after myocardial infarction and coronary death: analysis of community coronary event register. *BMJ* 1997; 314:541

[42] Hallqvist J, Lundberg M, Didrichsen F, Ahlbom A: Socioeconomic differences in risk of myocardial infarction 1971-1994 in Sweden: time trends, relative risks and population attributable risks. *International Journal of Epidmiology* 1998; 27:410-415

[43] Eaker ED: Psychosocial factors in the epidmiology of coronary heart disease in women. *Psychiatr Clin North Am* 1989; 12:167-173

[44] Kuper H, Adami HO, Theorell T, Weiderpass E: Psychosocial determinants of coronary heart disease in middle-aged women: a prospective study in Sweden. *Am J Epidmiol* 2006; 164:349-357

[45] Wamala, SP, Lynch J, Kaplan GA: Women´s exposure to early and later life socioeconomic disadvantage and coronary heart disease risk: the Stockholm Female Coronary Risk Study. *International Journal of Epidmiology* 2001; 0:275-284

[46] Lawlor DA, Ebrahim S, Smith GD: Adverse socioeconomic position across the lifecourse increases coronary heart disease risk cumulatively: findings from the British women´s heart and health study. *J Epidmiol Community Health* 2005; 59:785-793

[47] Hart CL, Davey Smith G, Blane D: Inequalities in mortality by social class measured at three stages of the life course. *Am J Public Health* 1998; 88:471-474

[48] Marmot M, Bartley M: Social class and coronary heart disease. In: Stansfeld S, Marmot M, eds. Stress and the Heart. London: BMJ books; 2002:5-19

[49] Pekkanen J, Tuomilehto J, Uutela A, Vartiainen E, Nissinen A: Social class, health behaviour, and mortality among men and women in eastern Finland. *BMJ* 1995; 311:589-93

[50] Marmot MG, Bosma H, Hemingway H, Brunner E, Stansfeld S: Contribution of job control and other risk factors to social variations in coronary heart disease incidence. *Lancet* 1997; 350:235-239

[51] Peter R, Siegrist J: Psychosocial work environment and the risk of coronary heart disease. *Int Arch Occup Environ Health* 2000; 73 Suppl:41-45

[52] Bosma H, Marmot MG, Hemingway,H, Nicholsen AC, Brunner E, Stansfeld SA: Low job control and risk of coronary heart disease in Whitehall II (prospective cohort) study. *BMJ* 1997; 314:558-565

[53] Wamala SP, Mittleman MA, Horsten M, Schenck-Gustafsson K, Orth-Gómer K: Job stress and the occupational gradient in coronary heart disease risk in women. The Stockholm Female Coronary Risk Study. *Social Science and Medicine* 2000; 51:481-489

[54] Chandola T, Brunner E, Marmot M: Chronic stress at work and the metabolic syndrome: prospective study. *BMJ* 2006; 332:521-525

[55] Eaker ED, Sullivan LM, Kelly-Hayes M, D´Agostino RB Sr, Benjamin EJ: Does job strain increase the risk for coronary heart disease or death in men and women? The Framingham Offspring Study. *Am J Epidemiol* 2004; 159:950-958

[56] Peter R, Hammarstrom A, Hallqvist J, Siegrist J, Theorell T, SHEEP Study Group: Does occupational gender segregation influence the association of effort-reward imbalance with myocardial infaction in the SHEEP study? *Int J Behav Med* 2006; 13:34-43

[57]   La Rosa JH: Women, work, and health: employment as a risk factor for coronary heart disease. *Am J Obstet Gynecol* 1988; 158:1597-1602

[58]   Haynes SG, Feinleib M, Kennel WB: The relationship of psychosocial factors to coronary heart disease in the Framingham Study. III. Eight-year incidence of coronary heart disease. *Am J Epidemiol* 1980; 111:37-58

[59]   Orth-Gómer K, Leineweber C: Multiple stressors and coronary disease in women. The Stockholm Female Coronary Risk Study. *Biological Psychology* 2005; 69:57-66

[60]   Orth-Gómer K, Wamala SP, Horsten M, Schenck-Gustafsson K, Schneiderman N, Mittleman MA: Marital stress worsens prognosis in women with coronary heart disease: The Stockholm Female Coronary Risk Study. *JAMA* 2000; 284:3008-3014

[61]   Lee S, Colditz G, Berkam L, Kawachi I: Caregiving to children and grandchildren and risk of coronary heart disease in women. *Am J Public Health* 2003; 93:1939-44

[62]   Hall EM: Double exposure: the combined impact of the home and work environments on psychosomatic strain in Swedish women and men. *Int J Health Serv* 1992; 22:239-60

[63]   Theorell T, Tsutsumi A, Hallqvist J, Reuterwall C, Hogstedt C, Fredlund P et al: Decision latitude, job strain, and myocardial infarction: a study of working men in Stockholm. The SHEEP Study Group. Stockholm Heart Epidemiology Program. *Am J Public Health* 1998; 88:382-388

[64]   Lett HS, Blumenthal JA, Babyak MA, Strauman TJ, Robins C, Sherwood A: Social Support and coronary heart disease: epidmiologic evidence and implications for treatment. *Psychosomatic Medicine* 2005; 67:869-878

[65]   Hammar N, Alfredsson L, Johnson JV: Job strain, social support at work, and incidence of myocardial infarction. *Occup Environ Med* 1998; 55:548-553

[66]   Orth-Gómer K, Johnson JV: Social network interaction and mortality. A six year follow-up study of a random sample of the Swedish population. *J Chronic Dis* 1987; 40:949-57

[67]   Kaplan GA, Salonen JT, Cohen RD, Brand RJ, Syme SL, Puska P: Social connections and mortality from all causes and from cardiovascular disease: prospective evidence from eastern Finland. *Am J Epidemiol.* 1988; 128:370-380

[68]   Young LE, Cunningham SL, Buist DS: Lone mothers are at higher risk for cardiovascular disease compared with partnered mothers. Data from the National Health and Nutrition Examination Survey III (NHANES III). *Health Care Women Int* 2005; 26:604-21

[69]   Chandra V, Szklo M, Goldberg R, Tonascia J: The impact of marital status on survival after an acute myocardial infarction: a population-based study. *Am J Epidemiol* 1983; 117:320-325

[70]   Williams RB, Barefoot JC, Califf RM, Haney TL, Saunders WB. Pryor DB et al: Prognostic importance of social and economic resources among medically treated patients with angiographically documented coronary artery disease. *JAMA* 1992; 267:520-524

[71]   Hildingh C, Fridlund B: Social network and experiences of social support among women 12 months after their first myocardial infarction. *International Journal of Rehabilitation and Health* 1997; 3:131-142

[72] Rose GL, Suls J, Green PJ, Lounsbury P, Gordon E: Comparison of adjustment, activity, and tangible social support in men and women patients and their spouses during the six months pst-myocardial infarction. *The Society of Behavioral Medicine* 1996; 18:264-272.

[73] Strike PC, Steptoe A: Psychosocial factors in the development of coronary artery disease. *Prog Cardiovasc Dis* 2004; 46:337-347

[74] Haas DC, Chaplin WF, Shimbo D, Pickering TG, Burg M, Davidson KW: Hostility is an independent predictor of recurrent coronary deart disease events in men but not women: results from a population based study. *Heart* 2005; 91:1609-1610

[75] Lahad A, Heckbert SR, Koepsell TD, Psaty BM, Patrick LD: Hostility, aggression and the risk of nonfatal myocardial infarction in postmenopausal women. *J Psychosom Res* 1997; 43:183-195

[76] Chaput LA, Adams SH, Simon JA, Blumenthal RS, Vittinghoff E, Lin F, Loh E, Matthews KA: Hostility predicts recurrent events among post-menopausal women with coronary heart disease. *Am J Epidemiol* 2002; 126:1092-1096

[77] Doris A, Ebmeier K, Shajahan P: Depressive illness. *Lancet* 1999; 54:1369-1375

[78] Murray CJ, Lopez AD: Global mortality, disability, and the contribution of risk factors: Global Burden of Disease Study. *Lancet* 1997; 349:1436-142

[79] Weissman MM, Bland R, Joyce PR, Newman S, Wells JE, Wittchen HU: Sex differences in rates of depression: cross national perspectives. *J Affect Disord* 1993; 29: 77-84

[80] Kessler RC, McGonagle KA, Swartz M, Blazer DG, Nelson CB: Sex and depression in the National Comorbidity Survey. I: Lifetime prevalence, chronicity and recurrence. *J Affect Disord* 1993; 2-3: 85-96

[81] Mojtabai R, Olfson M: Major depression in community-dwelling middle-aged and older adults: prevalence and 2- and 4-year follow-up symptoms. *Psychological Medicine* 2004; 34:623-634

[82] Kühner C: Gender differences in unipolar depression: an update of epidemiological findings and possible explanations. *Acta Psychiatr Scand* 2003; 108:163-174

[83] Rudisch B, Nemeroff CB: Epidemiology of comorbid coronary artery disease and depression. *Biol Psychiatry* 2003; 54:227-240

[84] Rugulies R: Depression as a predictor for coronary heart disease. *Am J Prev Med* 2002; 23:51-61

[85] Sørensen C, Brandes A, Hendricks O, Thrane J, Friis-Hasche E, Haghfelt T, Bech P: Psychosocial predictors of depression in patients with acute coronary syndrome. *Acta Psychiatr Scand* 2005; 111:116-124

[86] Feinstein RE, Blumenfield M, Orlowski B, Frishman WH, Ovanessian S: A national survey of cardiovascular physicians' beliefs and clinical care practices when diagnosing and treating depression in patients with cardiovascular disease. *Cardiol Rev* 2006; 14:164-169

[87] Wassertheil-Smoller S, Shumaker S, Ockene J, Tavalera GA, Greeland P, Cochrane B, et al: Depression and cardiovascular sequelae in postmenopausal women. The Women´s Health Initiative (WHI). *Arch Intern Med* 2005; 164:289-298

[88] Ferketich Ak, Schwatzaum JA, Frid DJ, Moeschberger ML: Depression as an antecedent to heart disease among women and men in the NHANES I study. National Health and Nutrition Examination Survey. *Arch Intern Med* 2000; 160:1261-1268

[89] Mendes de Leon CF, Krumholz HM, Seeman TS, Vaccarino V, Williams CS, Kasl SV, Berkman LF: Depression and risk of coronary heart disease in elderly men and women: New Haven EPESE, 1982-1991. Established Populations for the Epidemiologic Studies of the Elderly. *Arch Intern Med* 1998; 158:2341-2348

[90] Penninx BWJH, Guralnik JM, Mendes de Leon CF, Pahor M, Visser M, Corti MC, Wallace RB: Cardiovascular events and mortality in newly and chronically depressed persons > 70 years of age. *Am J Cardiol* 1998; 81:988-994

[91] Williams SA, Kasl SV, Heiat A, Abramson JL, Krumholz HM, Vaccarino V: Depression and risk of deart failure among the elderly: a prospective community-based study. *Psychosomatic Medicine* 2002; 64:6-12

[92] Anderson RJ, Freedlan KE, Clouse RE, Lustman PJ: The prevalence of comorbid depression in adults with diabetes: a metanalysis. *Diabetes Care* 2001; 24:1069-1078

[93] Clouse RE, lustman PJ, Freedland KE, Griffith LS, McGill JB, Carney RM: Depression and coronary heart disease in women with diabetes. *Psychosomatic Medicine* 2003; 65:376-383

[94] Batten SV, Aslan M, Maciejewski PK, Mazure CM: Childhood maltreatment as a risk factor for adult cardiovascular disease and depression. *J Clin Psychiatry* 2004; 65:249-254

[95] Frasure-Smith N, Lesperance F: Reflections on depression as a cardia risk factor. *Psychosomatic Medicine* 2005; 67suppl1:19-25

[96] Drory Y, Kravetz S, Hirschberger G, Israel Study Group on First Acute Myocardial Infarction: Long-term mental health of women after a first acute myocardial infarction. *Arch Phys Med Rehabil* 2003; 84:1492-1498

[97] Frasure-Smith N, Lesperance F, Talajic M.: Depression and 18-month prognosis after myocardial infarction. *Circulation* 1995; 91:999-1005

[98] Bjerkeset O, Nordahl HM, Mykletun A, Holmen J, Dahl AA: Anxiety and depression following myocardial infarction: gender differences in a 5-year prospective study. *J Psychosom Res* 2005; 58:153-61

[99] Mallik S, Spertus JA, Reid KJ, Krumholz HM, Runsfeld JS, Weintraub WS et al: Depressive symptoms after acute myocardial infarction: evidence for highest rates in younger women. *Arch Intern Med* 2006; 166:876-883

[100] Frasure-Smith N, Lesperance F, Juneau M, Talajic M, Bourassa MG: Gender, depression, and one-year prognosis after myocardial infaction. *Psychosomatic Medicine* 1999; 61:2 6-37

[101] Ahnlund K, Frodi A: Gender differences in the development of depression. *Scand J Psychol* 1996; 37:229-237

[102] Kiecolt-Glaser JK, Newton TL: Marriage and health: his and hers. *Psychological Bulletin* 2001; 127:472-503

[103] Horsten M, Mittleman MA, Wamala SP, Schenck-Gustafsson K, Orth-Gómer K: Depressive symptoms and lack of social integration in relation to prognosis of CHD in middle-aged women. The Stockholm Female Coronary Risk Study. *European Heart Journal* 2000; 21:1072-1080.

In: Psychological Factors and Cardiovascular Disorders   ISBN: 978-1-60456-871-4
Editor: Leo Sher   © 2008 Nova Science Publishers, Inc.

Chapter III

DEPRESSION AS A RISK FACTOR FOR THE DEVELOPMENT OF HEART DISEASE

Tye Dawood and Gavin Lambert

Baker IDI Heart and Diabetes Institute, Melbourne, Australia.

"… …from the brain, and from the brain only, arise our pleasures, joys, … …as well as our sorrows, pains, grief, and tears. It is the same organ which makes us mad or delirious, inspires us with dread and fear, brings sleeplessness … …and aimless anxiety." *Hippocrates 400 BC*

ABSTRACT

Major depressive disorder is a complex disorder with a lifetime prevalence of approximately 20%, affecting people of any age, gender and background. It is projected that by the year 2020, MDD will be the 2nd leading contributor of the global burden of disease, second only to cardiovascular disease. Not only can the symptoms experienced affect an individual's day-to-day activities, with suicide being the ultimate misfortune, but there is now clear evidence to suggest that major depressive disorder is a risk factor for cardiovascular disease. As yet, the mechanism of increased cardiac risk attributable to depressive illness is uncertain, although several hypotheses have been proposed. These include modification of the activity of the autonomic nervous system, exaggerated platelet reactivity, endothelial dysfunction and inflammatory-mediated atherogenesis.

INTRODUCTION

Over countless generations and throughout different civilisations, the relationship between affect and the heart was not formally documented even though the (general public's) awareness of the link between grief and sadness and heart disease was well recognised. The association between mental health and cardiovascular health did not emerge until early in the twentieth century when Malzberg reported high mortality rates in hospital inpatients with depression [1]. It was not until 50 years later that evidence from prospective trials indicated that affective disorders participated in the development of cardiovascular disease. In a recent study that used health data collected prior to and up to three years following the September 11 terrorist attacks, acute stress reactions to the attacks predicted the onset of cardiovascular events over the follow-up period [2]; thereby, providing presumptive and convincing support of a link between stress and the heart.

There is now good evidence that patients with major depressive disorder (MDD) are at increased risk of developing coronary heart disease (CHD) [3-7]. This elevated risk is independent of the usual, established risk factors such as smoking, obesity, hypercholesterolemia, diabetes and hypertension. The association exists in both genders, across different age groups and in subjects living in different countries [7,8]. The CHD risk is increased 1.5-2 fold in those with minor depression and 3-4.5 fold in subjects with more severe depression. Based on these observations, the relative risk of developing CHD is, in fact, proportional to the severity of the depression.

At present the mechanism of increased cardiac risk attributable to depressive illness remains to be clearly established, but activation of the sympathetic nervous system, altered vagal activity and/or inflammatory-mediated atherogenesis are likely to be of major importance. Additionally, elevated cardiac risk may also be further compromised by co-existing lifestyle factors such as increased incidence of tobacco smoking [9], co-morbid obesity [10], reduced levels of exercise [11] and non-compliance with therapeutic medications [12].

MECHANISM OF RISK 1:
ACTIVATION OF THE SYMPATHETIC NERVOUS SYSTEM

The sympathetic nervous system is on centre stage in cardiovascular medicine. Increased stimulation of the cardiac sympathetic outflow has been demonstrated to contribute to myocardial infarction [13], the development of ventricular tachycardia and ventricular fibrillation outside hospital [14], and the neurohumoral features of myocardial stunning due to sudden emotional stress [15]. In heart failure there is similarly a high level of stimulation of the cardiac sympathetic nerves, which has been directly linked to the development of ventricular arrhythmias and sudden death [16]. Interestingly, in healthy subjects, laboratory mental stress is associated with a specific activation of the cardiac sympathetic nervous outflow [17]. In addition to blood pressure elevation, sympathetically mediated neural vasoconstriction may also exert metabolic effects, in skeletal muscle impairing glucose delivery to muscle [18], causing insulin resistance and hyperinsulinaemia, and in the liver retarding postprandial clearing of lipids [19], contributing to hyperlipidaemia. A trophic effect of sympathetic activation on cardiovascular growth can also occur, contributing to the development of left ventricular hypertrophy [20].

Sympathetic nervous responses are regionalised, making it difficult to draw meaningful conclusions based on simple venous norepinephrine plasma concentrations. A number of studies have reported low plasma, CSF or urinary norepinephrine in patients with depressive illness [21-24]. Contrary to these investigations, and suggestive of increased sympathetic activity in patients with depression following myocardial infarction, investigators in the Heart and Soul Study documented an association between carriage of the *short* allele in the promoter region of a serotonin transporter polymorphism (5-HTTLPR) and elevated urinary norepineprine levels [25]. This is a significant observation and may explain the increased cardiac risk in patients with MDD. Moreover, high plasma levels of noradrenaline and its metabolite 3-methoxy-4-hydroxyphenylglycol (MHPG) [26], and increased rates of spillover of noradrenaline to plasma [27-29] have also been documented in some patients with MDD. Using norepinephrine isotope dilution methodology [30] we were able to demonstrate that a sub-group of patients with MDD, who were otherwise healthy and not on any medication, had extraordinarily high whole body and cardiac sympathetic nervous activity [29]. Although we do not have evidence that these patients are at increased risk of developing coronary heart disease, the levels of sympathetic activity observed are of a similar magnitude to the levels observed in patients with essential hypertension [20] and patients unexpectedly developing ventricular arrhythmias [14].

The importance of hypertension in the development of left ventricular hypertrophy, myocardial infarction, heart failure and sudden death is well established [reviewed in Esler *et al.* (1990) [31]]. Indeed, over 90% of patients with heart failure in the Framingham study had a history of hypertension [32]. The longitudinal studies of Timio and colleagues, examining hypertension development and cardiovascular morbidity and mortality in cloistered nuns, provides evidence linking daily life stress to the development of high blood pressure [33]. Similarly, a recent study examining the effects of acute stress on the prediction of cardiovascular events over two years following the terrorist attacks of 9/11 demonstrated that high levels of stress immediately after the attacks were associated with increased diagnoses of hypertension and other cardiovascular-related problems [2]. Furthermore, the Specialist Medical Review Council of Australia concluded that stress was an initiating factor in the development of essential hypertension [34]. They based their finding on the observation that a rise in blood pressure is initiated and maintained by activation of the sympathetic nervous system, a phenomenon also observed in stress [34].

The association between depressive illness and blood pressure remains discordant. Several studies have investigated the relationship between the two disorders, with conflicting conclusions. One study in middle-aged subjects with depressive disorder and hypertension found no relationship between blood pressure and depression [35]. In elderly patients, high depression levels were associated with low systolic pressure at 3-4 years following the initial diagnosis of depressive illness, but no predictive relationship was established [36]. Furthermore, low diastolic blood pressure at baseline or decreases in blood pressure between the initial and follow-up measurements were predictive of depressive illness within the two-year study period, in the elderly [37]. In conflict with these findings, anxiety and depressive illness correlated with incidence of hypertension in 25-64 year old subjects, 7-16 years following baseline measurements [38]. Similarly, in young patients with depressive illness, the risk of developing hypertension within a five-year follow-up was significantly increased compared with subjects who did not have depression [39]. On balance, it remains to be proven that patients with MDD exhibit disproportionately elevated levels of blood pressure.

MECHANISM OF RISK 2: VAGAL ACTIVITY

Baroreflex Function

The cardiac baroreflex regulates heart rate and peripheral vascular resistance on a beat-to-beat basis to safeguard against changes in blood pressure [40]. When acute rises in blood pressure occur, consequent reflex reduction in heart rate and arterial tone are observed. This is the result of an increase in vagal activity accompanied by a decrease in sympathetic efferent activity [40]. The opposite occurs with acute reductions in blood pressure.

Arterial baroreflex dysfunction is directly linked to incidence rates for acute cardiac events in conditions such as hypertension [41], diabetes [42] and heart failure [43]. Following myocardial infarction, baroreflex sensitivity, a measure of the baroreflex gain, is reduced [40]. The reduction in baroreflex sensitivity enhances sympathoexcitation, which in turn reduces the baroreflex sensitivity even further. Moreover, in the Autonomic Tone and Reflexes After Myocardial Infarction (ATRAMI) study, baroreflex and heart rate variability were significant predictors of mortality following myocardial infarction independent of left ventricular ejection fraction and ventricular arrhythmias [44].

Conflicting results have been obtained in relation to baroreflex function in depressive illness. In patients with combined depressive illness and coronary heart disease, a 30% reduction in baroreflex sensitivity was observed compared to patients with coronary heart disease but without depressive illness [45]. However, a study by the same group showed that baroreflex function was not impaired in patients with depressive illness, in comparison with non-depressed patients, approximately six days post-myocardial infarction [46]. Nevertheless, the study showed a significant correlation between high anxiety and reduced baroreflex sensitivity in these patients. In contrast, Pitzalis et al. found reduced baroreflex sensitivity in depressed compared with non-depressed patients post-myocardial infarction [47]. Measurements were obtained 5-12 days following a first episode of myocardial infarction. Patients were not taking β-blockers. Although the study was not specifically designed to distinguish between those taking β-blockers and those not taking these medications, the authors noted that depressive illness did not affect baroreflex function in patients taking β-blockers [47]. Yet another study showed that a history of depressive illness with no cardiovascular disease, regardless of whether the patients were currently on treatment or not, was associated with reduced baroreflex sensitivity as compared with healthy controls [48]. The patients were all euthymic at study time and none had cardiac disease or other conventional cardiac risk factors. Patients with depressive illness were divided into three groups, those not on medication, those on SSRIs and those taking other antidepressants, including tricyclics, serotonin/noradrenaline reuptake inhibitors or monoamine oxidase inhibitors. The authors found no significant differences between these groups in baroreflex sensitivity. However, only 9 patients were in the non-medication group and 12 in the SSRI group, with baroreflex sensitivity being 21.2 ± 3.7 (mean $\pm$ SEM) ms/mmHg and 17.9 ± 2.4 ms/mmHg, respectively. Whether the power of the study was sufficient to detect a significant difference is debatable. There is a possibility that if more patients in each group were included the difference may have become significant. In other words, a significant reduction in baroreflex sensitivity in patients taking SSRIs would have been observed. Control subjects had a baroreflex sensitivity of 25.4 ± 1.7 ms/mmHg. Our own results indicated that cardiac baroreflex function in unmedicated patients with MDD, with no conventional cardiovascular risk factors, was not significantly impaired [49]. However, the clinical improvement observed in these patients following SSRI administration was accompanied by a substantial reduction in the slope of the cardiac baroreflex [49].

Heart Rate Variability

Heart rate variability (HRV), put simply, is the fluctuation in the R-R interval between consecutive heart beats [50]. While heart rate is influenced by both sympathetic and parasympathetic activity, at rest, heart rate is predominantly dependent on vagal tone [51].

Reduced heart rate variability has been proposed as one of the mechanisms by which depressive illness is associated with increased mortality in patients following a myocardial infarction. In the large multi-centre trial, Enhancing Recovery in Coronary Heart Disease (ENRICHD), reduced heart rate variability was significantly associated with depressive illness, as measured with the Beck Depression Inventory (BDI), in patients following a myocardial infarction [52]. Similarly, Frasure-Smith *et al.* followed the progress of patients post-myocardial infarction over a six month period and reported that patients with depressive illness had a 5-fold increase in mortality rate when compared with non-depressed patients [53]. It was proposed that increased mortality in the former patients was due to decreased heart rate variability and subsequent generation of fatal arrhythmias. Furthermore, the association between depressive illness, reduced vagal activity and increased mortality persisted 18 months following myocardial infarction [54]. In those with depressive illness, and without coronary heart disease, heart rate variability does not appear to be modified [49]. Similar to the decrease of the cardiac baroreflex function, treatment with an SSRI resulted in a significant decrease in heart rate variability [49].

MECHANISM OF RISK 3: ENDOTHELIAL DYSFUNCTION

Endothelial dysfunction can lead to enhanced plaque vulnerability, trigger plaque rupture and promote thrombus formation, culminating in atherosclerosis, unstable angina and myocardial infarction [55]. Studies investigating endothelial function indicated that patients with MDD have impaired endothelial function. In young adults with untreated depression, Rajagopalan and colleagues (2001) reported impairment in endothelial function when compared to the healthy control group [56]. There were no significant differences between the groups in endothelium-independent vasodilation. Similarly, a study investigating endothelial function in postmenopausal women with and without a history of depression, and with no apparent conventional cardiovascular risk factors and antidepressant-free, concluded that women with a history of depression had impaired endothelial function compared to women without a history of depression [57]. Furthermore, the number of previous depressive episodes correlated with the severity of endothelial dysfunction. Data from Broadley *et al.* (2002) supported the findings of this study, demonstrating that endothelial dysfunction persisted in patients with depression following treatment with antidepressants [58]. However, the investigators did not control for the antidepressants used, perhaps incorrectly concluding that all types of antidepressants do not improve endothelial function in depressed patients.

MECHANISM OF RISK 4: PLATELET REACTIVITY

There is evidence to suggest that psychological factors, including depression and mental stress, can have an effect on platelet function by increasing platelet reactivity and thrombus formation [59,60] and culminating in acute cardiac events [61,62]. Musselman *el al.* (1996) observed that depressed patients, not on any form of medication, were found to have higher platelet reactivity compared to the healthy group, at rest and following orthostatic challenge, with no differences in platelet counts [63]. Furthermore, a significant increase in binding of PAC1, a murine monoclonal antibody specific for the activated glycoprotein IIb/IIIa complex, and anti-LIBS1, a monoclonal antibody specific for ligands such as fibrinogen-induced binding sites on glycoprotein IIIa, was observed in depressed patients following orthostatic challenge. Similarly, Shimbo *et al.* (2002) showed that 5-HT-mediated platelet reactivity in patients with depression is significantly higher than in control subjects [64]. Moreover, there were no differences between the two groups with respect to adenosine diphosphate, a non-5-HT agonist.

P-Selectin

The properties of P-selectin render it a prime candidate in the development of atherosclerosis. Its overexpression in the endothelium on atherosclerotic plaques contributes to its adverse effects [65]. P-selectin on platelets was found to be higher in patients with MDD compared with control subjects [59]. However, no correlation was observed between the severity of depressive illness, as measured using the Hamilton Depression scale, and P-selectin. Contrary to this report, Musselman *et al.* demonstrated that resting P-selectin expression on platelets in subjects with depressive illness was comparable to that of controls [63]. Although these authors observed higher procoagulation at rest in MDD than in controls, the monoclonal antibody binding of GE12, which is specific for P-selectin, was similar in the two groups [63]. Yet another study demonstrated higher P-selectin fluorescence intensity, at baseline, in healthy controls in comparison with patients with MDD [60]. In agreement with platelet P-selectin results, soluble P-selectin concentrations in plasma in unmedicated subjects with depression, but otherwise healthy, were significantly elevated compared with matched controls [66].

MECHANISM OF RISK 5:
INFLAMMATORY-MEDIATED ATHEROGENESIS

Inflammation has been implicated in the initiation, progression and complications of atherosclerosis [67]. There has been conflicting evidence as to whether inflammatory markers are one of the mechanisms involved in the link between cardiovascular disease and depressive illness. Penninx and colleagues (2003) investigated the link between inflammatory markers and depressed mood in older people. They concluded that depressed elderly individuals had higher levels of interleukin (IL)-6, tumor necrosis factor (TNF)-α and C-reactive protein (CRP) [68]. When demographic variables and health were adjusted for, depressed mood was associated with high levels of at least two of the inflammatory markers. The link was bidirectional, demonstrating that individuals with high levels of at least two of the inflammatory markers exhibited an increased risk of depressed mood. When levels of CRP, IL-6, TNF-α, fibrinogen, IL-1 receptor antagonist and T- and B-lymphocytes were evaluated in middle-aged men and women with and without depressive symptoms, however, there appeared to be no association between depressed mood and hopelessness and high levels of inflammatory markers or immune activation [69].

CRP is part of a group of acute phase proteins manufactured by the body in response to trauma or infection [70]. It is secreted from the liver in response to IL-6 stimulation, while other factors such as IL-1 and glucocorticoids work in association with IL-6 to augment its effects [71]. CRP is not only a marker of inflammation but it actively participates in all stages of atherosclerotic lesion formation [72].

CRP is regarded as a risk marker for cardiovascular disease and also a prognostic indicator for cardiovascular disease development in patients with existing coronary syndromes. Several studies have demonstrated the significance of CRP as a prognostic indicator in both the short- and long-term [73-75]. There is a large body of evidence documenting the importance of CRP as a strong independent predictor of future cardiovascular disease events. This risk is present regardless of gender [76,77], ethnicity [78,79] and age [76,77].

A number of large-scale studies have been conducted to examine the association between depressive symptoms and CRP plasma concentrations. Tiemeier *et al.* found that there was no significant correlation between CRP and depressive disorders in subjects over 60 years when adjustment for age, gender and body mass index were taken into account [80]. However, the majority of studies showed a positive relationship between depressive symptoms and CRP levels. The Health ABC study (elderly participants) and the Cardiovascular Health Study (elderly participants free of cardiovascular disease), both demonstrated a significant association between depressive symptoms and CRP concentrations [68,81]. In a study of 18-89 year old cardiovascular disease-free participants, inflammatory markers, including CRP, were associated with depressive symptoms [82]. Furthermore, in young healthy subjects (18-39 years of age), a strong association was observed between CRP and a history of major depressive episode in men, but not in women [83]. This association was stronger for men who had experienced major depressive episodes in the preceding six months. Similarly, plasma concentrations of CRP were elevated in unmedicated, cardiovascular-free depression, where a significant positive relationship existed between the number of previous depressive episodes and CRP concentrations [49]. Following SSRI administration, CRP plasma concentrations were further elevated, in some patients to levels associated with increased cardiac risk [49].

CONCLUSION

A number of lifestyle factors can contribute to the increased risk of coronary artery disease following depressive illness. Non-adherence to treatment, which has been shown in patients with depressive disorder [84], is significantly associated with lower survival rates in patients with coronary artery disease [85], suggesting a possible link between the two. A correlation has been found between depressive illness and smoking [86], large quantities of alcohol consumption [87] and physical inactivity [88], all bona fide risk factors for cardiovascular disease development. Furthermore, depressive illness coupled with at least one of these factors, smoking, excessive alcohol consumption or physical inactivity, is associated with a greater risk of developing coronary artery disease [89].

The underlying mechanisms that render major depressive disorder a risk factor for the development of cardiovascular disease are most likely multi-factorial in origin. These include the autonomic nervous system, platelet activation, thrombogenesis and endothelial dysfunction. Identifying the mechanisms at play could result in relatively simple therapeutic strategies (eg low-dose aspirin, β-blockers, centrally acting sympatholytic agents) to be administered in those with MDD in order to modify cardiac risk. Further studies are necessary to elucidate the exact mechanisms involved in order to tailor therapies to reduce the burden of depression and cardiovascular disease on the community.

REFERENCES

[1]   Malzberg B: Mortality among patients with involution melancholia. *American Journal of Psychiatry* 1937; 93:1231-1238.

[2]   Holman EA, Silver RC, Poulin M, Andersen J, Gil-Rivas V, McIntosh DN: Terrorism, acute stress, and cardiovascular health: a 3-year national study following the September 11th attacks. *Arch Gen Psychiatry* 2008; 65(1):73-80.

[3]   Musselman DL, Evans DL, Nemeroff CB: The relationship of depression to cardiovascular disease: epidemiology, biology, and treatment. *Arch Gen Psychiatry* 1998; 55(7):580-92.

[4]   Glassman AH, Shapiro PA: Depression and the course of coronary artery disease. *Am J Psychiatry* 1998; 155(1):4-11.

[5]   Hemingway H, Marmot M: Evidence based cardiology: psychosocial factors in the aetiology and prognosis of coronary heart disease. Systematic review of prospective cohort studies. *BMJ* 1999; 318(7196):1460-7.

[6]   Bunker SJ, Colquhoun DM, Esler MD, Hickie IB, Hunt D, Jelinek VM, Oldenburg BF, Peach HG, Ruth D, Tennant CC, Tonkin AM: "Stress" and coronary heart disease: psychosocial risk factors. *Med J Aust* 2003; 178(6):272-6.

[7]   Rosengren A, Hawken S, Ounpuu S, Sliwa K, Zubaid M, Almahmeed WA, Blackett KN, Sitthi-amorn C, Sato H, Yusuf S: Association of psychosocial risk factors with risk of acute myocardial infarction in 11119 cases and 13648 controls from 52 countries (the INTERHEART study): case-control study. *Lancet* 2004; 364(9438):953-62.

[8]   Harris PA: The impact of age, gender, race, and ethnicity on the diagnosis and treatment of depression. *J Manag Care Pharm* 2004; 10(2 Suppl):S2-7.

[9]   Lasser K, Boyd JW, Woolhandler S, Himmelstein DU, McCormick D, Bor DH: Smoking and mental illness: A population-based prevalence study. *JAMA* 2000; 284(20):2606-10.

[10]   Zoccali R, Bruno A, Muscatello MR, La Torre D, Paterniti A, Corica F, Damiano MC, Di Rosa AE, Meduri M: Panic-agoraphobic spectrum in obese binge eaters. *Eat Weight Disord* 2004; 9(4):264-8.

[11]   Broocks A, Meyer TF, Bandelow B, George A, Bartmann U, Ruther E, Hillmer-Vogel U: Exercise avoidance and impaired endurance capacity in patients with panic disorder. *Neuropsychobiology* 1997; 36(4):182-7.

[12]   Roy-Byrne P, Russo J, Dugdale DC, Lessler D, Cowley D, Katon W: Undertreatment of panic disorder in primary care: role of patient and physician characteristics. *J Am Board Fam Pract* 2002; 15(6):443-50.

[13]   Mann DL, Kent RL, Parsons B, Cooper Gt: Adrenergic effects on the biology of the adult mammalian cardiocyte. *Circulation* 1992; 85(2):790-804.

[14]   Meredith IT, Broughton A, Jennings GL, Esler MD: Evidence of a selective increase in cardiac sympathetic activity in patients with sustained ventricular arrhythmias. *N Engl J Med* 1991; 325(9):618-24.

[15]   Wittstein IS, Thiemann DR, Lima JA, Baughman KL, Schulman SP, Gerstenblith G, Wu KC, Rade JJ, Bivalacqua TJ, Champion HC: Neurohumoral features of myocardial stunning due to sudden emotional stress. *N Engl J Med* 2005; 352(6):539-48.

[16]   Kaye DM, Lefkovits J, Jennings GL, Bergin P, Broughton A, Esler MD: Adverse consequences of high sympathetic nervous activity in the failing human heart. *J Am Coll Cardiol* 1995; 26(5):1257-63.

[17]   Esler M, Jennings G, Lambert G: Measurement of overall and cardiac norepinephrine release into plasma during cognitive challenge. *Psychoneuroendocrinology* 1989; 14(6):477-81.

[18]   Julius S, Gudbrandsson T, Jamerson K, Andersson O: The interconnection between sympathetics, microcirculation, and insulin resistance in hypertension. *Blood Press* 1992; 1(1):9-19.

[19]   Esler M: Sympathetic nervous system: contribution to human hypertension and related cardiovascular diseases. *J Cardiovasc Pharmacol* 1995; 26 Suppl 2:S24-8.

[20]   Schlaich MP, Kaye DM, Lambert E, Sommerville M, Socratous F, Esler MD: Relation between cardiac sympathetic activity and hypertensive left ventricular hypertrophy. *Circulation* 2003; 108(5):560-5.

[21]   Schildkraut JJ, Orsulak PJ, Schatzberg AF, Gudeman JE, Cole JO, Rohde WA, LaBrie RA: Toward a biochemical classification of depressive disorders. I. Differences in

urinary excretion of MHPG and other catecholamine metabolites in clinically defined subtypes of depressions. *Arch Gen Psychiatry* 1978; 35(12):1427-33.

[22]   Sweeney DR, Maas JW: Specificity of depressive diseases. *Annu Rev Med* 1978; 29:219-29.

[23]   Linnoila M, Karoum F, Calil HM, Kopin IJ, Potter WZ: Alteration of norepinephrine metabolism with desipramine and zimelidine in depressed patients. *Arch Gen Psychiatry* 1982; 39(9):1025-8.

[24]   Schatzberg AF, Samson JA, Bloomingdale KL, Orsulak PJ, Gerson B, Kizuka PP, Cole JO, Schildkraut JJ: Toward a biochemical classification of depressive disorders. X. Urinary catecholamines, their metabolites, and D-type scores in subgroups of depressive disorders. *Arch Gen Psychiatry* 1989; 46(3):260-8.

[25]   Otte C, McCaffery J, Ali S, Whooley MA: Association of a serotonin transporter polymorphism (5-HTTLPR) with depression, perceived stress, and norepinephrine in patients with coronary disease: the Heart and Soul Study. *Am J Psychiatry* 2007; 164(9):1379-84.

[26]   Roy A, Pickar D, De Jong J, Karoum F, Linnoila M: Norepinephrine and its metabolites in cerebrospinal fluid, plasma, and urine. Relationship to hypothalamic-pituitary-adrenal axis function in depression. *Arch Gen Psychiatry* 1988; 45(9):849-57.

[27]   Esler M, Turbott J, Schwarz R, Leonard P, Bobik A, Skews H, Jackman G: The peripheral kinetics of norepinephrine in depressive illness. *Arch Gen Psychiatry* 1982; 39(3):295-300.

[28]   Veith RC, Lewis N, Linares OA, Barnes RF, Raskind MA, Villacres EC, Murburg MM, Ashleigh EA, Castillo S, Peskind ER, *et al.*: Sympathetic nervous system activity in major depression. Basal and desipramine-induced alterations in plasma norepinephrine kinetics. *Arch Gen Psychiatry* 1994; 51(5):411-22.

[29]   Barton DA, Dawood T, Lambert EA, Esler MD, Haikerwal D, Brenchley C, Socratous F, Kaye DM, Schlaich MP, Hickie I, Lambert GW: Sympathetic activity in major depressive disorder: identifying those at increased cardiac risk? *J Hypertens* 2007; 25(10):2117-24.

[30]   Esler M, Jackman G, Bobik A, Kelleher D, Jennings G, Leonard P, Skews H, Korner P: Determination of norepinephrine apparent release rate and clearance in humans. *Life Sci* 1979; 25(17):1461-70.

[31]   Esler M, Jennings G, Lambert G, Meredith I, Horne M, Eisenhofer G: Overflow of catecholamine neurotransmitters to the circulation: source, fate, and functions. *Physiol Rev* 1990; 70(4):963-85.

[32]   Kannel WB, Castelli WP, McNamara PM, McKee PA, Feinleib M: Role of blood pressure in the development of congestive heart failure. The Framingham study. *N Engl J Med* 1972; 287(16):781-7.

[33]   Timio M, Saronio P, Venanzi S, Gentili S, Verdura C, Timio F: Blood pressure in nuns in a secluded order: A 30-year follow-up. *Miner Electrolyte Metab* 1999; 25(1-2):73-9.

[34]   *Specialist Medical Review Council of Australia*, Statements of Principles Nos. 31 and 32 of 2001 Concerning Hypertension. 2002, Commonwealth of Australia Government Gazette: Australian Government Printer, Canberra.

[35] Simonsick EM, Wallace RB, Blazer DG, Berkman LF: Depressive symptomatology and hypertension-associated morbidity and mortality in older adults. *Psychosom Med* 1995; 57(5):427-35.

[36] Henderson AS, Korten AE, Jacomb PA, Mackinnon AJ, Jorm AF, Christensen H, Rodgers B: The course of depression in the elderly: a longitudinal community-based study in Australia. *Psychol Med* 1997; 27(1):119-29.

[37] Paterniti S, Verdier-Taillefer MH, Geneste C, Bisserbe JC, Alperovitch A: Low blood pressure and risk of depression in the elderly. A prospective community-based study. *Br J Psychiatry* 2000; 176:464-7.

[38] Jonas BS, Franks P, Ingram DD: Are symptoms of anxiety and depression risk factors for hypertension? Longitudinal evidence from the National Health and Nutrition Examination Survey I Epidemiologic Follow-up Study. *Arch Fam Med* 1997; 6(1):43-9.

[39] Davidson K, Jonas BS, Dixon KE, Markovitz JH: Do depression symptoms predict early hypertension incidence in young adults in the CARDIA study? Coronary Artery Risk Development in Young Adults. *Arch Intern Med* 2000; 160(10):1495-500.

[40] Schwartz PJ, Billman GE, Stone HL: Autonomic mechanisms in ventricular fibrillation induced by myocardial ischemia during exercise in dogs with healed myocardial infarction. An experimental preparation for sudden cardiac death. *Circulation* 1984; 69(4):790-800.

[41] Parati G, Di Rienzo M, Bertinieri G, Pomidossi G, Casadei R, Groppelli A, Pedotti A, Zanchetti A, Mancia G: Evaluation of the baroreceptor-heart rate reflex by 24-hour intra-arterial blood pressure monitoring in humans. *Hypertension* 1988; 12(2):214-22.

[42] Ziegler D, Laude D, Akila F, Elghozi JL: Time- and frequency-domain estimation of early diabetic cardiovascular autonomic neuropathy. *Clin Auton Res* 2001; 11(6):369-76.

[43] Grassi G, Seravalle G, Bertinieri G, Turri C, Stella ML, Scopelliti F, Mancia G: Sympathetic and reflex abnormalities in heart failure secondary to ischaemic or idiopathic dilated cardiomyopathy. *Clin Sci (Lond)* 2001; 101(2):141-6.

[44] La Rovere MT, Bigger JT, Jr., Marcus FI, Mortara A, Schwartz PJ: Baroreflex sensitivity and heart-rate variability in prediction of total cardiac mortality after myocardial infarction. ATRAMI (Autonomic Tone and Reflexes After Myocardial Infarction) Investigators. *Lancet* 1998; 351(9101):478-84.

[45] Watkins LL, Grossman P: Association of depressive symptoms with reduced baroreflex cardiac control in coronary artery disease. *Am Heart J* 1999; 137(3):453-7.

[46] Watkins LL, Blumenthal JA, Carney RM: Association of anxiety with reduced baroreflex cardiac control in patients after acute myocardial infarction. *Am Heart J* 2002; 143(3):460-6.

[47] Pitzalis MV, Iacoviello M, Todarello O, Fioretti A, Guida P, Massari F, Mastropasqua F, Russo GD, Rizzon P: Depression but not anxiety influences the autonomic control of heart rate after myocardial infarction. *Am Heart J* 2001; 141(5):765-71.

[48] Broadley AJ, Frenneaux MP, Moskvina V, Jones CJ, Korszun A: Baroreflex sensitivity is reduced in depression. *Psychosom Med* 2005; 67(4):648-51.

[49] Dawood T, Lambert EA, Barton DA, Laude D, Elghozi JL, Esler MD, Haikerwal D, Kaye DM, Hotchkin EJ, Lambert GW: Specific serotonin reuptake inhibition in major depressive disorder adversely affects novel markers of cardiac risk. *Hypertens Res* 2007; 30(4):285-93.

[50] Task Force of the European Society of Cardiology and the North American Society of Pacing and Electrophysiology: Heart rate variability: standards of measurement, physiological interpretation and clinical use. *Circulation* 1996; 93(5):1043-65.

[51] Chess GF, Tam RM, Calaresu FR: Influence of cardiac neural inputs on rhythmic variations of heart period in the cat. *Am J Physiol* 1975; 228(3):775-80.

[52] Carney RM, Blumenthal JA, Stein PK, Watkins L, Catellier D, Berkman LF, Czajkowski SM, O'Connor C, Stone PH, Freedland KE: Depression, heart rate variability, and acute myocardial infarction. *Circulation* 2001; 104(17):2024-8.

[53] Frasure-Smith N, Lesperance F, Talajic M: Depression following myocardial infarction. Impact on 6-month survival. *JAMA* 1993; 270(15):1819-25.

[54] Frasure-Smith N, Lesperance F, Talajic M: Depression and 18-month prognosis after myocardial infarction. *Circulation* 1995; 91(4):999-1005.

[55] Bonetti PO, Lerman LO, Lerman A: Endothelial dysfunction: a marker of atherosclerotic risk. *Arterioscler Thromb Vasc Biol* 2003; 23(2):168-75.

[56] Rajagopalan S, Brook R, Rubenfire M, Pitt E, Young E, Pitt B: Abnormal brachial artery flow-mediated vasodilation in young adults with major depression. *Am J Cardiol* 2001; 88(2):196-8, A7.

[57] Wagner JA, Tennen H, Mansoor GA, Abbott G: History of major depressive disorder and endothelial function in postmenopausal women. *Psychosom Med* 2006; 68(1):80-6.

[58] Broadley AJ, Korszun A, Jones CJ, Frenneaux MP: Arterial endothelial function is impaired in treated depression. *Heart* 2002; 88(5):521-3.

[59] Piletz JE, Zhu H, Madakasira S, Pazzaglia P, Lindsay DeVane C, Goldman N, Halaris A: Elevated P-selectin on platelets in depression: response to bupropion. *J Psychiatr Res* 2000; 34(6):397-404.

[60] Lederbogen F, Baranyai R, Gilles M, Menart-Houtermans B, Tschoepe D, Deuschle M: Effect of mental and physical stress on platelet activation markers in depressed patients and healthy subjects: a pilot study. *Psychiatry Res* 2004; 127(1-2):55-64.

[61] Lip GY, Blann AD, Zarifis J, Beevers M, Lip PL, Beevers DG: Soluble adhesion molecule P-selectin and endothelial dysfunction in essential hypertension: implications for atherogenesis? A preliminary report. *J Hypertens* 1995; 13(12 Pt 2):1674-8.

[62] Mizia-Stec K, Zahorska-Markiewicz B, Mandecki T, Janowska J, Szulc A, Jastrzebska-Maj E: Serum levels of selected adhesion molecules in patients with coronary artery disease. *Int J Cardiol* 2002; 83(2):143-50.

[63] Musselman DL, Tomer A, Manatunga AK, Knight BT, Porter MR, Kasey S, Marzec U, Harker LA, Nemeroff CB: Exaggerated platelet reactivity in major depression. *Am J Psychiatry* 1996; 153(10):1313-7.

[64] Shimbo D, Child J, Davidson K, Geer E, Osende JI, Reddy S, Dronge A, Fuster V, Badimon JJ: Exaggerated serotonin-mediated platelet reactivity as a possible link in depression and acute coronary syndromes. *Am J Cardiol* 2002; 89(3):331-3.

[65]   Johnson-Tidey RR, McGregor JL, Taylor PR, Poston RN: Increase in the adhesion molecule P-selectin in endothelium overlying atherosclerotic plaques. Coexpression with intercellular adhesion molecule-1. *Am J Pathol* 1994; 144(5):952-61.

[66]   Leo R, Di Lorenzo G, Tesauro M, Razzini C, Forleo GB, Chiricolo G, Cola C, Zanasi M, Troisi A, Siracusano A, Lauro R, Romeo F: Association between enhanced soluble CD40 ligand and proinflammatory and prothrombotic states in major depressive disorder: pilot observations on the effects of selective serotonin reuptake inhibitor therapy. *J Clin Psychiatry* 2006; 67(11):1760-6.

[67]   Plutzky J: Inflammatory pathways in atherosclerosis and acute coronary syndromes. *Am J Cardiol* 2001; 88(8A):10K-15K.

[68]   Penninx BW, Kritchevsky SB, Yaffe K, Newman AB, Simonsick EM, Rubin S, Ferrucci L, Harris T, Pahor M: Inflammatory markers and depressed mood in older persons: results from the Health, Aging and Body Composition study. *Biol Psychiatry* 2003; 54(5):566-72.

[69]   Steptoe A, Kunz-Ebrecht SR, Owen N: Lack of association between depressive symptoms and markers of immune and vascular inflammation in middle-aged men and women. *Psychological Medicine* 2003; 33:667-674.

[70]   Ridker PM: Cardiology Patient Page. C-reactive protein: a simple test to help predict risk of heart attack and stroke. *Circulation* 2003; 108(12):e81-5.

[71]   Szalai AJ, van Ginkel FW, Wang Y, McGhee JR, Volanakis JE: Complement-dependent acute-phase expression of C-reactive protein and serum amyloid P-component. *J Immunol* 2000; 165(2):1030-5.

[72]   Woollard KJ: Soluble bio-markers in vascular disease: much more than gauges of disease? *Clin Exp Pharmacol Physiol* 2005; 32(4):233-40.

[73]   Morrow DA, Rifai N, Antman EM, Weiner DL, McCabe CH, Cannon CP, Braunwald E: C-reactive protein is a potent predictor of mortality independently of and in combination with troponin T in acute coronary syndromes: a TIMI 11A substudy. Thrombolysis in Myocardial Infarction. *J Am Coll Cardiol* 1998; 31(7):1460-5.

[74]   Heeschen C, Hamm CW, Bruemmer J, Simoons ML: Predictive value of C-reactive protein and troponin T in patients with unstable angina: a comparative analysis. CAPTURE Investigators. Chimeric c7E3 AntiPlatelet Therapy in Unstable angina REfractory to standard treatment trial. *J Am Coll Cardiol* 2000; 35(6):1535-42.

[75]   Lindahl B, Toss H, Siegbahn A, Venge P, Wallentin L: Markers of myocardial damage and inflammation in relation to long-term mortality in unstable coronary artery disease. FRISC Study Group. Fragmin during Instability in Coronary Artery Disease. *N Engl J Med* 2000; 343(16):1139-47.

[76]   Ridker PM, Cushman M, Stampfer MJ, Tracy RP, Hennekens CH: Inflammation, aspirin, and the risk of cardiovascular disease in apparently healthy men. *N Engl J Med* 1997; 336(14):973-9.

[77]   Ridker PM, Hennekens CH, Buring JE, Rifai N: C-reactive protein and other markers of inflammation in the prediction of cardiovascular disease in women. *N Engl J Med* 2000; 342(12):836-43.

[78] Kuller LH, Tracy RP, Shaten J, Meilahn EN: Relation of C-reactive protein and coronary heart disease in the MRFIT nested case-control study. Multiple Risk Factor Intervention Trial. *Am J Epidemiol* 1996; 144(6):537-47.

[79] Lowe GD, Yarnell JW, Rumley A, Bainton D, Sweetnam PM: C-reactive protein, fibrin D-dimer, and incident ischemic heart disease in the Speedwell study: are inflammation and fibrin turnover linked in pathogenesis? *Arterioscler Thromb Vasc Biol* 2001; 21(4):603-10.

[80] Tiemeier H, Hofman A, van Tuijl HR, Kiliaan AJ, Meijer J, Breteler MM: Inflammatory proteins and depression in the elderly. *Epidemiology* 2003; 14(1):103-7.

[81] Kop WJ, Gottdiener JS, Tangen CM, Fried LP, McBurnie MA, Walston J, Newman A, Hirsch C, Tracy RP: Inflammation and coagulation factors in persons > 65 years of age with symptoms of depression but without evidence of myocardial ischemia. *Am J Cardiol* 2002; 89(4):419-24.

[82] Panagiotakos DB, Pitsavos C, Chrysohoou C, Tsetsekou E, Papageorgiou C, Christodoulou G, Stefanadis C: Inflammation, coagulation, and depressive symptomatology in cardiovascular disease-free people; the ATTICA study. *Eur Heart J* 2004; 25(6):492-9.

[83] Danner M, Kasl SV, Abramson JL, Vaccarino V: Association between depression and elevated C-reactive protein. *Psychosom Med* 2003; 65(3):347-56.

[84] DiMatteo MR, Lepper HS, Croghan TW: Depression is a risk factor for noncompliance with medical treatment: meta-analysis of the effects of anxiety and depression on patient adherence. *Arch Intern Med* 2000; 160(14):2101-7.

[85] Horwitz RI, Viscoli CM, Berkman L, Donaldson RM, Horwitz SM, Murray CJ, Ransohoff DF, Sindelar J: Treatment adherence and risk of death after a myocardial infarction. *Lancet* 1990; 336(8714):542-5.

[86] Lerman C, Audrain J, Orleans CT, Boyd R, Gold K, Main D, Caporaso N: Investigation of mechanisms linking depressed mood to nicotine dependence. *Addict Behav* 1996; 21(1):9-19.

[87] Regier DA, Farmer ME, Rae DS, Locke BZ, Keith SJ, Judd LL, Goodwin FK: Comorbidity of mental disorders with alcohol and other drug abuse. Results from the Epidemiologic Catchment Area (ECA) Study. *JAMA* 1990; 264(19):2511-8.

[88] Camacho TC, Roberts RE, Lazarus NB, Kaplan GA, Cohen RD: Physical activity and depression: evidence from the Alameda County Study. *Am J Epidemiol* 1991; 134(2):220-31.

[89] Panagiotakos DB, Pitsavos C, Chrysohoou C, Stefanadis C, Toutouzas P: Risk stratification of coronary heart disease through established and emerging lifestyle factors in a Mediterranean population: CARDIO2000 epidemiological study. *J Cardiovasc Risk* 2001; 8(6):329-35.

In: Psychological Factors and Cardiovascular Disorders   ISBN: 978-1-60456-871-4
Editor: Leo Sher   © 2008 Nova Science Publishers, Inc.

Chapter IV

DEPRESSION IN PATIENTS WITH MYOCARDIAL INFARCTION

Abebaw Mengistu Yohannes

Faculty of Health, Psychology and Social Care, Manchester Metropolitan University, Manchester, United Kingdom.

ABSTRACT

Chronic heart disease is a major cause of morbidity and mortality in old age. Depression is common in patients admitted with the myocardial infarction (MI). Untreated depression in MI patients is associated with poor compliance with medical treatment, increased health care utilization, decreased social interaction and self-efficacy, and impaired quality of life. The benefits of antidepressant therapy have been well documented. However, not all MI patients can take part because of contraindications to antidepressants therapy and patient's fear of side effects and stigma attached to depression. Currently, the efficacy of cardiac rehabilitation in the treatment of depression is inconclusive. A well-designed cardiac rehabilitation programmes that include psychosocial education and cognitive behavioural therapy are needed.

INTRODUCTION

Coronary Heart Disease (CHD) is a common cause of hospital admission, morbidity and disability in old age. Depression is a commonly reported as the co-morbid illness in patients with CHD [1]. Major depression and cardiovascular disease are the leading causes of disability in old age [2]. The prevalence of major depression following myocardial infarction estimated between 15% to 45% [3-6]. Despite its high prevalence, depression is often under-recognised and under-treated. Untreated depression is associated with increasing cardiovascular morbidity and mortality [3,5,7] and poor compliance with medical treatment [8]. The chapter aims to provide guidance for identifying and treating depression in patients post myocardial infarction and the impact of depression on physical, psychological and health related quality of life (HRQoL). It will also discuss the effectiveness of rehabilitation including antidepressants and the efficacy of cardiac rehabilitation in the treatment of depression.

PREVALENCE OF DEPRESSION IN POST MYOCARDIAL INFARCTION (MI)

The National Institute for Health and Clinical Excellence (NICE) guidelines for CHD recently published on the management of depression in acute and secondary care and gave the point prevalence of depression amongst 16 to 65 year olds in the UK as 17 per 1,000 for males and 25 per 1,000 for females [9]. The US data combined from 2004/2005 extracted from the Office of Applies Studies found that 76 per 1000 of the US adults (>18 years) experienced at least one major depressive episode in the past year [10].

Older age, over 65 years, is an independent risk factor for mortality in post-MI patients [11-14]. It has been argued that this is due to the greater prevalence of other co-morbid diseases such as diabetes and hypertension in patients with MI. However, Maggioni *et al.* [13], in a larger survey (N= 9720 MI patients) using a multiple regression analysis older age was a predictor of mortality after controlling for hypertension and diabetes and infarct size. A previous study also found that those patients identified with major depression during hospital index for MI were 4 times the risk of dying within the preceding 4 months post discharge [14]. Post-MI depressed patients are reportedly less compliant in following recommendations (such as dietary recommendations, smoking cessation and activity levels) than post-MI patients without depression to reduce cardiac events [11]. This non-compliance may go some way to explain the higher mortality rates seen in depressed post-MI patients. The prevalence of depression is higher in women compared with men [15-17] and especially in those patients categorised within a lower socioeconomic status [15, 18,19].

A recent American College of Cardiology acute MI practice guidelines [20] recommend that the psychosocial status of patients should be evaluated, "including enquiries regarding symptoms of depression" as a matter of routine. Montano [21] reported that diagnosis of depression might be missed in approximately 50% of cases in primary care. Within the post-MI population, the presence of somatic complaints such as sleep disturbance, fatigue, weight loss and lethargy may mimic depressive symptoms following a cardiac event. It may be quite natural for patients to be depressed or anxious in the aftermath of a cardiac event and therefore appropriate screening is required periodically in post-MI patients to report whether low mood symptoms are persisting or not.

In large population surveys and meta-analysis [17-19], depression was associated with female gender, low socioeconomic status, and older age in post MI patients. In summary, the variables associated with the post MI depression are complex as listed in Table 1. A multimodal approach is needed to treat depression effectively in post MI patients.

DEPRESSION AND MORTALITY IN MI

The relationship between depression and earlier death after MI well documented. Several studies have reported that depression is associated with increased mortality after MI [3,5,8]. There is a steadily growing number of studies and reviews have shown that untreated depression is a risk factor for elevated cardiovascular morbidity and mortality following MI [8,12]. The association between depression and post-MI mortality and patient outcomes is complex because of co-morbidity. Co-morbidity coupled with depression and anxiety have been reported to increase post MI mortality [14, 19, 24]. There has since been an increasing focus on mood disturbance in patients recovering after MI. In addition more recent studies (>1992) appear to show a less pronounced association between mortality and depression [8] in post-MI patients and this may be partially due to a better understanding and early identification of depressive symptoms within the patient's care pathway. In contrast, a recent study by Dickens *et al.* [22] found that when depression was measured immediately preceding MI and at 12 months post-MI, depression was not related to mortality [22]. Therefore, the prognostic value of depression in post-MI remains uncertain.

Table 1. Risk factors associated with depression in patients with MI

Older age
Female gender
Lower socioeconomic status
Stressful life events
Active smoking
Personality type
Social isolation
Cardiovascular diseases
Co-morbid diseases e.g. diabetes
Elevated cholesterol level
Endothelial dysfunction
Atheroscleriosis

SCREENING TOOLS FOR DEPRESSION

The screening tools that have been used in pos-MI depression are listed in Table 2 [23-38]. Of these, the Beck Depression Inventory (BDI) and the Hospital Anxiety and Depression Scale (HADS) were the most commonly identified depression assessment tools in a review of the literature on post-MI depression by Thombs *et al.* [5]. A BDI score >10 is regarded as a 'case' for clinical depression and a HADS score of 8-10 border line and ≥ 11 considered as a 'case' for clinical depression respectively. These thresholds are important when investigating levels of depression present and considering the impact on post-MI mortality. In a prospective study Bush *et al.* [12] examined the presence of depression (2-5 days in post-MI patients) those patients identified with a clinical depression (BDI >10) had a higher 4-month mortality rates in comparison to patients with BDI <10 [12]. Although the difference was not statistically significant (p=0.06). The association of depressive symptoms (BDI < 10) of depression with mortality risk after MI is a new finding that warrants further investigation. This raises a question whether a BDI's cut off score < 10 might be too high to detect those patients suffering with underlying depression.

Table 2. Screening tools used for depression in patients with myocardial infarction

Measurement Tool	Psychometric Properties	Cardiac Studies used
Hospital Anxiety and Depression Scale (HADS)	23	22,24
Beck Depression Inventory (BDI)	25-27	12,14,28-31
Patient Health Questionnaire – 9 (PHQ-9)	32,33	1,3,34
Centre for Epidemiologic Studies Depression Scale (CES-D)	35,36	1
Hamilton Depression Scale (HAM-D)	37	38

A recent meta-analysis [8] that investigated the prognostic value of post-MI depression with cardiovascular outcomes (e.g. mortality and number of cardiovascular events). The findings revealed that post-MI depression was associated with a 2-2.5 fold increased with the risk of adverse cardiovascular outcomes.

When evaluating studies that investigated the prognostic value depression has on patient outcomes, the time point that depression is measured relative to MI is an important factor to consider. Studies to date have used a variety of time points relative to hospital index for MI in the assessment of depression that may account for some differences in findings. Depression following an MI may be an adjustment reaction and the body's response to a stressful situation and therefore may or may not have the potential to influence patient outcome dependent on if the depression is persistent or if it undergoes spontaneous remission [4]. Approximately 50% of post-MI depression undergoes spontaneous remission without treatment and the other percentage will persist or remit, only to relapse within a year [7]. Parasher et al. [4] conducted a prospective study (N = 1873 subjects) investigating the prognostic importance of depression on a number of outcomes including re-hospitalisation or mortality, and health status (as measured by the Seattle Angina Questionnaire, which looks at symptom burden, functional status and quality of life) [4]. The study reported that irrespective of whether the depressive symptoms have subsided since the baseline measures during hospitalisation, or newly developed or persist to the month after hospitalisation, there was a statistically significant (p <0.05) association with worse outcomes post-MI. This begs the close monitoring of patients with depression, for example, watchful waiting, telephone contacts post MI patients after discharge.

IMPACT OF DEPRESSION ON QUALITY OF LIFE

Quality of life (QoL) is defined as in a variety of ways and there is ongoing debate about the meaning of the concept and what it should measure. Health related quality of life (HRQoL) is a more disease-specific concept, which broadly encompasses the impact of disease and medical treatment on patients overall function and well-being [39]. The principle components of HRQoL are psychological and physical function [40]. There are a number of condition specific [41] and generic outcome measures available. The cardiac condition specific measures of HRQoL may include: Quality of life after myocardial infarction (QLMI) [42,43], Quality of life Index – Cardiac Version [41], Angina Pectoris Quality of Life Questionnaire [41] and the Seattle Angina Questionnaire [44].

Bush *et al.* [12] investigated the impact of depression on survival and HRQoL in patients following MI. Their findings showed that patients who had high level of depressive symptoms (BDI >10) at baseline coupled with elevated left ventricular ejection and older age (>65 years) at four months, had the odds ratio of 4 times more likely to die compared to non-depressed patients. They have also reported significant impairment in their HRQoL.

MI patients reported a significant decrease in HRQoL [39] although only some aspects of the changes in HRQoL occur more frequently among this population in comparison to normal population data. HRQoL changes over time in this population show men and women reporting improved HRQoL scores at 1 year in comparison to a short term 5 month follow-up [45]. In comparison to normative data, a number of the function and well-being scales did not reach normative levels in both men and women at 1 year post-MI, thus it may be argued that post-MI patients have a lower HRQoL than the population norm data.

The impact of MI on patients reported HRQoL on gender difference is quiet evident. Women reported to have poorer physical health, decreased physical function, increased bodily pain and reduced social function than men at 5 months follow-up post-MI [46]. However, in this study, there was no gender difference in the mental health component of SF-36 [46]. This is in contrast, to other studies findings that women reported to have a higher prevalence of depression [3,15-17]. In addition, early assessment of fatigue and depression post-MI may be a useful indicator of HRQoL at 1-year [45].

REHABILITATION IN THE POST-MI POPULATION

Psychological distress, including low mood has been identified as a predictor of health care utilisation following a cardiac event. It has been identified psychologically distressed MI patients are most likely to accrue four times the healthcare costs than non-distressed patients (47). It is, therefore, important to design appropriate interventions to reduce the distress of cardiac patients experience in order to reduce costs and improve quality of life.

TREATMENT OF DEPRESSION POST-MI

There are a number of interventions available in the treatment of depression and have the potential to improve outcomes, such as HRQoL of the post-MI population. Early screening for the presence of depression should take place to identify those with depression to design appropriate interventions and improve quality of care in patients admitted with acute MI in Table 2. The cardiovascular prognosis of depressed MI patients has been found not to be affected by the treatment of depression following an acute MI in two large randomised controlled studies [12,38].

Glassman *et al.* [38] evaluated the safety and efficacy of Sertraline antidepressant treatment of major depression in 369 patients (mean age: 57.1years), hospitalised for MI or unstable angina. The treatment had no significant effect on the primary outcome measure depression. However, the left ventricular ejection fraction in the Sertraline group significantly reduced from the baseline measure mean (SD), 54% (10), to week 16, 15% (11) compared with the placebo: baseline 52% (13) to, week 16, 53% (13). This suggests that Sertraline is a safe cardiovascular treatment choice in this population. The study was conducted in 40 outpatient cardiology centres and psychiatry clinics in seven different countries and subjects were randomised to 24 weeks double blind treatment of either placebo or Sertraline treatment. Sub-analysis of the findings indicate that patients with a prior history of major depressive disorder responded positively to Sertraline using a Clinical Global Impression Improvement scale without a change with the severity of depression. The clinical efficacy is unclear. Patients without prior history of episode of depression before their present post-MI depressive episode showed no evidence improvement in the drug efficacy compared with the placebo. This study has a number of limitations. The findings might not be generalisable due to the large number of potential subjects that were excluded (n= 11177); the sample size was not adequate to identify rare adverse events or drug-drug interactions and the treatment was not initiated until an average of 34 days post MI. Arguably, the subjects within this study had more contact with the healthcare professionals compared with the normal post-MI patients receive and this may have had an effect on the remission of depression in the sub-sample of this patient group.

The second multi-centre, randomised controlled clinical trial was the Enhancing Recovery in Coronary Heart Disease (ENRICHD) study [12], which examined whether treatment of depression and perceived social support following an MI reduced the risk of recurrent infarction and mortality. The intervention arm consisted of up to 6 months individual, and when feasible, group cognitive behavioural therapy (CBT) sessions and Sertraline for those patients identified with severe depression at enrolment and when improvement of at least 50% was not achieved on BDI < 10 scores after 5 sessions of CBT. 1,165 subjects were randomly assigned to either the usual care arm or intervention arm of the study. From the data generated, there was no evidence to suggest that the intervention has no effect on mortality. There was, however, a reported significant relationship between change in depression score and late mortality *within* the intervention arm. Patients whose depression did not improve with treatment were at higher risk of mortality than patients who responded to treatment. This is an important clinical finding as patients that do not respond to treatment should be more closely monitored and intervention for other modifiable risk factors should be considered. In the study, subjects had at least, one prior episode of depression prior to MI to be included; therefore, the finding might not be generalisable to the post-MI depressed population and as not all patients will have had a prior history of depressive episode.

Cardiac Rehabilitation

Cardiac rehabilitation is a part of routine medical management following MI. It forms a bridge for the patients from dependence as an in-patient to relative independence in the community. It is a multifactorial programme, which includes: exercise and psychological/educational aspects of intervention should form a component of comprehensive cardiac rehabilitation. The World Health Organisation define cardiac rehabilitation as 'the sum of activity to ensure them the best possible physical, mental and social conditions so that they by their own efforts, regain as normal as possible a place in the community and lead an active productive life' [48]. There are four phases of cardiac rehabilitation programme and each represents the stages in the patients cardiac care pathway:

Phase 1 – inpatient stage
Phase 2 – early post-discharge period
Phase 3 – Psycho-educational training combined with exercise training
Phase 4 – long-term maintenance

The British Association of Cardiac Rehabilitation (BACR) guidelines emphasise the importance of follow-up cardiac care [49] and may be used as the spine to which individual treatment programmes are tailored. Outcome measures to test whether cardiac rehabilitation was effective or not were traditionally mortality rates and/or re-infarction and other longer-term measures such as health care utilisation. In more recent years, it has become more widely accepted that HRQoL, risk-factor status, adherence to therapeutic regimes and lifestyle modifications are appropriate measures of the effectiveness of interventions both in the short-term and long-term follow-up respectively.

Exercise Intervention

The physiological benefits of regular exercise in cardiovascular health have been well-documented [50]. It includes increasing exercise tolerance, reduction in body weight, reduction in blood pressure and positive impact on reducing cholesterol levels. Assessment of functional capacity and a clinical risk stratification of the individual should take place prior to commencement of the programme and guidelines have been published from a number of internationally recognised professional bodies [49, 51] that address these needs.

Exercise forms an important component of cardiac rehabilitation as physical deconditioning so commonly occurs following a cardiac event. A Cochrane Review in 2001, examined the effectiveness of exercise-only cardiac rehabilitation in men and women of all ages with previous MI, revascularisation or angina patients [52]. All-cause mortality was reduced by 27%, cardiac mortality was reduced by 31% and combined end-point of mortality, non-fatal MI and revascularisation of 19% accrued over an average of 2.4 years. There were no additional benefits gained when a comprehensive cardiac rehabilitation programme added in the analysis (i.e. one that included a psycho-educational element). This may be partially explained as within the exercise-only cardiac rehabilitation programmes, a psycho-educational aspect may be taking place but in a non-structured/non-measurable format. The converse might be that the poor methodological design of the studies may have compromised the efficacy of the CR programmes.

In the United Kingdom, aerobic circuit training is the traditional method for group exercise training [53]. In this format the frequency, intensity and duration of the activity can be modified to meet individual desired training effects. The studies evaluated within the Cochrane Review [52] incorporated aerobic exercise (such as walking, cycling, jogging, and rowing) however for patients wanting to return to a fully independent active lifestyle, muscle strength is important in addition to aerobic endurance and resistance training. These exercises are safe to be undertaken by low-to- moderate risk patients with supervision [49].

Early trials of cardiac rehabilitation included 3 sessions of in-hospital exercise training per week [52]. However, a study by Kugler *et al.* [54] found that the completion of one in-hospital session and two home-based sessions per week is as effective as in-hospital training thrice weekly. This finding is encouraging as it promotes self-management and moves the locus of control towards the patient as they incorporate exercise activity into their lifestyle, which is important for the long-term maintenance.

EDUCATION INTERVENTION

Education forms part of a psychosocial intervention and is provided as part of a cardiac rehabilitation programme in approximately 70-80% of programmes [55,56]. However these interventions are diverse in nature and are not fully described in the literature causing difficulty when evaluating the effectiveness of such interventions. The intervention may include group and/or individual education to improve knowledge about heart function, risk factors for MI and risk factor modification. Education on modifiable risk factors such as smoking cessation, exercise and activity levels, dietary advice and the importance of compliance, aim to produce positive changes in behaviour and lifestyle. For these changes to take place information should be consistent, adequate and accurate. A checklist with the healthcare professional present may be helpful to clarify patients understanding what they are being educated on, especially as an estimated 30-78%, do not understand patient education material [57]. Misconceptions about their condition may prevent the patient from returning to their normal activities and/or participating in the rehabilitation programme and can affect compliance. By identifying, and where appropriate addressing, patients health beliefs with consistent advice and the option of educational leaflets, the patients misconceptions may be alleviated and thus reduce patient's anxiety. A further method of alleviating patient's misconceptions may be the provision of The Heart Manual [58] to the patient. This is a 6-week CBT tool that emphasises self-management and is designed to alleviate cardiac patient's misconceptions. A randomised control trial that carried out by Lewin *et al.* (59)

evaluated the earlier edition of The Heart Manual in 176 subjects aged <80 years admitted to a coronary care unit. Their findings showed that improved emotional state, fewer contacts with GPs and fewer hospital readmissions at 6-months post-MI in the intervention arm compared with the control arm. Cowen and colleagues [60] in a large ranmomised controlled trial identified treatment of depression in patients with MI may include better communication skills with patients, supprting patients to actively engage with cognitive behavioural therapy and adherence with homework assignments may enhance better health outcomes and social supprt. Therefore, a greater emphsis is needed on 'home work assignments' to show the efficacy of cognitive behavioural therapy.

A large meta-analysis by Dusseldorp *et al.* [61] of 8,988 subjects in 37 clinical trials found that cardiac rehabilitation programmes with an educational/psychological component produced a 34% reduction in cardiac mortality and 29% reduction in recurrent MI in up to 10 year follow-up. The largest response to treatment intervention resulted in the largest decrease in cardiac mortality and recurrent MI. However, in terms of psychological outcome; no significant effects of psycho-educational programmes on the treatment of anxiety or depression were seen. This may be partially due to the inclusion of two large trails [62,63] that produced negative results for psychological outcome, which may have skewed the results of the meta-analysis. An earlier meta-analysis by Linden *et al.* [64] that identified 43 relevant randomised controlled trials concluded the support for inclusion of psychological intervention alongside the usual care for post-MI patients receive. Therefore, the literature is suggestive for the inclusion of a psycho-educational as a component of cardiac rehabilitation programme. However, the findings are not conclusive at this stage. The benefits of psycho-education in the treatment of depression in post MI patients require further investigation.

A smoking cessation should be advocated as a part of the educational programme of CR. A recent meta-analysis [65] that investigated the effects of smoking cessation programme on mortality after myocardial with a follow-up duration of 2 to 10 years. The findings showed that smoking cessation reduced mortality. The relative risk reductions in all the studies ranged from 15% to 61%. They also revealed that continuing smoking is associated with a 20% increase in cardiac related deaths. Therefore a smoking cessation programme for MI patients should be encouraged at all times during the CR.

CARDIAC REHABILITATION IN OLDER PATIENTS

Depression is a risk factor for cardiac mortality and morbidity in post-MI patients in old age. Despite this, older patients are commonly excluded from cardiac rehabilitation research trials [65,66]. Even though research shows that older patients can benefit from the cardiac rehabilitation programme. A randomised controlled study by Stahle *et al.* [67] included 101 subjects (aged >65 years) recovering from a cardiac event. The authors have reported increasing exercise tolerance and improved QoL in the intervention group (n=50) compared with the control group (n=51). Follow-up data at 3 months in the intervention group showed that significant improvement in QoL and exercise tolerance, though, not maintained at 12-month follow-up. . The subjects not making behavioural changes and incorporating the exercise activity into their lifestyles after the post-intervention may explain this. Therefore, it is important to provide periodically supervised and maintenance exercise training may be necessary within this patient group to reduce a further decline in the improvements gained during the rehabilitation period.

MODEL OF CARE FOR DEPRESSION WITHIN MI POPULATION

The model of care for MI patients with depression may include:

- Use of valid screening tools which are sensitive and specific in the diagnosis of depression.
- It is important to complete the assessment for depression at the time appropriate when the MI is stable.
- Those identified with the screening tool for depression require further assessment by the qualified healthcare professionals using the Diagnostic Structured Manual IV criteria.
- There are effective interventions for the treatment of depression. Therefore, once the patient identified with depression appropriate treatment should be offered to the patient.
- Coordinated patient care aiming to empower the patient with increased access to information and education is worthy consideration.
- The long-term benefits of comprehensive cardiac rehabilitation programme that includes exercise and psychological/educational aspects of intervention require further investigation.
- The Figure 1 below shows the guidance and pathway for the identification of depression and treatment after post MI.

CONCLUSION

Depression is common following MI. Depression is under-recognized and untreated in post MI patients. It is an independent risk factor for cardiovascular morbidity and mortality. There are implications for assessing post-MI depression and these include the method of assessment (use of interview and/or questionnaire) and the time the assessment is undertaken relative to the MI. Cardiac rehabilitation improves exercise capacity and quality of life in patients with MI. A few studies have demonstrated the benefits of antidepressant alongside CBT in the treatment of depression. Cardiac rehabilitation for the post-MI population should be multifactorial which include exercise and psychological/educational aspects of intervention should form a large component of the CR programme. The inclusion of a psychological intervention alongside an exercise component is the best practice for the management of depression in post MI patients. The impact of cardiac rehabilitation on

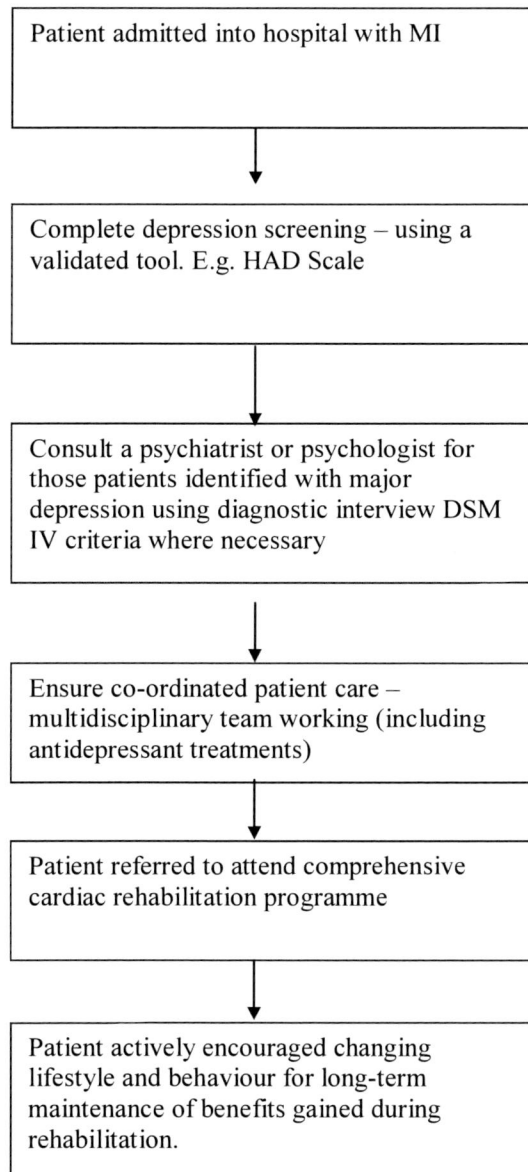

Figure 1. demonstrates patient's assessment and care pathway following MI.

depression and cardiovascular mortality and morbidity is inconclusive. Further investigation is needed into the timing of treatment within the post-MI population whether earlier intervention may improve prognosis and in turn reduce health care utilisation and costs.

REFERENCES

[1]   McManus D, Pipkin SS, Whooley MA. Screening for depression in patients with Coronary Heart Disease. *American Journal of Cardiology* 2005; 96:1076-1081.

[2]   Murray CJ, Lopez AD. Alternative projections of mortality and disability by cause 1990-2020: Global burden of disease study. *Lancet* 1997;349:1498-1504.

[3]   Office for National Statistics, Prevalence of treated depression per 1000 patients, by age, sex and calendar year: 1994 – 98 Office for National Statistics (ONS) Key Health Statistics from General Practice 1998. Table 5A7

[4]   Parashar S, Rumsfeld JS, Spertus JA, Reid KJ, Wenger NK, Krumholz HM, Amin A, Weintraub WS, Lichtman J. and Dawood D. Time Course of Depression and Outcome of Myocardial Infarction. *Archives of Internal Medicine*. 2006; 166:2035-2043

[5]   Thombs BD, Bass EB, Ford DE, Stewart KJ, Tsilidis KK, Patel U, Fauerbach JA, Bush DE and Ziegelstein RC. Prevalence of Depression in Survivors of Acute Myocardial Infarction, Review of the Evidence. *General Internal Medicine* 2006; 21:30–38.

[6]   Frasure-Smith N, Lesperance F, and Talajic M. Depression following myocardial infarction. Impact on 6 month survival. *Journal of the American Medical Association* 1993; 270:1819-1825

[7]   Schleifer SJ, Macari-Hinson MM, Coyle DA. The nature and course of depression following myocardial infarction. *Archives of Internal Medicine* 1989; 149:1785-1789.

[8]   van Melle JP, de Jonge P, Spijkerman TA, Tussen JGP, Ormel J, van Veldhuisen DJ, van den Brink RHS, van den Berg MP. Prognostic Association of Depression following Myocardial Infarction with Mortality and Cardiovascular Events: A Meta-Analysis. *Psychosomatic Medicine* 2004; 66:814–822

[9]   National Clinical Practice Guideline Number23; Depression: Management of depression in primary and secondary care. National Collaborating Centre for Mental Health Commissioned by the National Institute for Clinical Excellence; NICE 23

[10]   Substance Abuse and Mental Health Services Administration, Office of Applied Studies. (June 11, 2007). The NSDUH Report: State Estimates of Depression: 2004 and 2005. Rockville, MD.

[11]   Ziegelstein RC, Fauerbach JA, Stevens SS. Depressed patients are less likely to follow recommendations to reduce cardiac risk following myocardial infarction. *Circulation* 2000; 91: 999-1005

[12]   Bush DE, Ziegelstein RC, Tayback M, Richter D, Stevens S, Zahalsky H, Fauerbach JA. Even Minimal Symptoms of Depression Increase Mortality Risk After Acute Myocardial Infarction. *American Journal of Cardiology* 2001; 88:337–341

[13]   Maggioni AP, Maseri A, Fresco C. Age-related increase in mortality among patients with first myocardial infarction treated with thromboysis. The Investigators of the Gruppo Italiano per lo Studio della Sopravvivenza nell'Infarto Miocardico (GISSI-2). *New England Journal of Medicine* 1993; 329:1442-1448

[14]   Romanelli J, Fauerbach J, Bush DE, and Ziegelstein RC. The significance of Depression in Older Patients after myocardial infarction. *Journal of American Geriatrics Society* 2002; 50:817-822

[15]   Wade TJ, Cairney J, Pevalin DJ. Emergence of gender differences in depression during adolescence: national panel results from three countries. *Journal of the American Academy of Child & Adolescent Psychiatry* 2002; 41:190-198.

[16] Kornstein SG, Schatzberg AF, Thase ME, Yonkers KA, McCullough JP, Keitner GI, Gelenberg AJ, Ryan CE, Hess AL, Harrison W. Gender differences in chronic major and double depression. *Journal of Affective Disorders*, 2000; 60:1-11.

[17] Offord DR, Boyle MH, Campbell D, Goering P, Lin E, Wong M, Racine YA. One-year prevalence of psychiatric disorder in Ontarians 15 to 64 years of age. *Canadian Journal of Psychiatry*, 1996; 41:559-563.

[18] Eaton WW, Muntaner C, Bovasso G, Smith C. Socioeconomic status and depressive syndrome: the role of inter- and intragenerational mobility, government assistance, and work environment. *Journal of Health and Social Behaviour* 2001; 42:277-294.

[19] Lorant V, Deliege D, Eaton W, Robert A, Philippot P, Ansseau M. Socioeconomic inequalities in depression: A meta-analysis. *American Journal of Epidemiology*, 2003; 157:98-112

[20] Antman EM, Anbe DT, Armstrong PW. ACC/AHA guidelines for the management of patients with ST-elevation myocardial infarction; A report of the American College of Cardiology/American Heart Association Task Force on Practice Guidelines (committee to revise the 1999 guidelines for the management of patients with acute myocardial infarction). *Journal American College of Cardiology*. 2004; 44:1–211.

[21] Montano CB. Recognition and treatment of depression in a primary care setting. *Journal of Clinical Psychiatry* 1994; 12:18-34

[22] Dickens C, McGowan L, Percival C, Tomenson B, Cotter L, Heagerty A, Creed F. Depression Is a Risk Factor for Mortality After Myocardial Infarction. Fact or Artifact? *Journal of the American College of Cardiology* 2007; 49:18

[23] Herrmann C. International experiences with the Hospital Anxiety and Depression Scale: a review of validation data and clinical results. *Journal of Psychosomatic Research* 1997; 42:17–41.

[24] Mayou RA, Gill D, Thompson DR, Day A, Hicks N, Volmink J, and Neil A. Depression and Anxiety as Predictors of Outcome after Myocardial Infarction. *Psychosomatic Medicine* 2000; 62:212–219

[25] Beck AT, Steer RA, Garbin MG. Psychometric properties of the Beck Depression Inventory: twenty five years of evaluation. *Clinical Psychology Review* 1988; 8: 77–100.

[26] Strik JJMH, Honig A, Lousberg R, Denollet J. Sensitivity and specificity of observer and self rating questionnaires in depression following myocardial infarction. *Psychosomatics* 2001; 42:423–428.

[27] Beck AT, Steer RA. *Beck depression inventory manual*. San Antonio (TX): The Psychological Corporation, Harcourt-Brace-Jovanovich; 1987

[28] Carney RM, Blumenthal JA, Freedland KE, Youngblood M, Veith RC, Burg RM, Cornell C, Saab PG, Kaufmann PG, Czajkowski SM, Jaffe AS. Depression and Late Mortality after Myocardial Infarction in the Enhancing Recovery in Coronary Heart Disease (ENRICHD) study. *Psychosomatic medicine* 2004; 66:466–474

[29] Drory Y, Kravetz S, Hirschberger G. Long-Term Mental Health of Men After a First Acute Myocardial Infarction. *Archives of Physical Medicine and Rehabilitation* 2002; 83

[30] Lauzon C, Beck CA, Huynh T, Dion D, Racine N, Carignan S, Diodati JG, Charbonneau F, Dupuis F, Pilote L. Depression and prognosis following hospital admission because of acute myocardial infarction. *Canadian Medical Association Journal* 2003; 168(5):547

[31] Ruo B, Rumsfeld JS, Hlatky MA, Liu H, Browner WS, Whooley MA. Depressive symptoms and Health-Related Quality of Life, The Heart and Soul Study. *Journal of American Medical Association.* 2003; 290(2):215-221

[32] Kroenke K, Spitzer RL, Williams JB. The PHQ-9: validity of a brief depression severity measure. *General Internal Medicine* 2001; 16:606–613.

[33] Spitzer RL, Kroenke K, Williams JB. Validation and utility of a self-report version of PRIME-MD: the PHQ primary care study: Primary Care Evaluation of Mental Disorders: Patient Health Questionnaire. *Journal of the American Medical Association* 1999; 282:1737-1744.

[34] Spertus JA, Peterson E, Rumsfeld JS, Jones PG, Decker C. and Krumholz H. The Prospective Registry Evaluating Myocardial Infarction: Events and Recovery (PREMIER)—Evaluating the impact of myocardial infarction on patient outcomes. *American Heart Journal* 2006; 151:589-97

[35] Andresen EM, Malmgren JA, Carter WB, Patrick DL. Screening for depression in well older adults: evaluation of a short form of the CES-D (Center for Epidemiologic Studies Depression Scale). *American Journal of Preventative Medicine* 1994; 10:77–84.

[36] Irwin M, Artin KH, Oxman MN. Screening for depression in the older adult: criterion validity of the 10-item Center for Epidemiological Studies Depression Scale (CES-D). *Archives of Internal Medicine* 1999; 159:1701–1704.

[37] Jamerson BD, Krishnan KRR, Roberts J, Krishen A, Modell JG. Effect of buproprion SR on specific symptom clusters of depression: analysis of the 31-item Hamilton Rating Scale for Depression. *Psychopharmacology Bulletin* 2003; 37(2):67– 78.

[38] Glassman AH, O'Connor CM, Califf RM, Swedberg K, Schwartz P, Bigger JT, Ranga Rama Krishman K *et al.* Sertaline Treatment of major depression in patients with acute MI or unstable angina. *Journal of the American Medical Association* 2002; 288(6):701-709

[39] Mendes de Leon CF, Krumholz HM, Vaccarino VV, Williams CS, Glass TA, Berkman LF and Kas SV. A population based perspective of changes in health-related quality of life after myocardial infarction in men and women. *Journal of Clinical Epidemiology* 1998; 51:609-616

[40] Ware JE, Gandek B. Overview of the SF-36 health survey and the international quality of life assessment (IQOLA) project. *Journal of Clinical Epidemiology* 1998; 51:903-312

[41] Dempster M and Donnelly M. Measuring the health related quality of life of people with ischemic heart disease. *Heart* 2000; 83:641-644

[42] Lim LL-Y, Valenti LA, Knapp JC, et al. A self administered quality of life questionnaire after acute myocardial infarction. *Journal of Clinical Epidemiology* 1993;46:1249–56.

[43] Valenti L, Lim L, Heller RF, *et al*. An improved questionnaire for assessing quality of life after acute myocardial infarction. *Quality of Life Research* 1996; 5:151–61.

[44] Spertus JA, Winder TA, Dewhurst RA, Deyo J, Prodzinski M, McDonell SD. Development and evaluation of the Seattle Angina Questionnaire: a new functional status measure for coronary artery disease. *Journal American College of Cardiology* 1995; 25(2):333-41

[45] Brink E, Grankvist G, Karlson BW, Hallberg LR-M. Health-related quality of life in women and men one year after acute myocardial infarction. *Quality of Life Research* 2005; 14:749-757

[46] Brink E, Karlson BW, Hallberg LR-M. Health experiences of first-time myocardial infarction: factors influencing women's and men's health-related quality of life after five months. *Psychology, Health and Medicine* 2002; 7:5-16.

[47] Levin LA, Perk J, Hedback B. Cardiac Rehabilitation – a cost analysis. *Journal of Internal Medicine* 1991; 230:427-434

[48] World Health Organisation, Rehabilitation of patients with cardiovascular disease: Report of WHO Expert Committee. *Technical report series 270*. Geneva: WHO, 1964

[49] Scottish Intercollegiate Guidelines Network. Cardiac Rehabilitation, a national clinical guideline, Edinburgh: 2002.

[50] Myers J. Exercise and Cardiovascular Health *Circulation* 2003; 107:2-5

[51] Wenger NK, Froelicher ES, Smith LK, *et al*. Cardiac Rehabilitation. Clinical Practice Guideline No. 17. Rockville, MD: U.S. Department of Health and Human Services, Public Health Service, Agency for Health Care Policy and Research and the National Heart, Lung, and Blood Institute. AHCPR Publication No. 96-0672. 1995.

[52] Jolliffe JA, Rees K, Taylor RS, Thompson D, Oldridge N, Ebrahim S. Exercise-based rehabilitation for coronary heart disease. Cochrane Database of Systematic Reviews 2001, Issue 1.

[53] Chartered Society of Physiotherapy. Standards for the exercise component of phase III cardiac rehabilitation. London: The Chartered Society of Physiotherapy, 1999

[54] Kugler J, Dimsdale J, Hartley L and Sherwood J. Hospital supervised vs home exercise in cardiac rehabilitation: effects on aerobic fitness, anxiety, and depression. *Archives of Physical Medicine and Rehabilitation* 1990; 71(5):322 -325

[55] Thompson DR, Bowman GS, Kitson AL *et al*. Cardiac rehabilitation services in England and Wales: a national survey. *International Journal of Cardiology* 1997; 59:299–304.

[56] Campbell NC, Grimshaw JM, Ritchie LD *et al*. Outpatient cardiac rehabilitation: are the potential benefits being realised? *Journal of Royal College of Physicians London* 1996; 30:514–519.

[57] Duryee R. The efficacy of inpatient education after myocardial infarction. *Heart and Lung* 1992; 21:217–225.

[58] Lothian Primary Care NHS Trust. *The Heart Manual*, 2nd ed. Edinburgh; 2002.

[59] Lewin B, Robertson IH, Cay EL, Irving JB and Campbell M. Effects of self-help post myocardial-infarction rehabilitation on psychological adjustment and use of health services. *Lancet* 1992; 339:1036-1040

[60] Cowan MJ, Freedland KE, Burg MM, Saab PG, Marsten E, Youngblood ME, Cornell CE, Powell LH, Czaajkowski SM, for the ENRICHED investigators. Predictors of treatment response for depression and inadequate social support – The ENRICHD Randmised Clinial Trial. *Psychotherapy Psychosomatics* 2008;77:27-37.

[61] Dusseldorp E, van Elderen T, Maes S, Meulman J, Kraaij V. A meta-analysis of psychoeducational programmes for coronary heart disease patients. *Health Psychology* 1999; 18:506-519

[62] Jones DA and West RR. Psychological rehabilitation after myocardial infarction: multicentre randomised controlled trial. *British Medical Journal* 1996; 313:1517-1521

[63] Frasure-Smith N, Lesperance F, Prince RH, Verrier P, Garber RA and Juneau M. Randomised trial of home-based psychosocial nursing intervention for patients recovering from myocardial infarction. *Lancet* 1997; 350:473-479

[64] Linden W, Stossel C, Maurice J. Psychosocial interventions for patients with coronary artery disease a meta-analysis. *Archives of Internal Medicine* 1996; 156:745-752.

[65] Wilson K, Gibson N, Willan A, Cook D. Effect of smoking cessation on mortality after myocardial infarction: meta-analysis of cohort studies. *Arch Intern Med* 2000;160:939-944.

[66] West R. Cardiac rehabilitation of older patients. *Reviews in Clinical Gerontology* 2004;13:241-255.

[67] Stahle A, Mattsson E, Ryden L, Unden AL and Nordlander R. Improved physical fitness and quality of life following training of elderly patients after acute coronary events. *European Heart Journal* 1999; 20:1475–1484

In: Psychological Factors and Cardiovascular Disorders   ISBN: 978-1-60456-871-4
Editor: Leo Sher   © 2008 Nova Science Publishers, Inc.

Chapter V

DEPRESSIVE SYMPTOMS AND ATHEROSCLEROSIS

Mohammed F. Faramawi

Preventive Medicine, Epidemiology and Biostatistics Department, Menufiya University, Shibin El Kom, Egypt.

ABSTRACT

Depression and cardiovascular disease are prevalent public health problems. Several epidemiological studies have shown that depression is a strong predictor of adverse cardiovascular outcomes such as coronary artery disease and heart failure. Little is known about the role of atherosclerosis as an important mechanism responsible for the link between depressive symptoms and adverse cardiovascular outcomes.

INTRODUCTION

Depressive symptoms affect people of all races, incomes and ages [1]. It is three to five times more common in the elderly than in young. The prevalence of depressive symptoms in subjects aged 65 years and older in the United States ranges from 11% to 20% [1]. Clinical depression affects about 19 million Americans annually. About 5%-10% of women and 2%-5% of men will experience at least one major depressive episode during their adult life.

Atherosclerosis begins in childhood with the development of fatty streaks [2]. The clinical manifestations of the disease increase with age through the fifth and sixth decades of life [2]. In the United States, approximately, 30% of persons above 50 years have some evidence of carotid artery disease. Atherosclerosis is the leading cause of death in the developed world. In the USA, atherosclerosis is responsible for more than half of the yearly mortality and more than 500,000 people die annually of myocardial infarction alone [3]. The treatment of cardiovascular disease in the USA costs more than $100 billion a year. In the developing countries, atherosclerosis will be an important cause of mortality in the coming decades [4-7].

Little is known about the role of atherosclerosis as an important mechanism responsible for the link between depressive symptoms and adverse cardiovascular outcomes [8,9]. Few epidemiologic studies have examined the association between depressive symptoms and atherosclerosis of peripheral arteries such as carotid arteries. In the previous studies, the indicators of the arterial wall atherosclerosis were the increase in the wall stiffness, intima media thickness, detection of calcium deposition or plaques [8-11]. In the following chapter the light will be shed on the relationship between depressive symptoms and carotid artery atherosclerosis.

THE RELATIONSHIP OF DEPRESSION WITH CAROTID ARTERY ATHEROSCLEROSIS

Doppler Ultrasonography and Carotid Artery Atherosclerosis

Doppler ultrasonography has been used as a diagnostic tool for carotid artery abnormalities [12]. Ultrasound examination of carotid arteries can provide information about carotid intima-media thickness (CIMT), total cross-sectional area of carotid plaques, or severity of arterial stenosis. Although these phenotypes are atherosclerosis indicators, they represent different stages of atherogenesis which is a complex multi-step process that has many physical , biochemical, molecular and genetic determinants [13].

Atherosclerosis can be viewed as a gradual process from thickening to plaques. Among carotid ultrasound determinations, intima media thickness reflects a hypertrophic response of arterial intimal and medial cells to lipid infiltration [14]. Arterial plaques represent a later stage of atherogenesis related to inflammation, oxidation, endothelial dysfunction, and/or smooth muscle cell proliferation [15]. In summary, CIMT, total carotid plaque area, and carotid stenosis provide information about the different stages of atherosclerosis.

How are Depressive Symptoms Detected in the Epidemiological Studies?

Epidemiological studies have used depression scores obtained from different screening tests as a measure for depressive symptoms while exploring the association of depressive symptoms with the increased risk of developing CVD. There are many screening tests that have been validated against a gold standard diagnostic tool such as the Structured Clinical Interview for DSM-IV Disorders (SCID) [16] to detect depressive symptoms. The following depressive symptoms screening tests are recommended by the U.S. Preventive Services Task Force (USPSTF) [17,18].

- The Self Report Center for Epidemiologic Studies Depression Scale (CES-D) is a 20-item instrument used to measure the presence and severity of depressive symptoms [19]. It has been reported that 11% of elderly men and 19% of elderly women score above the cutoff point for being at high risk of clinical depression on this scale. A CES-D (10-item) version was developed. The reliability of the 10-item CES-D version is comparable to that reported for the 20-item version.

- The Zung Depression scale is a 20-item self-rating scale. It takes less than 5 minutes to complete. It has been used in multiple chronic illnesses, including different types of cancers and hepatitis [20].
- The Montgomery-Asberg Depression Rating Scale is a self-administered questionnaire which is effective in detecting depressive symptoms in those who have chronic illness [21]. Nevertheless, it is not specifically recommended by the USPSTF for screening in the general population since it has fewer somatic items.
- Beck Depression Inventory (BDI) is a common screening tool for depression in the dialysis population [22]. It measures cognitive-affective symptoms and attitudes, impaired performance and somatic symptoms.
- The Geriatric Depression Scale (GDS) is a 30-item self-report questionnaire designed to detect depression in the elderly [23]. The answer to these items may be yes or no. The simple yes/no responses are more easily used than the graduated responses found on other standard assessment scales such as the Beck Depression Inventory, and the Zung self-rating depression scale. The GDS is recommended as a routine part of a comprehensive geriatric assessment. A short version of the GDS containing 15 questions has been developed [24,25].

Literature shows that two study designs were used to explore the association between depressive symptoms and carotid artery atherosclerosis

A) Cross-Sectional Design

The Rotterdam study, a population-based cross-sectional study conducted in the Netherlands to study the association between carotid artery atherosclerotic and depression [11]. Carotid ultrasonography was used to detect carotid artery stiffness as an indicator of atherosclerosis. This study showed that arterial stiffness was more prevalent in depressed elderly [11]. The Rotterdam study was a cross-sectional study. Therefore it could not show the temporal relationship between carotid artery stiffness and depressive symptoms i.e. whether carotid artery stiffness preceded depressive symptoms [11].

B) Prospective (Longitudinal) Design

Haas et al tested the relationship between depressive symptoms and carotid artery plaque [10]. Information about the baseline self-reported depressive symptoms and the carotid plaque at 10-year follow-up were assessed. After adjusting for the important covariates such as age, race, cholesterol level and blood pressure participants with elevated depression scores at baseline were more than 2 times as likely as those with no depressive symptoms to have carotid plaque [10]. Because the carotid ultrasonography was not performed at the baseline assessment, the investigators could not exclude the possibility that participants with depressive symptoms at baseline had existing atherosclerosis.

The second study was conducted by Everson et al. [3]. They examined the association between high levels of hopelessness as an indicator for depressive symptoms and progression of carotid atherosclerosis in the participants of the Kuopio Ischemic Heart Disease Study [8]. This population-based study included middle-aged men from Eastern Finland. The investigators reported that the carotid atherosclerosis progression was greatest among men reporting high levels of hopelessness at both baseline and follow-up [8]. Finally, the Cardiovascular Health Study (CHS), a population-based longitudinal study showed that the presence of depressive symptoms at baseline was associated with larger CIMT as an indicator for atherosclerosis in the elderly [9]. The adjusted relative risks of developing abnormal CIMT over 3 years due to the presence of depressive symptoms at baseline ranged from 1.21 to 1.30.

The CHS had characteristics, which distinguished it from the previous two studies. Persons who had an abnormal CIMT were excluded at the baseline [9]. This gave a better chance to establish temporality between depressive symptoms and CIMT as an indicator for atherosclerosis. Also, the repeated measures of depressive symptoms and carotid artery atherosclerosis gave a better assessment of the association between depressive symptoms and carotid artery atherosclerosis. This is because depressive symptoms vary from time to time.

PATHWAYS LINK DEPRESSION AND ATHEROSCLEROSIS

Some investigators believe that depressive symptoms precede carotid artery atherosclerosis [8-10]. These investigators proposed several mechanisms which could link depressive symptoms with atherosclerosis. Depressive symptoms are associated with bad eating habits and sedentary behavior which lead to weight gain [26]. Individuals with major depression may have high levels of inflammatory markers such as C-reactive protein. This could be due to increased release of the inflammatory mediators from the adipose tissue and white blood cells [26,27]. These markers are associated with atherosclerosis. Additionally, an increase in autonomic nervous system discharge as well as platelet activation in depressed people could contribute significantly to the pathway which links depressive symptoms with the occurrence of atherosclerosis process [28,29].

Other investigators think that atherosclerosis starts before depressive symptoms. Atherosclerosis leads to reduction in cerebral blood flow and alteration in cerebral metabolism [11]. These changes may lead to structural changes in the brain which may lead to depression (Vascular depression hypothesis) [30]. A study conducted by Mlekusch et al; supported this hypothesis [31]. In this study a significantly higher prevalence of depressive symptoms was found in patients with carotid artery stenosis than in control subjects at baseline (33.6% versus 16.7%,). At follow-up, a significant reduction of depressive symptoms was observed in patients who underwent carotid artery stent (33.6% versus 9.8%). The frequency of depressive symptoms remained unaffected in control subjects (16.7% versus 13.0%). Mlekusch el al; concluded that depressive symptoms in patients with carotid artery stenosis may improve after successful endovascular revascularization therapy [31].

FUTURE STUDIES

Future studies need to focus on developing the proper interventions which could alleviate depressive symptoms. Alleviation of such symptoms not only can prevent adverse cardiovascular outcomes such as CAD and atherosclerosis but it may also improve the quality of life. Exercise could be one of the tools used to alleviate depressive symptoms. In Maastricht Aging Study participants engaged in physical exercise were .56 times less likely to develop depressed mood [32]. Researchers have reported substantial benefits of exercise training programs in reducing depressive symptoms [33]. Exercise training decreases depressive symptoms as effectively as antidepressant medication [33].

In summary, depressive symptoms are associated with adverse outcomes such as CVD. Atherosclerosis could be an important mechanism responsible for the link between depressive symptoms and adverse cardiovascular outcomes. There is a great need for health care practitioners to monitor and alleviate depressive symptoms in healthy as well as diseased populations to prevent the adverse cardiovascular outcomes.

REFERENCES

[1]   Djernes JK. Prevalence and predictors of depression in populations of elderly: a review. *Acta Psychiatr Scand* 2006;113(5):372-87.

[2]   Daniels SR. Cardiovascular disease risk factors and atherosclerosis in children and adolescents. *Curr Atheroscler Rep* 2001;3(6):479-85.

[3]   Naghavi M, Falk E, Hecht HS, Jamieson MJ, Kaul S, Berman D, et al. From vulnerable plaque to vulnerable patient--Part III: Executive summary of the Screening for Heart Attack Prevention and Education (SHAPE) Task Force report. *Am J Cardiol* 2006;98(2A):2H-15H.

[4]   Prevalence of coronary artery calcium among asymptomatic men and women in a developing country: comparison with the USA data. *Atherosclerosis* 2005;183(1):141-5.

[5]   Coronary artery disease in the developing world. *Am H J* 2004;148(1):7-15.

[6]   Coronary heart disease risk factor profile of children in a country with developing economy--an issue that needs prompt attention.[comment]. *JPMA - Journal of the Pak Med Assoc* 2004;54(12):642.

[7]   The global epidemic of atherosclerotic cardiovascular disease. *Medical Principles & Practice* 2002;11 Suppl 2:3-8.

[8]   Everson SA, Kaplan GA, Goldberg DE, Salonen R, Salonen JT. Hopelessness and 4-year progression of carotid atherosclerosis. The Kuopio Ischemic Heart Disease Risk Factor Study. *Arterioscler Thromb Vasc Biol* 1997;17(8):1490-5.

[9]   Faramawi MF, Gustat J, Wildman RP, Rice J, Johnson E, Sherwin R. Relation between depressive symptoms and common carotid artery atherosclerosis in American persons > or =65 years of age. *Am J Cardiol* 2007;99(11):1610-3.

[10]   Haas DC, Davidson KW, Schwartz DJ, Rieckmann N, Roman MJ, Pickering TG, et al. Depressive symptoms are independently predictive of carotid atherosclerosis. *Am J Cardiol* 2005;95(4):547-50.

[11]   Tiemeier H, van Dijck W, Hofman A, Witteman JC, Stijnen T, Breteler MM. Relationship between atherosclerosis and late-life depression: the Rotterdam Study. *Arch Gen Psychiatry* 2004;61(4):369-76.

[12]   Stapf C, Elkind MS, Mohr JP. Carotid artery dissection. *Annu Rev Med* 2000;51:329-47.

[13]   Spence JD, Hegele RA. Noninvasive phenotypes of atherosclerosis: similar windows but different views. *Stroke* 2004;35(3):649-53.

[14]   Cheng KS, Mikhailidis DP, Hamilton G, Seifalian AM. A review of the carotid and femoral intima-media thickness as an indicator of the presence of peripheral vascular disease and cardiovascular risk factors. *Cardiovasc Res* 2002;54(3):528-38.

[15]   Hegele RA. The pathogenesis of atherosclerosis. *Clin Chim Acta* 1996;246(1-2):21-38.

[16]   Tuunainen A, Langer RD, Klauber MR, Kripke DF. Short version of the CES-D (Burnam screen) for depression in reference to the structured psychiatric interview. *Psychiatry Res* 2001;103(2-3):261-70.

[17]   McQuaid JR, Stein MB, McCahill M, Laffaye C, Ramel W. Use of brief psychiatric screening measures in a primary care sample. *Depress Anxiety* 2000;12(1):21-9.

[18]   McCahill ME. Screening for depression. *Am Fam Physician* 2002;66(6):952, 955.

[19]   Lewinsohn PM, Seeley JR, Roberts RE, Allen NB. Center for Epidemiologic Studies Depression Scale (CES-D) as a screening instrument for depression among community-residing older adults. *Psychol Aging* 1997;12(2):277-87.

[20]   Zung WW. A Self-Rating Depression Scale. *Arch Gen Psychiatry* 1965;12:63-70.

[21]   Wang PL, Watnick SG. Depression: a common but underrecognized condition associated with end-stage renal disease. *Semin Dial* 2004;17(3):237-41.

[22]   Wilson B, Spittal J, Heidenheim P, Herman M, Leonard M, Johnston A, et al. Screening for depression in chronic hemodialysis patients: comparison of the Beck Depression Inventory, primary nurse, and nephrology team. *Hemodial Int* 2006;10(1):35-41.

[23]   Kurlowicz L. The geriatric depression scale (GDS). *Insight* 2000;25(1):18-9.

[24]   Greenberg SA. How to try this: the Geriatric Depression Scale: Short Form. *Am J Nurs* 2007;107(10):60-9; quiz 69-70.

[25]   Jongenelis K, Pot AM, Eisses AM, Gerritsen DL, Derksen M, Beekman AT, et al. Diagnostic accuracy of the original 30-item and shortened versions of the Geriatric Depression Scale in nursing home patients. *Int J Geriatr Psychiatry* 2005;20(11):1067-74.

[26]   Agatisa PK, Matthews KA, Bromberger JT, Edmundowicz D, Chang YF, Sutton-Tyrrell K. Coronary and aortic calcification in women with a history of major depression. *Arch Intern Med* 2005;165(11):1229-36.

[27]   Miller GE, Freedland KE, Carney RM, Stetler CA, Banks WA. Pathways linking depression, adiposity, and inflammatory markers in healthy young adults. *Brain Behav Immun* 2003;17(4):276-85.

[28] Musselman DL, Tomer A, Manatunga AK, Knight BT, Porter MR, Kasey S, et al. Exaggerated platelet reactivity in major depression. *Am J Psychiatry* 1996;153(10):1313-7.

[29] Glassman AH. Depression, cardiac death, and the central nervous system. *Neuropsychobiology* 1998;37(2):80-3.

[30] Jones DJ, Bromberger JT, Sutton-Tyrrell K, Matthews KA. Lifetime history of depression and carotid atherosclerosis in middle-aged women. *Arch Gen Psychiatry* 2003;60(2):153-60.

[31] Mlekusch W, Mlekusch I, Minar E, Haumer M, Kopp CW, Ahmadi R, et al. Is there improvement of "vascular depression" after carotid artery stent placement? *Radiology* 2006;240(2):508-14.

[32] van Gool CH, Kempen GI, Bosma H, van Boxtel MP, Jolles J, van Eijk JT. Associations between lifestyle and depressed mood: longitudinal results from the Maastricht Aging Study. *Am J Public Health* 2007;97(5):887-94.

[33] Lavie CJ, Milani RV. Cardiac rehabilitation, exercise training, and psychosocial risk factors. *J Am Coll Cardiol* 2006;47(1):212; author reply 212-3.

In: Psychological Factors and Cardiovascular Disorders   ISBN: 978-1-60456-871-4
Editor: Leo Sher   © 2008 Nova Science Publishers, Inc.

Chapter VI

PSYCHIATRIC DISORDERS AND CARDIOVASCULAR DISEASE ANXIETY, DEPRESSION AND HYPERTENSION

Simon J.C. Davies, Sean D. Hood, David Christmas and David J. Nutt

Psychopharmacology Unit, University of Bristol, Bristol, United Kingdom;
School of Psychiatry and Clinical Neurosciences, University of Western Australia, Queen Elizabeth II Medical Centre, Perth, Australia.

ABSTRACT

Whereas the association of depression with cardiovascular disease is well established, the literature relating to anxiety disorders and cardiovascular disease is much less developed. There have been several studies which have examined the association of anxiety disorders with cardiovascular diagnoses, in particular with hypertension, an independent risk factor both for myocardial infarction and for stroke.

Here mechanisms proposed for the association of depression and cardiovascular disease based on cytokines, platelets, the autonomic nervous system and illness behaviour are reviewed. The evidence linking anxiety disorders and cardiovascular disease is then examined.

Focussing more specifically on hypertension, data on the associations of abnormal blood pressure with anxiety disorders and with depression are reviewed. While there is considerable evidence for associations of hypertension with panic disorder and some evidence for associations of hypertension with generalized anxiety disorder and depression, associations of low blood pressure with measures of psychological dysfunction have also been reported.

Finally the evidence relating to the aetiology of the association of panic disorder with hypertension is explored, again relating to autonomic nervous system dysfunction, cytokines and platelets. A putative neurobiological model of panic and hypertension involving autonomic nervous system dysfunction modulated by the neurotransmitter serotonin is presented.

1. INTRODUCTION

The association of depression with cardiovascular disease is now well established in medical literature, having been reported in no fewer than seventeen independent studies (for example [1-6]. Depression is not only an independent risk factor for myocardial infarction [7-10] but also for cardiovascular mortality following a cardiac event [11-13] or following coronary artery bypass surgery [14,15]. Treatment of depression appears to improve cardiovascular outcomes [8,16]. The risk of cardiovascular mortality in the five years following myocardial infarction is linked to the intensity of depression around the time of the cardiac event, suggesting a dose-dependent effect of depressive symptoms even well below the threshold for a diagnosable depressive disorder [17].

The literature relating to anxiety disorders and cardiovascular disease is less developed, but there have been several studies which have examined the association of anxiety disorders with cardiovascular disease and in particular with hypertension, an independent risk factor both for myocardial infarction and for stroke.

In this chapter we will a) revise the mechanisms proposed for the established association of depression and cardiovascular disease b) review the evidence linking anxiety disorders and cardiovascular disease c) examine the data on the association of hypertension with anxiety disorders, in particular panic disorder, and with depression and d) explore the evidence relating to a neurobiological model of the association of panic disorder with hypertension, which may provide useful insights for future research.

2. MECHANISMS UNDERLYING THE ASSOCIATION OF DEPRESSION AND CARDIOVASCULAR DISEASE

Three putative mechanisms which may explain the mechanism underlying the association of depression and cardiovascular disease have been widely discussed and studied in the literature. a) inflammatory mediators and cytokines, b) platelet dysfunction, and c) dysfunction of catecholamines and the autonomic nervous system. A fourth possibility, relating to illness behaviour, such as the functional consequences of depressed mood on adherence to medication regimens for comorbid cardiovascular disease has also been given consideration [18,19]. The rationale for the first three of these mechanisms is discussed here.

2a. Inflammatory Mediators and Cytokines

Major depression is associated with raised inflammatory markers. Most consistently raised are IL-1, IL-2, IL-6, TNFα and CRP [20-22]. For a review of inflammatory markers and the proposal of an immunological aetiology of depression see Schiepers et al [23]. It has also been proposed that the pro-inflammatory state seen is secondary to psychological stress and sympathetic overactivity seen in depression [24].

Pro-inflammatory cytokines have been suggested to participate in atheroma and thrombus formation [25]. Preclinical studies have shown interleukin-1 (IL-1), interleukin-6 (IL-6) and tumour necrosis factor-alpha (TNFα) induce vascular cell adhesion molecule-1 (VCAM-1) expression on the vascular endothelium [26]. This increases the adhesion of leukocytes to the endothelium and has been proposed to initiate atheromatous plaque formation [27]. Further studies have also shown that TNFα has direct effects upon the myocardium (via TNF receptors 1 and 2); causing decreased contractility and increased apoptosis [28]. This work has been corroborated by clinical studies showing TNFα levels correlate with severity [29] and IL-6 levels predicted future mortality of heart failure [30]. Moreover, increased levels of C-reactive protein (CRP), a further marker of inflammation, predict future risk of coronary disease in healthy controls [31]. From this data it is not possible to determine the direction of this association. It could be that heart failure or impending coronary disease instigates the pro-inflammatory state observed rather than vice versa. However, further research is required to resolve this issue. This notwithstanding, inflammatory markers that are raised in major depression have been implicated in both preclinical and clinical studies as either directly deleterious to the cardiovascular system, or markers of poor cardiac outcome. This suggests an activated immune system could be another potential link between cardiovascular and mood disorders.

2b. Platelet Dysfunction

Platelet activation has long been associated with atheroma formation, acute coronary syndromes and myocardial infarction [32]. Platelets are activated by several mechanisms, several of which are associated with major depression. These include: altered serotonin functioning, increased catecholamines and mechanical sheer stress, platelet factor 4 and β-thromboglobulin.

Patients with major depression have been found to have increased platelet activity compared to controls by measuring monoclonal antibody binding prothrombinase complexes [33]. This finding is corroborated by using plasma levels of platelet factor 4 and β-thromboglobulin to determine platelet activity. Platelet factor 4 and β-thromboglobulin are stored within platelets. They are released during platelet activation and are potent enhancers of activation [34]. These two factors are only usually detectable in trace amounts in the circulation, therefore any increase in their levels would indicate an increase in platelet activation. It has been found that both platelet factor 4 and β-thromboglobulin are increased in patients with both ischaemic heart disease and depression compared with either ischaemic heart disease only, or healthy controls. Moreover, there were no differences between the ischaemic heart disease only group and healthy controls [35]. This suggests that there is greater platelet activation in depressed patients, therefore producing an increased risk of cardiovascular disease.

Serotonin dysfunction has been proposed as a mechanism of increased platelet activity both in depression and anxiety disorders. Platelets store serotonin in intracellular dense granules. When activated they release the dense granules (also containing activating substances adenosine diphosphate, calcium ions and thromboxane A2). The released serotonin acts on surrounding platelets via 5HT-2A receptors to activate them in a positive feedback loop. During an acute coronary syndrome serotonin increases thrombus stability and also increases ischaemia due to vasoconstriction [36,37]. Depressed patients have increased platelet 5HT-2A binding [38]. Therefore increased platelet sensitivity to serotonin activation could be one explanation of an increased risk of cardiovascular disease. Selective serotonin reuptake inhibitors (SSRIs) have been associated with reduced recurrent cardiac ischaemia, but increased gastrointestinal bleeding following acute coronary syndromes [39]. This appears counter-intuitive as an increase in available serotonin caused by SSRIs should produce a more thrombotic environ. This can be resolved by the fact that platelets are formed without any intracellular serotonin and so have to collect it by uptake from plasma [40]. SSRIs have high affinity for the membrane serotonin transporter [41]. By blocking this uptake, platelets are left with reduced stores of serotonin which reduces the positive feedback loop when they are activated [42], thus reduction in platelet activity may contribute to the cardio-protective action of SSRIs [41].

Catecholamines also stimulate platelet activation through α-2 adrenoceptors. This can be either indirect, though potentiation of other activating factors, or direct when in high concentrations [43]. Patients with depression have been found to have higher plasma levels of noradrenaline than controls [44], as will be discussed in the next section.

2c. Autonomic Nervous System Dysfunction

It has been suggested that cardiovascular disease and depression may be linked through dysfunction of the autonomic nervous system. Evidence uniting mood and cardiovascular disorders comes both from studies of catecholamine concentrations in plasma at rest or in response to stress. For instance, depression has been associated with sympathetic nervous system overactivity evidenced by elevated plasma norepinephrine [45] and excess catecholamine response to orthostatic challenge [46]. By contrast in one study plasma catecholamine concentrations were slightly higher in non-depressed controls than in subjects with depression [47].

Heart rate variability is a marker of autonomic nervous system dysfunction which may be a consequence of sympathetic nervous system overactivity or imbalance between the activity of the sympathetic and parasympathetic nervous systems. This is diminished in depression [48-50]. In cardiovascular disease diminished heart rate variability is associated with a worse prognosis for instance after myocardial infarction [51] or in heart failure [52], although the predictive value of heart rate variability on the prognosis of depression has yet to be established.

Changes in catecholamine concentration and autonomic concentrations reported in depression may represent a target for serotonin promoting treatments. In a healthy volunteer study [53] taking 50mg/day of the Selective Serotonin Reuptake Inhibitor (SSRI) antidepressant Sertraline for two days was associated with lower plasma norepinephrine appearance rates than use of placebo. This is also evidence that SSRI treatment can increase heart rate variability [54]. Both of these lines of evidence point towards a beneficial modulating role for serotonin in the autonomic dysfunction that may link depression and cardiovascular disease. However, cognitive therapy for depression has also been reported to increase heart rate variability [55], so recovery from illness may in itself be protective.

3. OVERVIEW OF DEPRESSION AND ANXIETY DISORDERS

Depression and anxiety disorders are overlapping diagnostic categories, demarcated by pharmacological dissection, expert consensus, and medicopolitical forces over recent decades. Refinement of the standard categorical classification systems (DSM, ICD) continues with the release of DSM-V expected in 2012 (Figure 1). DSM-IV provides definitions of several distinct, but related anxiety disorders, including generalized anxiety disorder, panic disorder, agoraphobia, social phobia (social anxiety disorder), specific phobia, obsessive-complusive disorder and post-traumatic stress disorder. Comorbidity (ie: the simultaneous presence of both depression and anxiety disorders) is common, and usually associated with increased symptoms, impairment and morbidity [56].

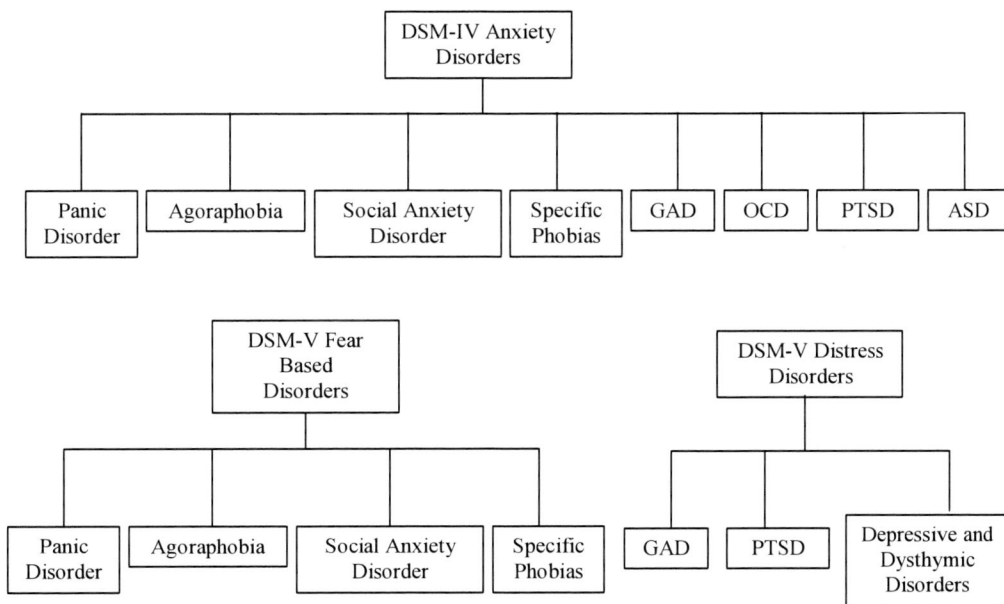

Figure 1. Existing DSM-IV Classification of Anxiety Disorders (upper panel), with possible DSM-V Classification (lower panels), illustrating the proposals for "Fear-based" and "Distress" disorders with Generalized Anxiety Disorder moving across to the "Distress Disorder" category. Adapted from Watson et al (2005) [56].

In the proposed DSM-V categorization, which is evolving through a consideration of epidemiological, clinical and biological evidence [57], it is expected that these disorders will be categorised differently. If current plans are adopted DSM-V may delineate panic disorder, agoraphobia, social phobia and specific phobias into a sub-category of "fear-based anxiety disorders" while generalized anxiety disorder and depressive disorders may be classified together occupying a separate sub-category, with both groups being listed together under "distress disorders". Meanwhile, obsessive-compulsive disorder may be moved away from the anxiety and mood disorders into a new categorization.

Panic Disorder

Of the various clinical anxiety disorders recognised in modern classification systems, Panic Disorder is of particular interest in a cardiovascular context. Panic disorder was first recognised as a discrete clinical entity in 1980 [58] and revised diagnostic criteria were published in the DSM-III-R system of 1987 [59]. Using DSM-III-R criteria, panic attacks are described as discrete episodes of fear or discomfort in which four or more recognised symptoms are experienced. The panic symptoms listed in DSM-III-R are i) shortness of breath (dyspnoea) or smothering sensations, ii) dizziness, unsteady feelings, or faintness, iii) palpitations or accelerated heart rate (tachycardia), iv) trembling or shaking, v) sweating, vi) choking, vii) nausea or abdominal distress, viii) depersonalization or derealization, ix) numbness or tingling sensations (paraesthesias), x) hot flushes or chills, xi) chest pain or discomfort, xii) fear of dying, xiii) fear of going crazy or doing something uncontrolled.

In DSM-III-R, panic disorder is diagnosed in individuals who have spontaneous panic attacks which come on suddenly, reach a peak quickly and are not attributable to any organic cause, and who experience at least four such attacks per month or one attack followed by a month of persistent fear of further attacks. In DSM-IV the criteria were revised slightly [59]. DSM-IV requires recurrent unexpected panic attacks, with at least one of the attacks followed by 1 month or more of either a) persistent concern about having additional attacks, b) worry about the implications of the attack or its consequences (e.g., losing control, having a heart attack, "going crazy") or c) a significant change in behaviour related to the attacks. As in DSM-III-R, attacks must not be due to any organic cause.

Panic Disorder is common in the general population [60,61] and even more common in hospital outpatient clinics [62,63] but is poorly recognised in medical settings [64]. People with panic attacks may present in the emergency department with chest pain, but recognition rates as low as 2% have been reported in this setting [65], despite the development of brief interview schedules which would allow physicians with no extra training to diagnose panic disorder reliably and initiate effective pharmacological treatment [66].

4. EVIDENCE FOR ASSOCIATION OF ANXIETY DISORDERS WITH CARDIOVASCULAR DISEASE

Published data on the association of anxiety disorders and cardiovascular disease is less extensive than that for depression. Several previous studies have shown associations of coronary heart disease with panic disorder or related anxiety disorders [67]. Two small studies reported an excess of cardiovascular mortality in patients with panic disorder [68] and its diagnostic fore-runner anxiety neurosis [69]. Using data derived from the Epidemiological Catchment Area study Weissman [70] reported a significant excess of cardiovascular conditions including history of "heart attack" which had an odds ratio of 4.54 in panic disorder compared to subjects with no psychiatric illness. In this study panic disorder was diagnosed by a structured psychiatric interview but cardiovascular endpoints were identified by self report and unsupported by physician verification. The authors acknowledged that patients with panic disorder may over-report cardiovascular illness because of hypochondriasis.

We reported that among 390 hypertensive patients attending a hospital clinic, those with a history of panic disorder or panic attacks had a significant excess of coronary heart disease compared with hypertensive patients who had not experienced panic attacks [64]. The odds ratios for coronary heart disease were 2.1 for all panic attacks and 3.0 for panic disorder. There was also an excess of myocardial infarction, with odds ratios of 2.5 for all panic attacks and 10.4 for panic disorder.

However, none of these studies succeeded in combining both a robust method for diagnosing panic disorder and a similarly robust method for diagnosing cardiovascular endpoints. Subsequently, using a managed care database in the US of 78,000 patients, Gomez-Caminero [71] also reported a 2 fold increased risk for cardiovascular disease in patients with panic disorder, independent of the presence of major depressive disorder. This study had the advantage of large numbers and a prospective design. Panic disorder and cardiovascular outcomes were obtained from clinical records, although these were based on the ICD-9 diagnostic system. In a further prospective study, of 3369 postmenopausal women, those reporting one or more panic attacks in the previous 6 months were at increased risk of subsequent cardiovascular events (fatal and nonfatal myocardial infarction and stroke) over the following 5.3 years [72].

The association of cardiovascular conditions and phobic anxiety symptoms has been examined in prospective and cross-sectional studies. In one study, phobic anxiety had relative risk of 3.8 for fatal coronary heart disease in men followed up for an average of 6.7 years [73]. In similar studies [74,75] of men free of coronary heart disease at baseline, phobic anxiety was associated with excess CHD mortality, which was entirely due to excess sudden deaths. A further study by the same authors [76] showed an association between baseline anxiety, and increased risk of sudden cardiac death over 32 years of follow up. In another prospective study, Watkins [77] reported associations of phobic anxiety and depressive symptomatology with ventricular arrhythmias. Fleet's review [78] concluded these forms of anxiety, which he termed "panic-like anxiety" appeared to be an independent risk factor for cardiovascular death.

In contrast, a number of studies have examined the association of cardiovascular disease with measures of anxiety more closely related to generalized anxiety disorder. A meta analysis of anxiety as a risk factor for cardiovascular disease in studies up to 2003 concluded that the evidence for generalized anxiety as a cardiovascular risk factor was relatively sparse [79], with several studies finding no association. More recently Herbst et al in a population based study of older adults found only a non-significant trend towards an association between lifetime prevalence of an anxiety disorder and coronary heart disease [6].

Positive associations between generalized anxiety and cardiovascular disease have been reported in several studies. In a large prospective study which focussed on worry, a cardinal symptom of generalized anxiety disorder, total worry score was associated with total coronary heart disease and with angina pectoris but not with non-fatal MI or with coronary heart disease mortality [67]. Using a cross-sectional design, Barger [80] reported that generalized anxiety disorder conferred a five-fold risk of CHD in the general population. Shibeshi [81] reported that a high level of anxiety (measured on Kellner's Symptom Questionnaire) which was maintained after diagnosis of coronary artery disease conferred a strong risk of death or myocardial infarction. Most recently both depression and generalized anxiety were predictors of mortality in a cohort of individuals with stable coronary heart disease [82].

It is notable in the light of the proposed DSM-V categorization of anxiety and depressive disorders, that there is a more consistent body of evidence to support associations of cardiovascular disease with the fear based anxiety disorders (panic disorder and the phobias) rather than with generalized anxiety disorder. The proposed categorization, if adopted, may be particularly helpful in signposting further research into the biological and other factors which are characteristic of fear based anxiety disorders and are associated with cardiovascular disease.

5. HYPERTENSION

Hypertension is a common disorder with increasing prevalence through the lifespan. In the United States more than half of those aged 60 to 69 years and three-quarters of those aged 70 years are hypertensive [83]. Despite the continuing development of antihypertensive drug treatments, the prevalence of hypertension in the U.S.A. increased significantly by 10% between data collection conducted between 1999-2004 and an earlier data collection between 1988-94 in adults age over sixty years [84].

The importance of recognising and treating hypertension lies in it being a strong prognostic factor for myocardial infarction, heart failure and stroke irrespective of other risk factors [85]. From the age of 40 to 89, every 20 mmHg increase in systolic blood pressure or 10 mm Hg in diastolic blood pressure confers a doubling of mortality from both ischemic heart disease and stroke [86]. However, this risk is modifiable since treatment through antihypertensive drugs either alone or in combinations may lower blood pressure below target values [87] and reduce the excess risks of cardiovascular disease in all age groups.

Traditionally hypertension was categorised as either being "essential", meaning of unknown aetiology or "secondary" to an identifiable cause such as Renal artery stenosis, Cushing's disease or phaeochromocytoma. The use of the term "essential" was related to a belief held widely until the 1930s that hypertension was simply a compensatory mechanism to ensure perfusion remained adequate when arteries became sclerosed in other words an "essential" response to maintain the perfusion [88]. The link between hypertension and cardiovascular disease established through the Framingham Heart Study [89] and other cohorts and the evidence that treating hypertension could reduce this risk confirmed that hypertension is not an "essential" homeostatic response but the term "essential hypertension" has persisted to the modern day. In addition, hypertension previously considered "essential" and therefore thought to have no identifiable cause can often now be linked to an associated pathology. For instance, mechanisms which have been identified in "essential" hypertension are insulin resistance, salt sensitivity, sleep apnoea and dysfunction of the sympathetic nervous system [90,91].

6. ASSOCIATIONS WITH HYPERTENSION

6a. Association of Panic Disorder with Hypertension

Several authors have demonstrated an epidemiological association of hypertension with panic disorder. Hypertension was more common in patients with panic disorder than in controls in two small studies [92,93]. In the first, a retrospective study of patients referred from primary care with panic disorder the prevalence of hypertension, 15%, was reported to be significantly higher than the prevalence of 9% in patients without panic disorder [92]. Patients with panic disorder developed hypertension more commonly than did a control group of surgical patients over five years of follow-up [94]. In an uncontrolled study of African-Americans with hypertension 36% had panic attacks, and 10% fulfilled the diagnostic criteria for panic disorder [95]. Kaplan [96] has described anxiety-related hyperventilation in a prospective but uncontrolled study of patients referred to a tertiary care clinic with hypertension that was difficult to manage. Hyperventilation is a common feature of panic attacks. Of 300 consecutive patients, 35% had symptoms suggestive of hyperventilation, and in 85% of these the symptoms were reproduced by forced hyperventilation. All of these studies, however, were small, or uncontrolled, or both.

Two larger controlled cross-sectional studies have provided evidence for an association of hypertension with panic attacks and panic disorder. The first was derived from the Epidemiological Catchment Area study [70] and the second was performed by our own group in Sheffield, United Kingdom [97]. We studied 891 patients in three groups – hypertensive patients in primary care, matched normotensive controls from the same primary care practice and hypertensive patients attending a hospital clinic. Thirty seven percent of the hypertensives had experienced panic attacks compared with 21% of normotensives, a significant difference (p<0.001). The association was observed for hypertensive patients in both the hospital clinic and primary care settings and could therefore not be attributed to selective referral. Panic disorder, defined by DSM-III-R criteria, was significantly more common in hypertensives studied in primary care than in matched normotensives. There was a similar albeit non-significant excess of panic disorder in hospital clinic hypertensives compared with normotensive controls.

6b. Association of other Anxiety Measures and of Depression with Hypertension

Other studies have examined the association of measures of anxiety and depression with hypertension. In both cases the picture is conflicting.

Anxiety measured by various instruments in both longitudinal [98-103] and cross-sectional designs [101,102] was reported to be associated with hypertension. While some of these studies used measures of "tension-anxiety" [100,102], others employed the Spielberger Anxiety Inventory which describes symptoms most similar to those in generalized anxiety disorder [98,101]. In contrast one large prospective study [104] showed no association of anxiety with the development of hypertension.

For depression, several studies, both those with a longitudinal design [103,105] and cross-sectional studies [106] have reported an association. . By contrast large cross-sectional studies [101,104,107] have reported no excess risk of hypertension with depression.

However, further inspection of the literature reveals a separate body of research in large epidemiological cohorts which has focussed on the low blood pressure with psychological endpoints. Low blood pressure was associated with psychological dysfunction measured by the GHQ questionnaire [108,109]. The North Trondelag Health study, a population based cohort study conducted in Norway [110] reported that participants in the lowest 5% centile for systolic blood pressure had significantly lower depression and anxiety scores measured by the HAD scale than those with systolic blood pressures between the 40 and 60% centiles.

In other words, depression and measures of anxiety have been associated both with low and high blood pressure. These two batches of literature have yet to be fully reconciled into one overarching model. One study [111] reported that men with diastolic blood pressure below 75mmHg and those with diastolic blood pressure above 85mmHg both had significantly higher scores on the Beck Depressive Inventory than those in the 75-85 mmHg range. The possibility of a J shaped or U shaped relation between blood pressure and depression and anxiety requires further exploration.

7. MECHANISMS IN THE ASSOCIATION OF HYPERTENSION AND PANIC DISORDER

Earlier we considered possible mechanisms which may underlie the association between depression and cardiovascular disease. Here we examine the evidence for these mechanisms (autonomic dysfunction, cytokines/inflammatory mediators and platelets) in the association of hypertension and the fear based anxiety disorders most specifically panic disorder. In addition there are a number of further mechanisms such as those involving the respiratory system, illness behaviour, labelling effects and the impact of white coat hypertension which are worthy of consideration.

7a. Autonomic Nervous System Dysfunction

Most interest in the mechanism underlying the association of panic disorder and hypertension to date has focussed on catecholamine function and the autonomic nervous system since central or peripheral catecholamine dysfunction has been described in both disorders. Despite the majority of cases of hypertension being classified as 'essential hypertension', implying unknown aetiology, there has been an acknowledgement that in many cases a dysfunction of the autonomic nervous system may be the underlying pathology [112]. It has been suggested that psychiatric disorders may impair regulation of the autonomic nervous system leading to increased blood pressure variability [113]. Evidence from Esler's [114] studies of clinical microneurography and measurement of noradrenaline spillover from cardiac nerve terminals suggest sympathetic dysfunction in hypertensives. Using similar techniques excess adrenaline spillover from the heart was reported during panic attacks [115]. There is also evidence of abnormal central catecholamine function in both disorders. Nutt [116] reported altered central alpha 2 adrenoceptor sensitivity in panic disorder, and excess catecholamine spillover from the brain has been seen in hypertension [117].

In addition, we have explored the role of autonomic dysfunction in the association between hypertension, panic attacks and panic disorder [118]. We analysed 346 questionnaires completed by patients with panic (268 hypertensives and 78 normotensives), examining frequency of different panic symptoms. We performed a factor analysis and examined associations of factors identified with hypertension. Sweating and flushes were significantly more common in hypertensive patients' attacks. The first factor identified by Factor analysis was dominated by autonomic symptoms, notably sweating, flushes, and also shaking. Only this autonomic dominated factor was associated significantly with hypertension. This suggests that a common autonomic dysfunction may contribute to the association of hypertension with panic.

Serotonin (5-HT) systems may somewhat explain the association among autonomic nervous system dysfunction, hypertension and panic disorder. Serotonin promoting antidepressants are first line treatments in all anxiety disorders, and transient depletion of serotonin by acute tryptophan depletion renders treated patients with a history of panic disorder more vulnerable to panic on stress challenge [119]. Serotonin promoting antidepressants appear to have a cardioprotective effect in patients with depression co-morbid with ischaemic heart disease [120]. Polyak's intriguing finding that SSRI antidepressants have an antihypertensive effect in hypertensive patients with co-morbid anxiety disorders is worthy of close scrutiny [121]. After three to six months' drug treatment, patients with co-morbid panic disorder and mild hypertension, experienced more pronounced blood pressure reduction if on treatment with the SSRI drug fluoxetine than those treated with the antihypertensive agent moxonidine. Significant reduction of heart rate and blood pressure variability was only seen in the fluoxetine group.

A role for 5-HT in autonomic nervous system dysfunction is supported by evidence from clinical and pre-clinical sources. Increasing CSF serotonin has been shown to be associated with a marked elevation in ventricular fibrillation threshold in the cat and significant reduction in efferent sympathetic activity from the heart [122,123]. There is substantial literature on reduction in heart rate variability in panic disorder [124,125] which is restored to normal by SSRIs [126].

Thus, lowering 5-HT concentrations using the acute tryptophan depletion technique [127] should alter both cardiovascular and psychological parameters relevant to these conditions. We have previously reported that in treated patients with social anxiety disorder or panic disorder acute tryptophan depletion led to significantly greater blood pressure and psychological responses to stress challenges than that seen under non-depleted conditions [128] (figure 2). This suggests that 5HT is having an anti-stress role in both psychological and cardiovascular domains. A lack of correlation of cardiovascular and psychological responses in the difference between tryptophan depleted and non-depleted conditions in this study is suggestive of distinct effects on these two domains.

Our group has constructed a model to illustrate possible neurochemical mechanisms and neuroanatomical pathways that may be involved in the association of panic and hypertension [129] (figure 3). Brainstem-mediated sympathetic activation may lead to hypertension, ischaemia, cardiac arrhythmias and sudden death [130]. Pathologically elevated levels of brainstem-mediated sympathetic activity could result from excess excitatory drive, a deficit in inhibitory control, or a combination of these. Stimulation of the midbrain ventrolateral periaqueductal gray (VLPAG), an integrative centre for autonomic and behavioural responses, induces hypotension and sympathoinhibition. This can be prevented by blockade of $5\text{-}HT_{1A}$ receptors in the rostral ventrolateral medulla (RVLM), a region of critical importance in maintenance of arterial pressure [131]. Thus, serotonergic neurons within the VLPAG may moderate the activity of RVLM neurones. The model also incorporates Richerson's evidence on serotonergic neurones in the medullary raphe [132]. Changes associated with exposure to carbon dioxide or decreases in extracellular pH may be detected in the medullary raphe or the VLPAG, activating these serotonin dependent chemosensors to exert a negative feedback effect on RVLM activation.

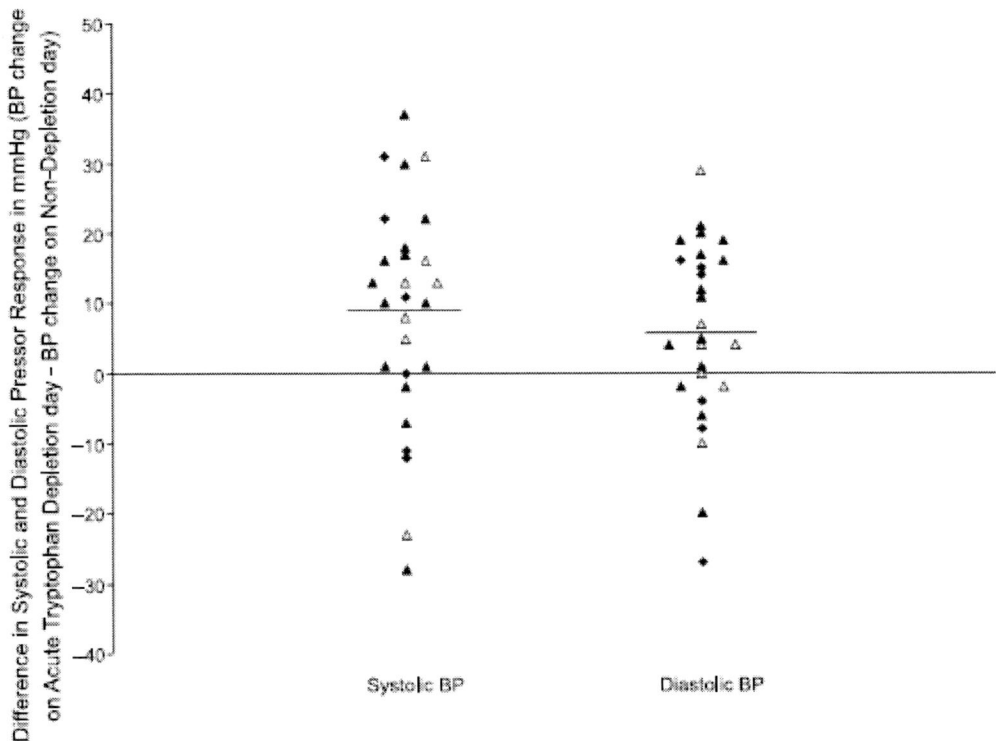

Figure 2. From Davies, Hood, Argyropoulos et al, J Clin Psychopharm 2006. [Ref 130]. Key: Closed triangles = Patients with panic disorder treated by SSRIs, Open Triangles = Patients with panic disorder treated by Cognitive Behaviour Therapy, Closed Diamonds = Patients with social anxiety disorder treated by SSRIs.

Decreased activity of serotonergic neurons in the VLPAG region could account for the association between hypertension and panic disorder (Figure 3). Serotonergic neurons within the VLPAG are thought to project to both the dorsal periaqueductal gray (DPAG) and the rostral ventrolateral medulla (reviewed by [133]). Activation of 5-HT1A and 5-HT2 receptors within the DPAG are thought to contribute to the inhibition of aversive behavioural responses [134,135], and this effect can be enhanced by chronic treatment with anti-panic medication imipramine [136]. Thus, VLPAG serotonin neurons are in a position to inhibit both the behavioural and autonomic components of panic responses. Neural systems underlying hypertension and behavioural and autonomic components of panic responses may therefore converge at the level of the brainstem. These brainstem structures are under inhibitory control by 5-HT neurons in the VLPAG, which serve as an important sympathomotor control system. If these neurons are compromised there may be vulnerability to both hypertension and the behavioural and autonomic symptoms of panic, which are alleviated by SSRIs and exacerbated by tryptophan depletion.

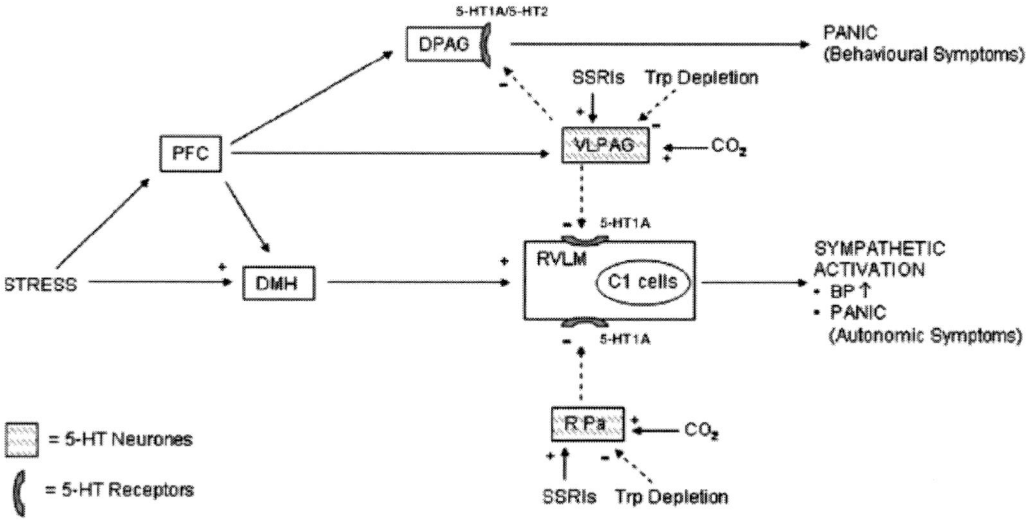

Figure 3. (From Davies, Lowry and Nutt, J Psychopharm 2007 [Ref 131].)

7b. Cytokines

As noted earlier there is considerable evidence linking depressive disorders to changes in concentrations of inflammatory markers, in particular IL-1, IL-2, IL-6, TNFα and CRP [21,137,138], and these markers are in turn associated with cardiovascular disease. Although increased anxiety symptoms have also been correlated with raised CRP, IL-6 and TNFα levels in one large study of 853 people free of cardiovascular disease [139], evidence for immune activation in specific anxiety disorders is relatively sparse. Focussing on panic disorder, interleukin-1β plasma concentrations were higher in patients with panic disorder than healthy controls both before and 1 month after treatment with alprazolam [140]. In a further study by the same group, there were no differences in TNFα concentrations between panic disorder patients and healthy controls [141]. Following a preliminary study reporting a modest increase in IL-2 in panic disorder patients compared with controls [142], another small study reported no excess of IL-2 production in patients having panic disorder with or without agoraphobia compared with healthy controls [143], but did note a negative correlation of IL-3 with state anxiety. At present therefore evidence of cytokine derangement in panic disorder is not well established and is insufficient to underpin the association with cardiovascular disease and in particular hypertension.

7c. Platelets

Dysfunction of the serotonin system is central to most current biochemical theories of the mechanisms of panic disorder [144]. Initial research focussed upon the functioning of platelet serotonin functions as a proxy for central nervous system functions. However, contradictory and equivocal evidence emerged with relation to changes in serotonin transporter [145-147], 5HT2 receptors [148,149], platelet monoaminoxidase content [150,151] and platelet serotonin content [152]. More recent work has focussed upon dysfunctional second messenger systems seen in platelets, initial studies have found decreased serotonin receptor coupling [153], decreased platelet cyclic adenosine monophosphate (cAMP) concentrations [154] and altered subunit ratios of protein kinase A [155]. Elevated platelet cAMP concentrations are known to inhibit platelet activation [156]. Therefore, it is possible that platelets are more aggregable in panic disorder - however previous studies have shown that platelets show less aggregation in response to serotonin challenge in panic disorder patients than controls [149]. Overall it remains unclear as to the degree of involvement platelets have in mediating the link between panic disorder and cardiovascular disease.

7d. Respiratory Mechanisms

Hyperventilation is a prominent component of panic attacks, and acute hyperventilation has a significant but short-lived pressor effect averaging 9/8 mmHg in normotensive subjects [157]. In Kaplan's study [96], anxiety-induced hyperventilation was thought to be present in 35% of patients with hypertension that was difficult to control, and in 85% of these patients symptoms were reproduced by hyperventilation.

Klein (1993) suggested that there are two main sub-types of panic attacks, the first due to "false suffocation alarms" and characterised by panics with a predominance of respiratory symptoms and the second group attributable to sympathetic nervous system or HPA axis deficits and not characterized by respiratory symptoms. In the factor analysis of panic attack symptoms in hypertensive and normotensive patients described earlier [128] we reported that the factor significantly associated with hypertension was the one comprising symptoms typical of sympathetic nervous system dysfunction. In fact, respiratory panic symptoms were no more common in hypertensives than normotensives and the factor dominated by respiratory symptoms had no association with hypertension.

7e. Illness Behaviour

Psychological symptoms may impair the ability of patients both to tolerate or adhere to medication regimes and to follow interventions that reduce cardiovascular risk after myocardial infarction. Panic attacks, anxiety and depression are associated with episodes of intolerance to antihypertensive agents [158]. When reported side effects were subdivided into those which would be considered as typical of the drugs implicated (drug-specific intolerance) and those which were not (non-specific intolerance), only intolerances due to non-drug specific side-effects were associated significantly with panic attacks and symptoms of depression and anxiety (figure 4). The number of episodes of non-specific intolerance was significantly associated with poor outcome in blood pressure control [158].

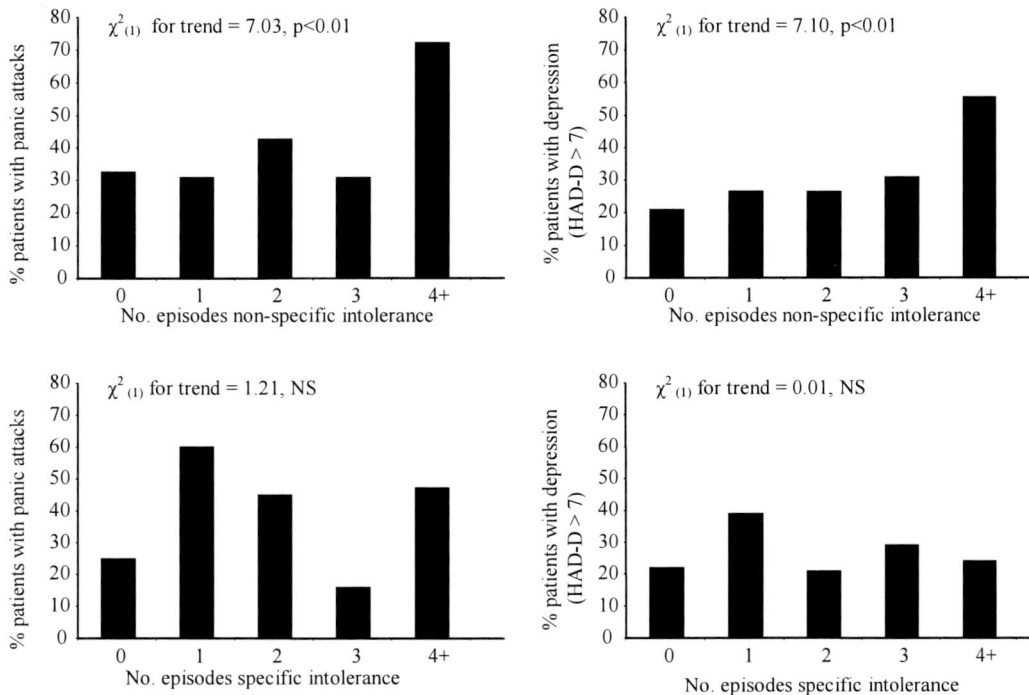

Figure 4. Relations of panic attacks and depression (HAD depression score >7) to non-specific intolerance episodes (upper panels) and to drug-specific intolerance episodes (lower panels). Note the significant relations of psychiatric morbidity to non-specific drug intolerance but not to drug-specific drug intolerance. (From Davies et al, Arch Int Med 2001 [ref 160].)

Depressed patients were less able to adhere to behaviour and lifestyle changes recommended after myocardial infarction [159]. Meta-analysis of anxiety and depression as a risk factor for non-compliance to medication across a range of medical disorders yields a clear effect for depression but a more complex picture for anxiety [160]. In most studies, however, the anxiety endpoint was measured using scales most related to the symptoms of generalized anxiety disorder. One study conducted in asthmatics which used a scale specifically measuring panic and fear reported an association between this endpoint and non-compliance [161].

7f. White Coat Hypertension & Labelling Effect

A simple explanation for reported associations of hypertension and panic disorder may be

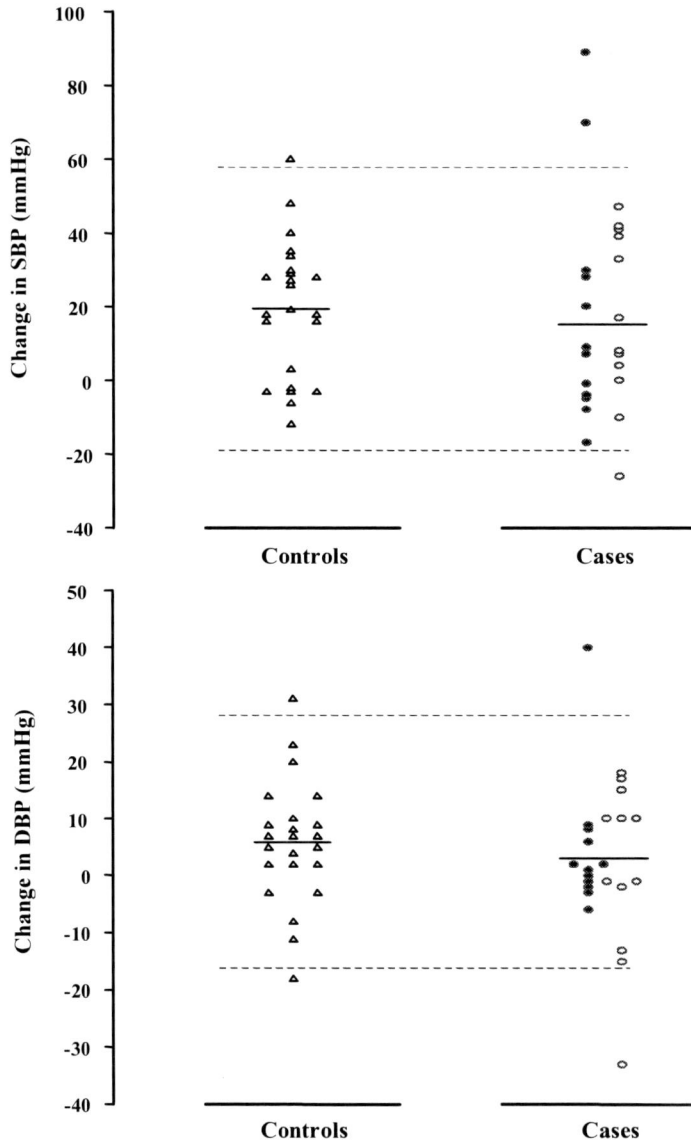

Figure 5. Scatter diagram of magnitude of white coat effect (clinic - mean daytime ambulatory blood pressure) in hypertensive patients, for systolic blood pressure (upper panel) and systolic blood pressure (lower panel). Key: Controls with no history of panic attacks (triangles), cases with panic disorder (black circles) or panic attacks (unshaded circles). From Davies et al, J Clin Hypertens 2003 [ref 165].

that patients with panic disorder appear artefactually to have higher blood pressures due to a greater 'white coat' (anxiety-induced hypertension) response compared with patients without panic disorder. Patients who are prone to panic attacks may perceive a primary care facility or hospital clinic as threatening, and could have a pressor effect as a conditioned response to these situations [162]. In an earlier clinical study we found no excess 'white coat effect' in patients with panic disorder and panic attacks making this explanation unlikely [163], (Figure 5).

One further possibility which cannot be excluded is that the association of panic disorder and hypertension might be due at least in part to a 'labelling effect'. Patients' awareness of a diagnosis of hypertension may lead to subsequent adverse effects on psychological well being [164] and to vulnerability to the development of panic disorder. Indeed, in the one study which examined the temporal relationship of the onset of panic attacks and hypertension [97], the diagnosis of hypertension preceded panic attacks significantly more often than vice versa (p<0.01).

8. FUTURE RESEARCH

An association between anxiety (especially panic disorder) and cardiovascular disease (especially hypertension) is intuitive and is well supported by existing scientific literature. Although our group and others have explored this relationship and posited autonomic dysfunction as an explanation, there are a number of additional areas worthy of research focus.

Firstly, the refinement of practical psychological and physiological tests that measure autonomic responses to stress, validated in both normal subjects and hypertensives would be a useful prerequisite to studies exploring neurobiological links between hypetension and panic disorder. Secondly, manipulation of serotonergic function via the acute tryptophan depletion technique in combination with the validated autonomic stress challenge platform would allow investigation of the ability of central serotonin to buffer the autonomic stress response in hypertensive patients and others. Exploration of adjunctive SSRI treatment in clinically hypertensive subjects, especially those with panic attacks featuring autonomic symptoms may be a therapeutic strategy worthy of further consideration.

Therefore, the development of reproducible and reliable tests that aid identification of a subset of hypertensive patients who may have co-morbid anxiety and autonomic dysfunction amenable to treatment with 5HT-promoting drugs such as SSRIs may be an ultimate goal of research in this area, broadening and refining the range of antihypertensive therapies available. Such outcomes would be of manifest benefit in the overall reduction of cardiovascular risk.

REFERENCES

[1]   Cohen HW, Madhavan S, Alderman MH. History of treatment for depression: risk factor for myocardial infarction in hypertensive patients. *Psychosom Med* 2001 Mar;63(2):203-9.

[2] Sawchuk CN, Roy-Byrne P, Goldberg J, Manson S, Noonan C, Beals J, et al. The relationship between post-traumatic stress disorder, depression and cardiovascular disease in an American Indian tribe. *Psychol Med* 2005 Dec;35(12):1785-94.

[3] Bunker SJ, Colquhoun DM, Esler MD, Hickie IB, Hunt D, Jelinek VM, et al. "Stress" and coronary heart disease: psychosocial risk factors. *Med J Aust* 2003 Mar 17;178(6):272-6.

[4] Rosengren A, Hawken S, Ounpuu S, Sliwa K, Zubaid M, Almahmeed WA, et al. Association of psychosocial risk factors with risk of acute myocardial infarction in 11119 cases and 13648 controls from 52 countries (the INTERHEART study): case-control study. *Lancet* 2004 Sep 11;364(9438):953-62.

[5] Rozanski A, Blumenthal JA, Davidson KW, Saab PG, Kubzansky L. The epidemiology, pathophysiology, and management of psychosocial risk factors in cardiac practice: the emerging field of behavioral cardiology. *J Am Coll Cardiol* 2005 Mar 1;45(5):637-51.

[6] Herbst S, Pietrzak RH, Wagner J, White WB, Petry NM. Lifetime major depression is associated with coronary heart disease in older adults: results from the National Epidemiologic Survey on Alcohol and Related Conditions. *Psychosom Med* 2007 Nov;69(8):729-34.

[7] Lesperance F, Frasure-Smith N, Juneau M, Theroux P. Depression and 1-year prognosis in unstable angina. *Arch Intern Med* 2000 May 8;160(9):1354-60.

[8] Glassman AH, Bigger JT, Gaffney M, Shapiro PA, Swenson JR. Onset of major depression associated with acute coronary syndromes: relationship of onset, major depressive disorder history, and episode severity to sertraline benefit. *Arch Gen Psychiatry* 2006 Mar;63(3):283-8.

[9] Kuper H, Marmot M, Hemingway H. Systematic review of prospective cohort studies of psychosocial factors in the etiology and prognosis of coronary heart disease. *Semin Vasc Med* 2002 Aug;2(3):267-314.

[10] Wulsin LR, Singal BM. Do depressive symptoms increase the risk for the onset of coronary disease? A systematic quantitative review. *Psychosom Med* 2003 Mar;65(2):201-10.

[11] Frasure-Smith N, Lesperance F, Talajic M. Depression following myocardial infarction. Impact on 6-month survival. *JAMA* 1993 Oct 20;270(15):1819-25.

[12] Welin C, Lappas G, Wilhelmsen L. Independent importance of psychosocial factors for prognosis after myocardial infarction. *J Intern Med* 2000 Jun;247(6):629-39.

[13] Carney RM, Blumenthal JA, Catellier D, Freedland KE, Berkman LF, Watkins LL, et al. Depression as a risk factor for mortality after acute myocardial infarction. *Am J Cardiol* 2003 Dec 1;92(11):1277-81.

[14] Connerney I, Shapiro PA, McLaughlin JS, Bagiella E, Sloan RP. Relation between depression after coronary artery bypass surgery and 12-month outcome: a prospective study. *Lancet* 2001 Nov 24;358(9295):1766-71.

[15] Blumenthal JA, Lett HS, Babyak MA, White W, Smith PK, Mark DB, et al. Depression as a risk factor for mortality after coronary artery bypass surgery. *Lancet* 2003 Aug 23;362(9384):604-9.

[16] Joynt KE, O'Connor CM. Lessons from SADHART, ENRICHD, and other trials. *Psychosom Med* 2005 May;67 Suppl 1:S63-S66.

[17] Lesperance F, Frasure-Smith N, Talajic M, Bourassa MG. Five-year risk of cardiac mortality in relation to initial severity and one-year changes in depression symptoms after myocardial infarction. *Circulation* 2002 Mar 5;105(9):1049-53.

[18] Gehi A, Haas D, Pipkin S, Whooley MA. Depression and medication adherence in outpatients with coronary heart disease: findings from the Heart and Soul Study. *Arch Intern Med* 2005 Nov 28;165(21):2508-13.

[19] Wang PS, Bohn RL, Knight E, Glynn RJ, Mogun H, Avorn J. Noncompliance with antihypertensive medications: the impact of depressive symptoms and psychosocial factors. *J Gen Intern Med* 2002 Jul;17(7):504-11.

[20] Pasic J, Levy WC, Sullivan MD. Cytokines in depression and heart failure. *Psychosomatic Medicine* 2003 Mar;65(2):181-93.

[21] Hayley S, Poulter MO, Merali Z, Anisman H. The pathogenesis of clinical depression: stressor- and cytokine-induced alterations of neuroplasticity. *Neuroscience* 2005;135(3):659-78.

[22] Miller GE, Stetler CA, Carney RM, Freedland KE, Banks WA. Clinical depression and inflammatory risk markers for coronary heart disease. *Am J Cardiol* 2002 Dec 15;90(12):1279-83.

[23] Schiepers OJ, Wichers MC, Maes M. Cytokines and major depression. *Progress in Neuro-Psychopharmacology and Biological Psychiatry* 2005 Feb;29(2):201-17.

[24] Kiecolt-Glaser JK, Glaser R. Depression and immune function: central pathways to morbidity and mortality. *J Psychosom Res* 2002 Oct;53(4):873-6.

[25] Libby P. Inflammation in atherosclerosis. *Nature* 2002 Dec 19;420(6917):868-74.

[26] Gidron Y, Gilutz H, Berger R, Huleihel M. Molecular and cellular interface between behavior and acute coronary syndromes. *Cardiovascular Research* 2002 Oct;56(1):15-21.

[27] Libby P. Inflammation in atherosclerosis. *Nature* 2002 Dec 19;420(6917):868-74.

[28] Pagani FD, Baker LS, Hsi C, Knox M, Fink MP, Visner MS. Left ventricular systolic and diastolic dysfunction after infusion of tumor necrosis factor-alpha in conscious dogs. *J Clin Invest* 1992 Aug;90(2):389-98.

[29] Torre-Amione G, Kapadia S, Benedict C, Oral H, Young JB, Mann DL. Proinflammatory cytokine levels in patients with depressed left ventricular ejection fraction: a report from the Studies of Left Ventricular Dysfunction (SOLVD). *J Am Coll Cardiol* 1996 Apr;27(5):1201-6.

[30] Tsutamoto T, Hisanaga T, Wada A, Maeda K, Ohnishi M, Fukai D, et al. Interleukin-6 spillover in the peripheral circulation increases with the severity of heart failure, and the high plasma level of interleukin-6 is an important prognostic predictor in patients with congestive heart failure. *J Am Coll Cardiol* 1998 Feb;31(2):391-8.

[31] Libby P. Inflammation in atherosclerosis. *Nature* 2002 Dec 19;420(6917):868-74.

[32] Markovitz JH, Matthews KA. Platelets and coronary heart disease: potential psychophysiologic mechanisms. *Psychosom Med* 1991 Nov;53(6):643-68.

[33]   Musselman DL, Tomer A, Manatunga AK, Knight BT, Porter MR, Kasey S, et al. Exaggerated platelet reactivity in major depression. *Am J Psychiatry* 1996 Oct;153(10):1313-7.

[34]   Nemeroff CB, Musselman DL, Evans DL. Depression and cardiac disease. *Depress Anxiety* 1998;8 Suppl 1:71-9.

[35]   Laghrissi-Thode F, Wagner WR, Pollock BG, Johnson PC, Finkel MS. Elevated platelet factor 4 and beta-thromboglobulin plasma levels in depressed patients with ischemic heart disease. *Biol Psychiatry* 1997 Aug 15;42(4):290-5.

[36]   Rentrop KP. Thrombi in acute coronary syndromes : revisited and revised. *Circulation* 2000 Apr 4;101(13):1619-26.

[37]   Benedict CR, Mathew B, Rex KA, Cartwright J, Jr., Sordahl LA. Correlation of plasma serotonin changes with platelet aggregation in an in vivo dog model of spontaneous occlusive coronary thrombus formation. *Circ Res* 1986 Jan;58(1):58-67.

[38]   Biegon A, Weizman A, Karp L, Ram A, Tiano S, Wolff M. Serotonin 5-HT2 receptor binding on blood platelets--a peripheral marker for depression? *Life Sci* 1987 Nov 30;41(22):2485-92.

[39]   Ziegelstein RC, Meuchel J, Kim TJ, Latif M, Alvarez W, Dasgupta N, et al. Selective serotonin reuptake inhibitor use by patients with acute coronary syndromes. *Am J Med* 2007 Jun;120(6):525-30.

[40]   Maurer-Spurej E. Serotonin reuptake inhibitors and cardiovascular diseases: a platelet connection. *Cell Mol Life Sci* 2005 Jan;62(2):159-70.

[41]   Sauer WH, Berlin JA, Kimmel SE. Effect of antidepressants and their relative affinity for the serotonin transporter on the risk of myocardial infarction. *Circulation* 2003 Jul 8;108(1):32-6.

[42]   Bakish D, Cavazzoni P, Chudzik J, Ravindran A, Hrdina PD. Effects of selective serotonin reuptake inhibitors on platelet serotonin parameters in major depressive disorder. *Biol Psychiatry* 1997 Jan 15;41(2):184-90.

[43]   Anfossi G, Trovati M. Role of catecholamines in platelet function: pathophysiological and clinical significance. *Eur J Clin Invest* 1996 May;26(5):353-70.

[44]   Veith RC, Lewis N, Linares OA, Barnes RF, Raskind MA, Villacres EC, et al. Sympathetic nervous system activity in major depression. Basal and desipramine-induced alterations in plasma norepinephrine kinetics. *Arch Gen Psychiatry* 1994 May;51(5):411-22.

[45]   Gold PW, Gabry KE, Yasuda MR, Chrousos GP. Divergent endocrine abnormalities in melancholic and atypical depression: clinical and pathophysiologic implications. *Endocrinol Metab Clin North Am* 2002 Mar;31(1):37-62, vi.

[46]   Maas JW, Katz MM, Koslow SH, Swann A, Davis JM, Berman N, et al. Adrenomedullary function in depressed patients. *J Psychiatr Res* 1994 Jul;28(4):357-67.

[47]   Carney RM, Freedland KE, Veith RC, Cryer PE, Skala JA, Lynch T, et al. Major depression, heart rate, and plasma norepinephrine in patients with coronary heart disease. *Biol Psychiatry* 1999 Feb 15;45(4):458-63.

[48] Stein PK, Carney RM, Freedland KE, Skala JA, Jaffe AS, Kleiger RE, et al. Severe depression is associated with markedly reduced heart rate variability in patients with stable coronary heart disease. *J Psychosom Res* 2000 Apr;48(4-5):493-500.

[49] Agelink MW, Boz C, Ullrich H, Andrich J. Relationship between major depression and heart rate variability. Clinical consequences and implications for antidepressive treatment. *Psychiatry Res* 2002 Dec 15;113(1-2):139-49.

[50] Carney RM, Blumenthal JA, Stein PK, Watkins L, Catellier D, Berkman LF, et al. Depression, heart rate variability, and acute myocardial infarction. *Circulation* 2001 Oct 23;104(17):2024-8.

[51] Kleiger RE, Miller JP, Bigger JT, Jr., Moss AJ. Decreased heart rate variability and its association with increased mortality after acute myocardial infarction. *Am J Cardiol* 1987 Feb 1;59(4):256-62.

[52] Nolan J, Fox KA. Heart rate variability and cardiac failure. *Heart* 1999 May;81(5):561.

[53] Shores MM, Pascualy M, Lewis NL, Flatness D, Veith RC. Short-term sertraline treatment suppresses sympathetic nervous system activity in healthy human subjects. *Psychoneuroendocrinology* 2001 May;26(4):433-9.

[54] Khaykin Y, Dorian P, Baker B, Shapiro C, Sandor P, Mironov D, et al. Autonomic correlates of antidepressant treatment using heart-rate variability analysis. *Can J Psychiatry* 1998 Mar;43(2):183-6.

[55] Carney RM, Freedland KE, Stein PK, Skala JA, Hoffman P, Jaffe AS. Change in heart rate and heart rate variability during treatment for depression in patients with coronary heart disease. *Psychosom Med* 2000 Sep;62(5):639-47.

[56] Nutt DJ, Argyropoulos S, Hood SD. *Clinician's Manual on Anxiety Disorders and Comorbid Depression.* London: Science Press; 2000.

[57] Watson D. Rethinking the mood and anxiety disorders: a quantitative hierarchical model for DSM-V. *J Abnorm Psychol* 2005 Nov;114(4):522-36.

[58] American Pyschiatric Association. *Diagnostic and Statistical Manual.* III ed. Washington DC: 1980.

[59] American Pyschiatric Association. *Diagnostic and Statistical Manual.* III-R ed. Washington DC: 1987.

[60] Eaton WW, Kessler RC, Wittchen HU, Magee WJ. Panic and panic disorder in the United States. *Am J Psychiatry* 1994 Mar;151(3):413-20.

[61] Katerndahl DA, Realini JP. Lifetime prevalence of panic states. *Am J Psychiatry* 1993 Feb;150(2):246-9.

[62] Chignon JM, Lepine JP, Ades J. Panic disorder in cardiac outpatients. *Am J Psychiatry* 1993 May;150(5):780-5.

[63] Beitman BD, Basha I, Flaker G, DeRosear L, Mukerji V, Lamberti JW. Major depression in cardiology chest pain patients without coronary artery disease and with panic disorder. *J Affect Disord* 1987 Jul;13(1):51-9.

[64] Davies SJ, Ghahramani P, Jackson PR, Hippisley-Cox J, Yeo WW, Ramsay LE. Panic attacks and panic disorder in hypertension, an important association often overlooked. Thirteenth Scientific Meeting of the American Society of Hypertension, New York. *Am J Hypertens* 1998;11(4 Suppl 2):21A.

[65]   Lynch P, Galbraith KM. Panic in the emergency room. *Can J Psychiatry* 2003 Jul;48(6):361-6.

[66]   Wulsin L, Liu T, Storrow A, Evans S, Dewan N, Hamilton C. A randomized, controlled trial of panic disorder treatment initiation in an emergency department chest pain center. *Ann Emerg Med* 2002 Feb;39(2):139-43.

[67]   Kubzansky LD, Kawachi I, Spiro A, III, Weiss ST, Vokonas PS, Sparrow D. Is worrying bad for your heart? A prospective study of worry and coronary heart disease in the Normative Aging Study. *Circulation* 1997 Feb 18;95(4):818-24.

[68]   Coryell W, Noyes R, Clancy J. Excess mortality in panic disorder. A comparison with primary unipolar depression. *Arch Gen Psychiatry* 1982 Jun;39(6):701-3.

[69]   Coryell W, Noyes R, Jr., House JD. Mortality among outpatients with anxiety disorders. *Am J Psychiatry* 1986 Apr;143(4):508-10.

[70]   Weissman MM, Markowitz JS, Ouellette R, Greenwald S, Kahn JP. Panic disorder and cardiovascular/cerebrovascular problems: results from a community survey. *Am J Psychiatry* 1990 Nov;147(11):1504-8.

[71]   Gomez-Caminero A, Blumentals WA, Russo LJ, Brown RR, Castilla-Puentes R. Does panic disorder increase the risk of coronary heart disease? A cohort study of a national managed care database. *Psychosom Med* 2005 Sep;67(5):688-91.

[72]   Smoller JW, Pollack MH, Wassertheil-Smoller S, Jackson RD, Oberman A, Wong ND, et al. Panic attacks and risk of incident cardiovascular events among postmenopausal women in the Women's Health Initiative Observational Study. *Arch Gen Psychiatry* 2007 Oct;64(10):1153-60.

[73]   Haines AP, Imeson JD, Meade TW. Phobic anxiety and ischaemic heart disease. *Br Med J (Clin Res Ed)* 1987 Aug 1;295(6593):297-9.

[74]   Kawachi I, Sparrow D, Vokonas PS, Weiss ST. Symptoms of anxiety and risk of coronary heart disease. The Normative Aging Study. *Circulation* 1994 Nov;90(5):2225-9.

[75]   Albert CM, Chae CU, Rexrode KM, Manson JE, Kawachi I. Phobic anxiety and risk of coronary heart disease and sudden cardiac death among women. *Circulation* 2005 Feb 1;111(4):480-7.

[76]   Kawachi I, Colditz GA, Ascherio A, Rimm EB, Giovannucci E, Stampfer MJ, et al. Prospective study of phobic anxiety and risk of coronary heart disease in men. *Circulation* 1994 May;89(5):1992-7.

[77]   Watkins LL, Blumenthal JA, Davidson JR, Babyak MA, McCants CB, Jr., Sketch MH, Jr. Phobic anxiety, depression, and risk of ventricular arrhythmias in patients with coronary heart disease. *Psychosom Med* 2006 Sep;68(5):651-6.

[78]   Fleet RP, Beitman BD. Cardiovascular death from panic disorder and panic-like anxiety: a critical review of the literature. *J Psychosom Res* 1998 Jan;44(1):71-80.

[79]   Suls J, Bunde J. Anger, anxiety, and depression as risk factors for cardiovascular disease: the problems and implications of overlapping affective dispositions. *Psychol Bull* 2005 Mar;131(2):260-300.

[80]   Barger SD, Sydeman SJ. Does generalized anxiety disorder predict coronary heart disease risk factors independently of major depressive disorder? *J Affect Disord* 2005 Sep;88(1):87-91.

[81]   Shibeshi WA, Young-Xu Y, Blatt CM. Anxiety worsens prognosis in patients with coronary artery disease. *J Am Coll Cardiol* 2007 May 22;49(20):2021-7.

[82]   Frasure-Smith N, Lesperance F. Depression and anxiety as predictors of 2-year cardiac events in patients with stable coronary artery disease. *Arch Gen Psychiatry* 2008 Jan;65(1):62-71.

[83]   Burt VL, Whelton P, Roccella EJ, Brown C, Cutler JA, Higgins M, et al. Prevalence of hypertension in the US adult population. Results from the Third National Health and Nutrition Examination Survey, 1988-1991. *Hypertension* 1995 Mar;25(3):305-13.

[84]   Ostchega Y, Dillon CF, Hughes JP, Carroll M, Yoon S. Trends in hypertension prevalence, awareness, treatment, and control in older U.S. adults: data from the National Health and Nutrition Examination Survey 1988 to 2004. *J Am Geriatr Soc* 2007 Jul;55(7):1056-65.

[85]   Collins R, Armitage J, Parish S, Sleigh P, Peto R. MRC/BHF Heart Protection Study of cholesterol-lowering with simvastatin in 5963 people with diabetes: a randomised placebo-controlled trial. *Lancet* 2003 Jun 14;361(9374):2005-16.

[86]   Lewington S, Clarke R, Qizilbash N, Peto R, Collins R. Age-specific relevance of usual blood pressure to vascular mortality: a meta-analysis of individual data for one million adults in 61 prospective studies. *Lancet* 2002 Dec 14;360(9349):1903-13.

[87]   Chobanian AV, Bakris GL, Black HR, Cushman WC, Green LA, Izzo JL, Jr., et al. The Seventh Report of the Joint National Committee on Prevention, Detection, Evaluation, and Treatment of High Blood Pressure: the JNC 7 report. *JAMA* 2003 May 21;289(19):2560-72.

[88]   White GW. THE NEW HAMPSHIRE ACADEMY OF SCIENCE. *Science* 1931 Jul 24;74(1908):98.

[89]   Kannel WB. Cardioprotection and antihypertensive therapy: the key importance of addressing the associated coronary risk factors (the Framingham experience). *Am J Cardiol* 1996 Feb 22;77(6):6B-11B.

[90]   Mancia G, Grassi G, Parati G, Zanchetti A. The sympathetic nervous system in human hypertension. *Acta Physiol Scand Suppl* 1997;640:117-21.

[91]   Esler M. The sympathetic system and hypertension. *Am J Hypertens* 2000 Jun;13(6 Pt 2):99S-105S.

[92]   Katon W. Panic disorder and somatization. Review of 55 cases. *Am J Med* 1984 Jul;77(1):101-6.

[93]   Katon W. Panic disorder: epidemiology, diagnosis, and treatment in primary care. *J Clin Psychiatry* 1986 Oct;47 Suppl:21-30.

[94]   Noyes R, Jr., Clancy J, Crowe R, Hoenk RP, Slymen DJ. The familial prevalence of anxiety neurosis. *Arch Gen Psychiatry* 1978 Sep;35(9):1057-74.

[95]   Bell CC, Hildreth CJ, Jenkins EJ, Carter C. The relationship of isolated sleep paralysis and panic disorder to hypertension. *J Natl Med Assoc* 1988 Mar;80(3):289-94.

[96]   Kaplan NM. Anxiety-induced hyperventilation. A common cause of symptoms in patients with hypertension. *Arch Intern Med* 1997 May 12;157(9):945-8.

[97] Davies SJ, Ghahramani P, Jackson PR, Noble TW, Hardy PG, Hippisley-Cox J, Yeo WW, Ramsay LE. Association of panic disorder and panic attacks with hypertension. *Am J Med* 1999 Oct;107(4):310-6.

[98] Gafarov VV, Gromova HA, Gagulin IV, Ekimova YC, Santrapinskiy DK. Arterial hypertension, myocardial infarction and stroke: risk of development and psychosocial factors. *Alaska Med* 2007;49(2 Suppl):117-9.

[99] Markovitz JH, Matthews KA, Wing RR, Kuller LH, Meilahn EN. Psychological, biological and health behavior predictors of blood pressure changes in middle-aged women. *J Hypertens* 1991 May;9(5):399-406.

[100] Markovitz JH, Matthews KA, Kannel WB, Cobb JL, D'Agostino RB. Psychological predictors of hypertension in the Framingham Study. Is there tension in hypertension? *JAMA* 1993 Nov 24;270(20):2439-43.

[101] Paterniti S, Alperovitch A, Ducimetiere P, Dealberto MJ, Lepine JP, Bisserbe JC. Anxiety but not depression is associated with elevated blood pressure in a community group of French elderly. *Psychosom Med* 1999 Jan;61(1):77-83.

[102] Perez LH, Gutierrez LA, Vioque J, Torres Y. Relation between overweight, diabetes, stress and hypertension: a case-control study in Yarumal--Antioquia, Colombia. *Eur J Epidemiol* 2001;17(3):275-80.

[103] Jonas BS, Franks P, Ingram DD. Are symptoms of anxiety and depression risk factors for hypertension? Longitudinal evidence from the National Health and Nutrition Examination Survey I Epidemiologic Follow-up Study. *Arch Fam Med* 1997 Jan;6(1):43-9.

[104] Shinn EH, Poston WS, Kimball KT, St Jeor ST, Foreyt JP. Blood pressure and symptoms of depression and anxiety: a prospective study. *Am J Hypertens* 2001 Jul;14(7 Pt 1):660-4.

[105] Davidson KW, Kupfer DJ, Bigger JT, Califf RM, Carney RM, Coyne JC, et al. Assessment and treatment of depression in patients with cardiovascular disease: National Heart, Lung, and Blood Institute Working Group Report. *Psychosom Med* 2006 Sep;68(5):645-50.

[106] Rabkin JG, Charles E, Kass F. Hypertension and DSM-III depression in psychiatric outpatients. *Am J Psychiatry* 1983 Aug;140(8):1072-4.

[107] Wiehe M, Fuchs SC, Moreira LB, Moraes RS, Pereira GM, Gus M, et al. Absence of association between depression and hypertension: results of a prospectively designed population-based study. *J Hum Hypertens* 2006 Jun;20(6):434-9.

[108] Wessely S, Nickson J, Cox B. Symptoms of low blood pressure: a population study. *BMJ* 1990 Aug 18;301(6748):362-5.

[109] Pilgrim JA, Stansfeld S, Marmot M. Low blood pressure, low mood? *BMJ* 1992 Jan 11;304(6819):75-8.

[110] Hildrum B, Mykletun A, Stordal E, Bjelland I, Dahl AA, Holmen J. Association of low blood pressure with anxiety and depression: the Nord-Trondelag Health Study. *J Epidemiol Community Health* 2007 Jan;61(1):53-8.

[111] Barrett-Connor E, Palinkas LA. Low blood pressure and depression in older men: a population based study. *BMJ* 1994 Feb 12;308(6926):446-9.

[112] Mann SJ. Neurogenic essential hypertension revisited: the case for increased clinical and research attention. *Am J Hypertens* 2003 Oct;16(10):881-8.

[113] Sloan RP, Shapiro PA, Bagiella E, Myers MM, Gorman JM. Cardiac autonomic control buffers blood pressure variability responses to challenge: a psychophysiologic model of coronary artery disease. *Psychosom Med* 1999 Jan;61(1):58-68.

[114] Esler M, Rumantir M, Kaye D, Jennings G, Hastings J, Socratous F, et al. Sympathetic nerve biology in essential hypertension. *Clin Exp Pharmacol Physiol* 2001 Dec;28(12):986-9.

[115] Wilkinson DJ, Thompson JM, Lambert GW, Jennings GL, Schwarz RG, Jefferys D, et al. Sympathetic activity in patients with panic disorder at rest, under laboratory mental stress, and during panic attacks. *Arch Gen Psychiatry* 1998 Jun;55(6):511-20.

[116] Nutt DJ. Altered central alpha 2-adrenoceptor sensitivity in panic disorder. *Arch Gen Psychiatry* 1989 Feb;46(2):165-9.

[117] Ferrier C, Cox H, Esler M. Elevated total body noradrenaline spillover in normotensive members of hypertensive families. *Clin Sci (Lond)* 1993 Feb;84(2):225-30.

[118] Davies SJ, Jackson PR, Lewis G, Hood SD, Nutt DJ. Panic attacks are more likely to include autonomic symptoms in patients with hypertension than in normotensives - a comparison of symptoms, and factor analysis. ECNP Workshop on Psychophamacology. Nice 2006. *Eur Neuropsychopharmacol* 2006;S94-S95.

[119] Bell C, Forshall S, Adrover M, Nash J, Hood S, Argyropoulos S, et al. Does 5-HT restrain panic? A tryptophan depletion study in panic disorder patients recovered on paroxetine. *J Psychopharmacol (Oxf)* 2002;16(1):5-14.

[120] Glassman AH, O'Connor CM, Califf RM, Swedberg K, Schwartz P, Bigger JT, Jr., et al. Sertraline treatment of major depression in patients with acute MI or unstable angina. *JAMA* 2002 Aug 14;288(6):701-9.

[121] Polyák J. How should we manage cardiovascular panic disorder accompanied by hypertension? *J Hypertens* 2001;19 (Suppl. 2):S64.

[122] Lown B, DeSilva RA. Roles of psychologic stress and autonomic nervous system changes in provocation of ventricular premature complexes. *Am J Cardiol* 1978 May 22;41(6):979-85.

[123] Lehnert H, Lombardi F, Raeder EA, Lorenzo AV, Verrier RL, Lown B, et al. Increased release of brain serotonin reduces vulnerability to ventricular fibrillation in the cat. *J Cardiovasc Pharmacol* 1987 Oct;10(4):389-97.

[124] Yeragani VK, Sobolewski E, Igel G, Johnson C, Jampala VC, Kay J, et al. Decreased heart-period variability in patients with panic disorder: a study of Holter ECG records. *Psychiatry Res* 1998 Mar 20;78(1-2):89-99.

[125] Friedman BH, Thayer JF. Autonomic balance revisited: panic anxiety and heart rate variability. *J Psychosom Res* 1998 Jan;44(1):133-51.

[126] Yeragani VK, Jampala VC, Sobelewski E, Kay J, Igel G. Effects of paroxetine on heart period variability in patients with panic disorder: a study of holter ECG records. *Neuropsychobiology* 1999 Sep;40(3):124-8.

[127] Hood SD, Bell C, Nutt DJ. Acute tryptophan depletion. Part I: Rationale and Methodology. *Aust N Z J Psychiatry* 2005;39:558-64.

[128] Davies SJ, Hood SD, Argyropoulos SV, Morris K, Bell C, Witchel HJ, et al. Depleting serotonin enhances both cardiovascular and psychological stress reactivity in recovered patients with anxiety disorders. *J Clin Psychopharmacol* 2006 Aug;26(4):414-8.

[129] Davies SJ, Lowry CA, Nutt DJ. Panic and hypertension: brothers in arms through 5-HT? *J Psychopharmacol* 2007 Aug;21(6):563-6.

[130] Grassi G, Kiowski W. Is the autonomic dysfunction the missing link between panic disorder, hypertension and cardiovascular disease? *J Hypertens* 2002 Dec;20(12):2347-9.

[131] Bago M, Dean C. Sympathoinhibition from ventrolateral periaqueductal gray mediated by 5-HT(1A) receptors in the RVLM. *Am J Physiol Regul Integr Comp Physiol* 2001 Apr;280(4):R976-R984.

[132] Richerson GB. Serotonergic neurons as carbon dioxide sensors that maintain pH homeostasis. *Nat Rev Neurosci* 2004 Jun;5(6):449-61.

[133] Johnson PL, Lightman SL, Lowry CA. A functional subset of serotonergic neurons in the rat ventrolateral periaqueductal gray implicated in the inhibition of sympathoexcitation and panic. *Ann N Y Acad Sci* 2004 Jun;1018:58-64.

[134] Beckett S, Marsden CA. The effect of central and systemic injection of the 5-HT1A receptor agonist 8-OHDPAT and the 5-HT1A receptor antagonist WAY100635 on periaqueductal grey-induced defence behaviour. *J Psychopharmacol* 1997;11(1):35-40.

[135] Nogueira RL, Graeff FG. Role of 5-HT receptor subtypes in the modulation of dorsal periaqueductal gray generated aversion. *Pharmacol Biochem Behav* 1995 Sep;52(1):1-6.

[136] Jacob CA, Cabral AH, Almeida LP, Magierek V, Ramos PL, Zanoveli JM, et al. Chronic imipramine enhances 5-HT(1A) and 5-HT(2) receptors-mediated inhibition of panic-like behavior in the rat dorsal periaqueductal gray. *Pharmacol Biochem Behav* 2002 Jul;72(4):761-6.

[137] Pasic J, Levy WC, Sullivan MD. Cytokines in depression and heart failure. *Psychosomatic Medicine* 2003 Mar;65(2):181-93.

[138] Miller GE, Stetler CA, Carney RM, Freedland KE, Banks WA. Clinical depression and inflammatory risk markers for coronary heart disease. *Am J Cardiol* 2002 Dec 15;90(12):1279-83.

[139] Pitsavos C, Panagiotakos DB, Papageorgiou C, Tsetsekou E, Soldatos C, Stefanadis C. Anxiety in relation to inflammation and coagulation markers, among healthy adults: the ATTICA study. *Atherosclerosis* 2006 Apr;185(2):320-6.

[140] Brambilla F, Bellodi L, Perna G, Bertani A, Panerai A, Sacerdote P. Plasma interleukin-1 beta concentrations in panic disorder. *Psychiatry Res* 1994 Nov;54(2):135-42.

[141] Brambilla F, Bellodi L, Perna G. Plasma levels of tumor necrosis factor-alpha in patients with panic disorder: effect of alprazolam therapy. *Psychiatry Res* 1999 Dec 13;89(1):21-7.

[142] Rapaport MH, Stein MB. Serum cytokine and soluble interleukin-2 receptors in patients with panic disorder. *Anxiety* 1994;1(1):22-5.

[143] Weizman R, Laor N, Wiener Z, Wolmer L, Bessler H. Cytokine production in panic disorder patients. *Clin Neuropharmacol* 1999 Mar;22(2):107-9.

[144] Argyropoulos S, Nutt DJ. The role of serotonin in panic: evidence from tryptophan depletion studies. *Acta Neuropsychiatrica* 2004;16:1-6.

[145] Norman TR, Judd FK, Gregory M, James RH, Kimber NM, McIntyre IM, et al. Platelet serotonin uptake in panic disorder. *J Affect Disord* 1986 Jul;11(1):69-72.

[146] Pecknold JC, Suranyi-Cadotte B, Chang H, Nair NP. Serotonin uptake in panic disorder and agoraphobia. *Neuropsychopharmacology* 1988 May;1(2):173-6.

[147] Nutt DJ, Fraser S. Platelet binding studies in panic disorder. *J Affect Disord* 1987 Jan;12(1):7-11.

[148] Norman TR, Judd FK, Staikos V, Burrows GD, McIntyre IM. High-affinity platelet [3H]LSD binding is decreased in panic disorder. *J Affect Disord* 1990 Jun;19(2):119-23.

[149] Butler J, O'Halloran A, Leonard BE. The Galway Study of Panic Disorder. II: Changes in some peripheral markers of noradrenergic and serotonergic function in DSM III-R panic disorder. *J Affect Disord* 1992 Oct;26(2):89-99.

[150] Gorman J, Liebowitz MR, Fyer AJ, Levitt M, Baron M, Davies S, et al. Platelet monoamine oxidase activity in patients with panic disorder. *Biol Psychiatry* 1985 Aug;20(8):852-7.

[151] Balon R, Rainey JM, Pohl R, Yeragani VK, Oxenkrug GF, McCauley RB. Platelet monoamine oxidase activity in panic disorder. *Psychiatry Res* 1987 Sep;22(1):37-41.

[152] Balon R, Pohl R, Yeragani V, Rainey J, Oxenkrug GF. Platelet serotonin levels in panic disorder. *Acta Psychiatr Scand* 1987 Mar;75(3):315-7.

[153] Dell'Osso L, Carmassi C, Palego L, Trincavelli ML, Tuscano D, Montali M, et al. Serotonin-mediated cyclic AMP inhibitory pathway in platelets of patients affected by panic disorder. *Neuropsychobiology* 2004;50(1):28-36.

[154] Marcourakis T, Gorenstein C, Brandao de Almeida PE, Ramos RT, Glezer I, Bernardes CS, et al. Panic disorder patients have reduced cyclic AMP in platelets. *J Psychiatr Res* 2002 Mar;36(2):105-10.

[155] Tardito D, Zanardi R, Racagni G, Manzoni T, Perez J. The protein kinase A in platelets from patients with panic disorder. *Eur Neuropsychopharmacol* 2002 Oct;12(5):483-7.

[156] Schwartz UR, Walter U, Eigenthaler M. Taming platelets with cyclic nucleotides. *Biochemical Pharmacology 62*, 1153-1161. 2001. Ref Type: Generic.

[157] Todd GP, Chadwick IG, Yeo WW, Jackson PR, Ramsay LE. Pressor effect of hyperventilation in healthy subjects. *J Hum Hypertens* 1995 Feb;9(2):119-22.

[158] Davies SJ, Jackson PR, Ramsay LE, Ghahramani P. Drug intolerance due to nonspecific adverse effects related to psychiatric morbidity in hypertensive patients. *Arch Intern Med* 2003 Mar 10;163(5):592-600.

[159] Ziegelstein RC. Depression in patients recovering from a myocardial infarction. *JAMA* 2001 Oct 3;286(13):1621-7.

[160] DiMatteo MR, Lepper HS, Croghan TW. Depression is a risk factor for noncompliance with medical treatment: meta-analysis of the effects of anxiety and depression on patient adherence. *Arch Intern Med* 2000 Jul 24;160(14):2101-7.

[161] Mawhinney H, Spector SL, Heitjan D, Kinsman RA, Dirks JF, Pines I. As-needed medication use in asthma usage patterns and patient characteristics. *J Asthma* 1993;30(1):61-71.

[162] Pickering TG, Devereux RB, Gerin W, James GD, Pieper C, Schlussel YR, et al. The role of behavioral factors in white coat and sustained hypertension. *J Hypertens Suppl* 1990 Dec;8(7):S141-S147.

[163] Davies SJ, Jackson PR, Ramsay LE, Ghahramani P, Palmer RL, Hippisley-Cox J. No evidence that panic attacks are associated with the white coat effect in hypertension. *J Clin Hypertens (Greenwich)* 2003 Mar;5(2):145-52.

[164] Macdonald LA, Sackett DL, Haynes RB, Taylor DW. Labelling in hypertension: a review of the behavioural and psychological consequences. *J Chronic Dis* 1984;37(12):933-42.

In: Psychological Factors and Cardiovascular Disorders   ISBN: 978-1-60456-871-4
Editor: Leo Sher   © 2008 Nova Science Publishers, Inc.

Chapter VII

CARDIOVASCULAR DISORDERS AND DEPRESSION WITH IRRITABILITY ANGER AND HOSTILITY

Renerio Fraguas and Dan V. Iosifescu

Department and Institute of Psychiatry, Faculty of Medicine, University of Sao Paulo,
Sao Paulo, Brazil;
Massachusetts General Hospital, Harvard Medical School, Boston, USA.

ABSTRACT

An increased prevalence of depression has been reported in patients suffering from several cardiac disorders. A large body of the literature supports the conclusion that depression is a risk factor for the development or aggravation of a cardiac disease. Similarly to depression, irritability/anger/hostility have also been associated with various cardiovascular conditions, including Coronary Heart Disease (CHD), hypertension, cardiac arrhythmias, cardiovascular risk factors, and cardiovascular mortality. Intriguingly, there is a high comorbidity between depression and irritability/anger/hostility. Actually, some studies have recently suggested that the presence of irritability/anger/hostility may define a special subtype of major depressive disorder with increased cardiovascular morbidity. In this chapter, we describe the studies that have addressed the association between depression with irritability/anger/hostility and cardiovascular conditions, particularly the cardiovascular risk factors. These studies support several related findings: 1) an association between major depressive disorder (MDD) with irritability and vascular disease; 2) an increased severity of subcortical white matter lesions in MDD with anger attacks; and 3) an association of anger attacks in MDD patients who are also smokers (with smoking history >11 years) and have high total serum cholesterol ($\geq$200mg/dL). Patients with MDD and cardiac disease were also reported to have increased sympathetic arousal and insomnia. Other studies however support the finding that patients with high depressive tendencies and lack of anger or hostility would represent an extremely severe form of exhaustion, also associated with an increased cardiovascular morbidity; suggesting that the relationship between depression with irritability/anger/hostility and cardiovascular disease is rather complex. In conclusion, the current literature reviewed here suggests the clinical subtype of depression accompanied by irritability/anger/hostility may be associated with high rates of cardiovascular disease and cardiac risk factors. Some studies suggest that vascular changes in the brain may be more characteristic for this depressive subtype and may represent the biological link explaining the association with cardiac disease. Establishing this clinical and biological subtype of depression could have significant clinical impact, allowing clinicians to define a population at risk which may need increased clinical attention, both from cardiologists and from psychiatrists.

INTRODUCTION

Depression and Cardiovascular Conditions

An increased prevalence of depression has been reported in several cardiac disorders such as cardiac arrhythmia [1,2], heart failure [3,4] and coronary heart disease (CHD); higher rates of depression were also found after myocardial revascularization [5,6] and in subjects with cardiovascular risk factors [7] and markers of cardiac morbidity [7], suggesting the association between depression and cardiovascular disease can occur in multiple ways. A large body of the literature supports the conclusion that depression is a risk factor for the development or aggravation of a cardiac disease. In line with this view, major depressive disorder (MDD), diagnosed using standard diagnostic criteria, has been associated in prospective studies with higher rates of myocardial infarction (MI) [8], cardiac mortality [9], and cardiac associated rehospitalization [10]. When using either a non-structured clinical diagnosis [11] or a threshold score on a depression severity scale to quantify depression, researchers have found depression to be associated in prospective studies with increased incidence of angina [12], CHD [11], heart failure [13], MI [11] and mortality [14]. Finally, depressive symptoms, regardless of the diagnosis of depression, have been associated with increased incidence of hypertension [15,16], MI [17], cardiac events [18,19], CHD [20,21], and all-cause mortality [20,22].

Irritability/Anger/Hostility and Cardiovascular Conditions

Similarly to depression, irritability/anger/hostility have also been associated with various cardiovascular conditions, including CHD [23-25], hypertension [26], cardiac arrhythmias [27], cardiovascular risk factors [26,28-30], and cardiovascular mortality [31].

Intriguingly, there is a high comorbidity between depression and irritability/anger/hostility. Actually, some studies have recently suggested that the presence of irritability/anger/hostility may define a special subtype of major depressive disorder [32,33]. In this chapter, we describe the studies that have addressed the association between depression with irritability/anger/hostility and cardiovascular conditions, particularly the cardiovascular risk factors. First we introduce a few considerations about depression with irritability/anger/hostility.

DEPRESSION WITH IRRITABILITY/ANGER/HOSTILITY

Since the initial description of a hostile depressive subtype in 1966 [34], the reported prevalence of irritability/anger/hostility in depression has ranged between 34% and 60% [35-37]. A particular form of irritable depression marked by recurrent anger attacks, spontaneous episodes characterized by feelings of rage and symptoms of physiologic arousal similar to panic attacks and accompanied by chronic irritability, has been reported to occur in 20-60% of patients with unipolar depression [38-41] and nearly two-thirds of patients with bipolar depression [42].

Currently, according with the DSM-IV criteria, irritability is considered a diagnostic feature of MDD in children and adolescents [43]. However, unfortunately, most standard rating scales of depressive symptom severity do not specifically measure irritability [44,45]. Notwithstanding, several studies have suggested that the presence of irritability/anger/hostility may be associated with greater morbidity in patients with mood disorder. Anger, irritability or hostility have been associated with treatment non-adherence [46,47], suicide attempts [46,48-53], violence [54] and accidents [52], higher prevalence of bipolarity [42], and higher rate or offspring with attentional problems [55]. In addition, there is some data suggesting that depression with anger may be associated with distinct abnormalities of subcortical white matter structure [56] and brain metabolism [57]; and a possible increased serotonergic dysfunction [58]. Taken together, theses studies suggest that the presence of irritability/anger/hostility may indicate a subtype of depression with distinct clinical and biological characteristics.

It should be noted that the concept of depression with irritability/anger/hostility has some non answered questions. For example, little is known about the distinction between irritable depression and depression with comorbid personality disorders or other psychiatric diagnoses associated with high rates of irritability. The interactions between temperament, personality and mood should be conceptualized as a complex phenomenon [59]. The nature of depressive symptoms may be influenced by personality traits; in this model, irritability may be one manifestation of sensitivity to negative stimuli [60], or interpersonal sensitivity [61]. Also, increased anxiety levels may define a specific subtype of MDD [62] and irritability is often manifested in the presence of increased anxiety (as an inadequate response of individuals overwhelmed by stress and anxiety); in a factor analysis, this continuum of symptoms in depression appeared to be best captured by a common anxiety/irritability factor [63]. One model posits that these symptoms represent markers of a trait sometimes referred to as negative affectivity – that is, hypersensitivity to negative stimuli [60].

DEPRESSION WITH IRRITABILITY/ANGER/HOSTILITY AND CARDIOVASCULAR DISEASE

Some studies have reported an association between cardiovascular conditions and depression with irritability/anger/hostility. About 70% of patients with MDD disorder and CHD submitted to myocardial revascularization surgery have been reported to have increased levels of irritability both pre and post-operatively [5]. Recently, Perlis et al. [64] investigated the baseline characteristics of MDD with irritability in 1456 subjects enrolled in the Sequenced Treatment Alternatives to Relieve Depression (STAR*D) study. Substantial levels of irritability were commonly found; present more than 50% of the time in at least 40% of the participants. The measurement was performed using the item "irritability" of the Inventory of Depressive Symptomatology (IDS) [65], which does not correspond to any used in previous studies. After controlling for differences in sex, age, and overall depression severity, depression with irritability was significantly associated with vascular disease, suggesting that the presence of irritability could confer a greater vascular morbidity.

Another study focusing on the association of depression with irritability/anger/hostility, investigated the association between brain white matter hyperintensities (WMH) and MDD with anger attacks [56]. In this study, 65 subjects meeting DSM-III-R criteria for MDD were administered brain magnetic resonance imaging scans at 1.5T to detect T2 WMH. The results showed that the severity of subcortical white matter lesions as well as total white matter lesions were significantly higher in MDD subjects with anger attacks compared with MDD subjects with no such attacks. Since brain WMHs have been correlated with cardiovascular risk factors [66], it is possible that these data indicate a correlation of depression with anger attacks and cardiovascular risk factors, consistent with reported correlations between cardiovascular risk factors and hostility [26,28-30] and with previous studies associating MDD with anger attacks with cardiovascular risk factors [67]. However, it is possible that the white matter lesions may be directly related to the biology of anger attacks, not mediated by cardiovascular risk factors, and that cardiovascular risk factors may independently cause brain white matter lesions and cardiovascular disease. The morphological changes in brain white matter described by Iosifescu et al. [56] and the reduced regional cerebral blood flow in the left ventromedial prefrontal cortex and left amygdala during anger induction reported by Dougherty et al. (2004) both suggest that vascular abnormalities associated with MDD with anger attacks may characterize a biologically different subtype distinct from other types of depression.

DEPRESSION WITH IRRITABILITY/ANGER/HOSTILITY AND CARDIOVASCULAR RISK FACTORS

The observed high prevalence of cardiovascular risk factors in patients with depression and in subjects with increased anger [68] has led to the conclusion this may be one of the mechanisms for the high rates of cardiovascular morbidity associated with these conditions. In fact, depression as well as irritability/anger/hostility have previously been independently associated with established cardiovascular risk factors, including smoking [69], high cholesterol levels [70], blood hypertension [71], and diabetes [72].

The independent association of depression and anger with high serum cholesterol levels has been described repeatedly over the past four decades, though definitions of anger and depression have varied. Studies from the early 1960s reported high cholesterol levels in patients experiencing feelings related to anger, such as irritation [73]. These initial studies have been supported by more recent data showing an association of increased levels of cholesterol with distinct measurements of anger including angry reaction [68] and irritable aspect of neuroticism [74]. Prospective studies have confirmed this association. For example, a cholesterol-lowering diet with increased fish intake for 5 years resulted in decreased hostility and depressive symptoms [75], and high levels of hostility in adolescence predicted high lipid ratios 21-23 years later [30].

The association of increased levels of cholesterol with depression is less consistent than that reported for anger and/or hostility. A study has indicated that levels of cholesterol may vary in accordance to the subtype of depression. Patients with melancholic depression have significantly higher levels of very low-density lipoprotein cholesterol (VLDL-C) than those with less severe depression (e.g. dysthymic disorder) [76].

Rahe et al., in 1971, were probably the first to hypothesize that anger and depression could be aspects of a common clinical entity highly associated with cardiovascular risk factors. Because they found positive correlations between serum cholesterol concentrations and feelings of depression and anger, they proposed that anger could be a dimension of depressive mood [77]. Fava et al. (1993), also reported an association between MDD with anger attacks and elevated levels of cholesterol [67].

Ravaja et al., have proposed that depression would be a moderator of the relationship between cardiovascular risk factors and anger [78]. They reported a negative association between hostility and cardiovascular risk factors in patients with high depressive tendencies. Patients with high depressive tendencies and lack of anger or hostility would represent the most severe form of exhaustion where the individual had "given-up" [78]. Other studies have also shown an association of low levels of cholesterol with depression [79] and hostility [80]. In contrast, our group has found that anger attacks in MDD patients were independently associated with smoking (for periods >11 years) and with total serum levels of cholesterol ≥200mg/dL, after adjusting for age, gender, BMI, and baseline severity of depression [81]. When we divided cholesterol levels in low (≤160mg/dL) [82] normal (>160mg/dL and <200mg/dL) and high levels (≥ 200mg/dL), we did not find an increased distribution of MDD patients with anger attacks in the group with low levels of cholesterol compared to the group with normal levels (p =.106), as would have been suggested by the previous results [72]. However, in that study, we did not measure the fractions of cholesterol, and it is possible that the relationship of cholesterol with anger might be different for different fractions of cholesterol. For example, high anger-out (angry temperament) has been associated with low levels of high-density lipoprotein cholesterol (HDL-C) and with high levels of low-density lipoprotein cholesterol (LDL-C) [83]. In addition, the relationship of anger with lipid profile may be different for different aspects of anger. For example, It has been reported that impulsive anger-out (angry temperament), as measured with the STAXI, but not the neurotic anger was associated with abnormal lipid profile [84].

Although confirmatory studies are needed, it is possible that the relationship of MDD with anger attacks and increased levels of cholesterol is mediated by homocysteine. Homocysteine is an important component of the one-carbon metabolism involved in energetic transfer at the level of mitochondria; and multiple studies suggest high homocysteine serum levels represent an important risk factor for and a target of therapeutic intervention in cardiovascular disease [85]. Increased levels of homocysteine have been positively associated with severity of depression and length of current depressive episode in patients with MDD and anger attacks but not in patients with MDD without anger attacks [86]. Homocysteine-induced endoplasmatic reticulum in human cultured hepatocytes has been associated with overproduction of lipid components including cholesterol [87]. Consequently, hypercholesterolemia in patients with MMD and anger attacks could at least in part be mediated via homocysteine-induced dysregulation of the cholesterol biosynthetic pathway in the liver.

Extending the complexity of the relationship between depression, cardiovascular risk factors and irritability/anger/hostility, it should be remembered that smoking [88] can mediate the relationship of depressive symptoms with increased mortality. Also, depression, anger, and hostility can increase cardiac morbidity and mortality through other mechanisms independently of smoking and cholesterol [9]. In addition, depressed patients with cardiovascular risk factors may experience lower response to antidepressant treatment compared to other subjects with MDD [89], which can further aggravate their prognosis.

CARDIOVASCULAR RISK FACTORS AND OTHER DEPRESSIVE SUBTYPES

Anxiety disorders frequently co-occur with depression and may contribute to the increased cardiac morbidity seen in depressed patients. Symptoms of anxiety have been associated with CHD [90] and fatal CHD [91]. In addition, panic disorder has been associated with increased mortality, particularly of cardiac causes [92]. However, few studies have investigated the cardiac impact of a concurrent anxiety disorder in depressed patients [22]. In 4,041 patients with MDD enrolled in the STAR*D study, cardiac disease at baseline was associated with symptoms of sympathetic arousal and early morning insomnia after adjustments for gender, age, ethnicity, employment status, and education [93].

The association between sympathetic arousal and cardiac disease is consistent with prior evidence of increased sympathetic (or decreased parasympathetic) central nervous activity as a potential link between depression and increased cardiac morbidity [94]. Sympathetic hyperreactivity, generally defined as a dispositional tendency to exaggerated heart rate and blood pressure responses in the face of challenging or aversive events, has been associated with more rapid progression of carotid atherosclerosis [95]. Insomnia has been prospectively associated with an increased risk of MI [96] and cardiac mortality [97]. Insomnia in MDD have been associated with increased levels of excreted norepinephrine, epinephrine, and dopamine [98]. The finding of an association between concurrent panic disorder in MDD patients and cardiac disease also suggests the relevance of increased sympathetic arousal, since patients with panic disorder have been reported to have increased sympathetic activation [99]. Although less extensively studied than depression, panic disorder has also been associated with cardiac morbidity and mortality [92]. High anxiety scores have previously been associated with cardiovascular risk factors [67]. However, since a prospective study did not find an association of trait-anxiety or state-anxiety and cardiac mortality [22], it is probably relevant to make the distinction between a chronic and moderate-intensity anxiety as seen in generalized anxiety disorder and an episodic high-intensity anxiety as seen in panic disorder when the objective is to evaluate the cardiovascular impact of anxiety [100]. Our own study of 4,041 patients enrolled in STAR* D did not evaluate negative affectivity, distressed personality, hostility, and anger, which is a limitation since such psychological/psychiatric factors may mediate the potential cardiac impact in individuals with MDD [101].

In conclusion, the current literature reviewed here supports the association of depression with anger/irritability with high rates of cardiovascular disease and cardiac risk factors. Some studies suggest that vascular changes in the brain may be more characteristic for this depressive subtype and may explain the association with cardiac disease. Such findings can have a significant clinical impact, allowing clinicians to define a population at risk which may need increased clinical attention, both from cardiologists and from psychiatrists.

REFERENCES

[1]   Carney RM, Freedland KE, Rich MW, Smith LJ, and Jaffe AS: Ventricular tachycardia and psychiatric depression in patients with coronary artery disease. *American Journal of Medicine* 1993; 95(1):23-8.

[2]   Sloan RP and Bigger JT, Jr.: Biobehavioral factors in Cardiac Arrhythmia Pilot Study (CAPS). Review and examination. *Circulation* 1991; 83(4 Suppl):II52-7.

[3]   Almeida JR, Alves TC, Wajngarten M, Rays J, Castro CC, Cordeiro Q, et al.: Late-life depression, heart failure and frontal white matter hyperintensity: a structural magnetic resonance imaging study. *Braz J Med Biol Res* 2005; 38(3):431-6.

[4]   Freedland KE, Rich MW, Skala JA, Carney RM, Davila-Roman VG, and Jaffe AS: Prevalence of depression in hospitalized patients with congestive heart failure. *Psychosom Med* 2003; 65(1):119-28.

[5]   Fraguas Junior R, Ramadan ZB, Pereira AN, and Wajngarten M: Depression with irritability in patients undergoing coronary artery bypass graft surgery: the cardiologist's role. *Gen Hosp Psychiatry* 2000; 22(5):365-74.

[6]   Ferketich AK, Schwartzbaum JA, Frid DJ, and Moeschberger ML: Depression as an antecedent to heart disease among women and men in the NHANES I study. National Health and Nutrition Examination Survey. *Arch Intern Med* 2000; 160(9):1261-8.

[7]   Carney RM, Freedland KE, Miller GE, and Jaffe AS: Depression as a risk factor for cardiac mortality and morbidity: a review of potential mechanisms. *Journal of Psychosomatic Research* 2002; 53(4):897-902.

[8]   Pratt LA, Ford DE, Crum RM, Armenian HK, Gallo JJ, and Eaton WW: Depression, psychotropic medication, and risk of myocardial infarction. Prospective data from the Baltimore ECA follow-up. *Circulation* 1996; 94(12):3123-9.

[9]   Frasure-Smith N, Lesperance F, and Talajic M: Depression and 18-month prognosis after myocardial infarction. *Circulation* 1995; 91(4):999-1005.

[10]   Fulop G, Strain JJ, and Stettin G: Congestive heart failure and depression in older adults: clinical course and health services use 6 months after hospitalization. *Psychosomatics* 2003; 44(5):367-73.

[11]   Ford DE, Mead LA, Chang PP, Cooper-Patrick L, Wang NY, and Klag MJ: Depression is a risk factor for coronary artery disease in men: the precursors study. *Arch Intern Med* 1998; 158(13):1422-6.

[12]   Borowicz L, Jr., Royall R, Grega M, Selnes O, Lyketsos C, and McKhann G: Depression and cardiac morbidity 5 years after coronary artery bypass surgery. *Psychosomatics* 2002; 43(6):464-71.

[13]   Williams SA, Kasl SV, Heiat A, Abramson JL, Krumholz HM, and Vaccarino V: Depression and risk of heart failure among the elderly: a prospective community-based study. *Psychosom Med* 2002; 64(1):6-12.

[14]   Lesperance F, Frasure-Smith N, Talajic M, and Bourassa MG: Five-year risk of cardiac mortality in relation to initial severity and one-year changes in depression symptoms after myocardial infarction. *Circulation* 2002; 105(9):1049-53.

[15]   Davidson K, Jonas BS, Dixon KE, and Markovitz JH: Do depression symptoms predict early hypertension incidence in young adults in the CARDIA study? Coronary Artery Risk Development in Young Adults. *Arch Intern Med* 2000; 160(10):1495-500.

[16]   Jonas BS, Franks P, and Ingram DD: Are symptoms of anxiety and depression risk factors for hypertension? Longitudinal evidence from the National Health and Nutrition Examination Survey I Epidemiologic Follow-up Study. *Arch Fam Med* 1997; 6(1):43-9.

[17]   Barefoot JC and Schroll M: Symptoms of depression, acute myocardial infarction, and total mortality in a community sample. *Circulation* 1996; 93(11):1976-80.

[18]   Wassertheil-Smoller S, Applegate WB, Berge K, Chang CJ, Davis BR, Grimm R, Jr., et al.: Change in depression as a precursor of cardiovascular events. SHEP Cooperative Research Group (Systoloc Hypertension in the elderly). *Arch Intern Med* 1996; 156(5):553-61.

[19]   Sesso HD, Kawachi I, Vokonas PS, and Sparrow D: Depression and the risk of coronary heart disease in the Normative Aging Study. *Am J Cardiol* 1998; 82(7):851-6.

[20]   Ariyo AA, Haan M, Tangen CM, Rutledge JC, Cushman M, Dobs A, et al.: Depressive symptoms and risks of coronary heart disease and mortality in elderly Americans. Cardiovascular Health Study Collaborative Research Group. *Circulation* 2000; 102(15):1773-9.

[21]   Empana JP, Sykes DH, Luc G, Juhan-Vague I, Arveiler D, Ferrieres J, et al.: Contributions of depressive mood and circulating inflammatory markers to coronary heart disease in healthy European men: the Prospective Epidemiological Study of Myocardial Infarction (PRIME). *Circulation* 2005; 111(18):2299-305.

[22]   Jiang W, Kuchibhatla M, Cuffe MS, Christopher EJ, Alexander JD, Clary GL, et al.: Prognostic value of anxiety and depression in patients with chronic heart failure. *Circulation* 2004; 110(22):3452-6.

[23]   Iribarren C, Sidney S, Bild DE, Liu K, Markovitz JH, Roseman JM, et al.: Association of hostility with coronary artery calcification in young adults: the CARDIA study. Coronary Artery Risk Development in Young Adults. *Jama* 2000; 283(19):2546-51.

[24]   Julkunen J, Salonen R, Kaplan GA, Chesney MA, and Salonen JT: Hostility and the progression of carotid atherosclerosis. *Psychosom Med* 1994; 56(6):519-25.

[25]   Matthews KA, Owens JF, Kuller LH, Sutton-Tyrrell K, and Jansen-McWilliams L: Are hostility and anxiety associated with carotid atherosclerosis in healthy postmenopausal women? *Psychosom Med* 1998; 60(5):633-8.

[26]   Yan LL, Liu K, Matthews KA, Daviglus ML, Ferguson TF, and Kiefe CI: Psychosocial factors and risk of hypertension: the Coronary Artery Risk Development in Young Adults (CARDIA) study. *Jama* 2003; 290(16):2138-48.

[27]   Eaker ED, Sullivan LM, Kelly-Hayes M, D'Agostino RB, Sr., and Benjamin EJ: Anger and Hostility Predict the Development of Atrial Fibrillation in Men in the Framingham Offspring Study. *Circulation* 2004.

[28]   Miller TQ, Smith TW, Turner CW, Guijarro ML, and Hallet AJ: A meta-analytic review of research on hostility and physical health. *Psychol Bull* 1996; 119(2):322-48.

[29]   Raikkonen K, Matthews KA, Flory JD, and Owens JF: Effects of hostility on ambulatory blood pressure and mood during daily living in healthy adults. *Health Psychol* 1999; 18(1):44-53.

[30]   Siegler IC, Peterson BL, Barefoot JC, and Williams RB: Hostility during late adolescence predicts coronary risk factors at mid-life. *American journal of epidemiology* 1992; 136(2):146-54.

[31]   Koskenvuo M, Kaprio J, Rose RJ, Kesaniemi A, Sarna S, Heikkila K, et al.: Hostility as a risk factor for mortality and ischemic heart disease in men. *Psychosom Med* 1988; 50(4):330-40.

[32]   Fava M, Anderson K, and Rosenbaum JF: "Anger attacks": possible variants of panic and major depressive disorders. *American Journal of Psychiatry* 1990; 147(7):867-70.

[33]   Fava M, Rosenbaum JF, Pava JA, McCarthy MK, Steingard RJ, and Bouffides E: Anger attacks in unipolar depression, Part 1: Clinical correlates and response to fluoxetine treatment. *American Journal of Psychiatry* 1993; 150(8):1158-63.

[34]   Overall JE, Hollister LE, Johnson M, and Pennington V: Nosology of depression and differential response to drugs. *Jama* 1966; 195(11):946-8.

[35]   Overall JE, Goldstein BJ, and Brauzer B: Symptomatic volunteers in psychiatric research. *J Psychiatr Res* 1971; 931-43.

[36]   Baker M, Dorzab J, Winokur G, and Cadoret RJ: Depressive disease: classification and clinical characteristics. *Compr Psychiatry* 1971; 12(4):354-65.

[37]   Snaith RP and Taylor CM: Irritability: definition, assessment and associated factors. *Br J Psychiatry* 1985; 147127-36.

[38]   Gould RA, Ball S, Kaspi SP, Otto MW, Pollack MH, Shekhar A, et al.: Prevalence and correlates of anger attacks: a two site study. *J Affect Disord* 1996; 39(1):31-8.

[39]   Morand P, Thomas G, Bungener C, Ferreri M, and Jouvent R: Fava's anger attacks questionnaire: Evaluation of the French version in depressed patients. *Journal of European Psychiatry* 1998; 13(1):41-45.

[40]   Fava M, Uebelacker LA, Alpert JE, Nierenberg AA, Pava JA, and Rosenbaum JF: Major depressive subtypes and treatment response. *Biol Psychiatry* 1997; 42(7):568-76.

[41]   Posternak MA and Zimmerman M: Anger and aggression in psychiatric outpatients. *J Clin Psychiatry* 2002; 63(8):665-72.

[42]   Perlis RH, Smoller JW, Fava M, Rosenbaum JF, Nierenberg AA, and Sachs GS: The prevalence and clinical correlates of anger attacks during depressive episodes in bipolar disorder. *Journal of Affective Disorders* 2004; 79(1-3):291-5.

[43]   First MB, Spitzer R, and Gibbon M, *Structured Clinical Interview for DSM-IV Axis I Disorders*. 1996, New York: Biometrics Research Department, New York State Psychiatric Institute.

[44]   Hamilton M: A rating scale for depression. *J Neurol Neurosurg Psychiatry* 1960; 2356-62.

[45]   Montgomery SA and Asberg M: A new depression scale designed to be sensitive to change. *Br J Psychiatry* 1979; 134382-9.

[46]   Weissman M, Fox K, and Klerman GL: Hostility and depression associated with suicide attempts. *Am J Psychiatry* 1973; 130(4):450-5.

[47]   Pugh R: An association between hostility and poor adherence to treatment in patients suffering from depression. *Br J Med Psychol* 1983; 56 (Pt 2)205-8.

[48]   Crook T, Raskin A, and Davis D: Factors associated with attempted suicide among hospitalized depressed patients. *Psychol Med* 1975; 5(4):381-8.

[49]   Seidlitz L, Conwell Y, Duberstein P, Cox C, and Denning D: Emotion traits in older suicide attempters and non-attempters. *J Affect Disord* 2001; 66(2-3):123-31.

[50]   Burch EA, Jr.: Suicide attempt histories in alcohol-dependent men: differences in psychological profiles. *Int J Addict* 1994; 29(11):1477-86.

[51]   Pendse B, Westrin A, and Engstrom G: Temperament traits in seasonal affective disorder, suicide attempters with non-seasonal major depression and healthy controls. *J Affect Disord* 1999; 54(1-2):55-65.

[52]   Romanov K, Hatakka M, Keskinen E, Laaksonen H, Kaprio J, Rose RJ, et al.: Self-reported hostility and suicidal acts, accidents, and accidental deaths: a prospective study of 21,443 adults aged 25 to 59. *Psychosom Med* 1994; 56(4):328-36.

[53]   Horesh N, Rolnick T, Iancu I, Dannon P, Lepkifker E, Apter A, et al.: Anger, impulsivity and suicide risk. *Psychother Psychosom* 1997; 66(2):92-6.

[54]   Asnis GM, Kaplan ML, van Praag HM, and Sanderson WC: Homicidal behaviors among psychiatric outpatients. *Hosp Community Psychiatry* 1994; 45(2):127-32.

[55]   Alpert JE, Petersen T, Roffi PA, Papakostas GI, Freed R, Smith MM, et al.: Behavioral and emotional disturbances in the offspring of depressed parents with anger attacks. *Psychotherapy and Psychosomatics* 2003; 72(2):102-6.

[56]   Iosifescu DV, Renshaw PF, Dougherty DD, Lyoo IK, Lee HK, Fraguas R, et al.: Major depressive disorder with anger attacks and subcortical MRI white matter hyperintensities. *J Nerv Ment* Dis 2007; 195(2):175-8.

[57]   Dougherty DD, Rauch SL, Deckersbach T, Marci C, Loh R, Shin LM, et al.: Ventromedial prefrontal cortex and amygdala dysfunction during an anger induction positron emission tomography study in patients with major depressive disorder with anger attacks. *Archives of General Psychiatry* 2004; 61(8):795-804.

[58] Fava M, Vuolo RD, Wright EC, Nierenberg AA, Alpert JE, and Rosenbaum JF: Fenfluramine challenge in unipolar depression with and without anger attacks. *Psychiatry Research* 2000; 94(1):9-18.

[59] Clark LA, Watson D, and Mineka S: Temperament, personality, and the mood and anxiety disorders. *J Abnorm Psychol* 1994; 103(1):103-16.

[60] Watson D and Clark LA: Negative affectivity: the disposition to experience aversive emotional states. *Psychol Bull* 1984; 96(3):465-90.

[61] Bagby RM, Kennedy SH, Dickens SE, Minifie CE, and Schuller DR: Personality and symptom profiles of the angry hostile depressed patient. *J Affect Disord* 1997; 45(3):155-60.

[62] Fava M, Alpert JE, Carmin CN, Wisniewski SR, Trivedi MH, Biggs MM, et al.: Clinical correlates and symptom patterns of anxious depression among patients with major depressive disorder in STAR*D. *Psychol Med* 2004; in press.

[63] Gullion CM and Rush AJ: Toward a generalizable model of symptoms in major depressive disorder. *Biol Psychiatry* 1998; 44(10):959-72.

[64] Perlis RH, Fraguas R, Fava M, Trivedi MH, Luther JF, Wisniewski SR, et al.: Prevalence and clinical correlates of irritability in major depressive disorder: a preliminary report from the Sequenced Treatment Alternatives to Relieve Depression study. *J Clin Psychiatry* 2005; 66(2):159-66; quiz 147, 273-4.

[65] Rush AJ, Gullion CM, Basco MR, Jarrett RB, and Trivedi MH: The Inventory of Depressive Symptomatology (IDS): psychometric properties. *Psychol Med* 1996; 26(3):477-86.

[66] Iosifescu DV, Renshaw PF, Lyoo IK, Lee HK, Perlis RH, Papakostas GI, et al.: Brain white-matter hyperintensities and treatment outcome in major depressive disorder. *Br J Psychiatry* 2006; 188180-5.

[67] Fava M, Abraham M, Pava J, Shuster J, and Rosenbaum J: Cardiovascular risk factors in depression. The role of anxiety and anger. *Psychosomatics* 1996; 37(1):31-7.

[68] Richards JC, Hof A, and Alvarenga M: Serum lipids and their relationships with hostility and angry affect and behaviors in men. *Health Psychology* 2000; 19(4):393-8.

[69] Brown C, Madden PA, Palenchar DR, and Cooper-Patrick L: The association between depressive symptoms and cigarette smoking in an urban primary care sample. *International journal of psychiatry in medicine* 2000; 30(1):15-26.

[70] Ledochowski M, Murr C, Sperner-Unterweger B, Neurauter G, and Fuchs D: Association between increased serum cholesterol and signs of depressive mood. *Clinical chemistry and laboratory medicine* 2003; 41(6):821-4.

[71] Davidson K, Jonas BS, Dixon KE, and Markovitz JH: Do depression symptoms predict early hypertension incidence in young adults in the CARDIA study? Coronary Artery Risk Development in Young Adults. *Archives of Internal Medicine* 2000; 160(10):1495-500.

[72] Deshields TL, Jenkins JO, and Tait RC: The experience of anger in chronic illness: a preliminary investigation. *International journal of psychiatry in medicine* 1989; 19(3):299-309.

[73]   Frideman M, Rosenman RH, and Carroll V: Changes in the serum cholesterol and blood clotting time in men subjected to cyclic variation of occupational stress. *Circulation* 1958; 17(5):852-61.

[74]   Goebel PN, Peter H, Mueller SK, and Hand I: Neuroticism, other personality variables, and serum lipid levels in patients with anxiety disorders and normal controls. *International journal of psychiatry in medicine* 1998; 28(4):449-62.

[75]   Weidner G, Connor SL, Hollis JF, and Connor WE: Improvements in hostility and depression in relation to dietary change and cholesterol lowering. The Family Heart Study. *Annals of internal medicine* 1992; 117(10):820-3.

[76]   Huang TL and Chen JF: Lipid and lipoprotein levels in depressive disorders with melancholic feature or atypical feature and dysthymia. *Psychiatry and clinical neurosciences* 2004; 58(3):295-9.

[77]   Rahe RH, Rubin RT, Gunderson EK, and Arthur RJ: Psychologic correlates of serum cholesterol in man. A longitudinal study. *Psychosomatic medicine* 1971; 33(5):399-410.

[78]   Ravaja N, Kauppinen T, and Keltikangas-Jarvinen L: Relationships between hostility and physiological coronary heart disease risk factors in young adults: the moderating influence of depressive tendencies. *Psychological Medicine* 2000; 30(2):381-93.

[79]   Morgan RE, Palinkas LA, Barrett-Connor EL, and Wingard DL: Plasma cholesterol and depressive symptoms in older men. *Lancet* 1993; 341(8837):75-9.

[80]   Niaura R, Banks SM, Ward KD, Stoney CM, Spiro A, 3rd, Aldwin CM, et al.: Hostility and the metabolic syndrome in older males: the normative aging study. *Psychosomatic Medicine* 2000; 62(1):7-16.

[81]   Fraguas R, Iosifescu DV, Bankier B, Perlis R, Clementi-Craven N, Alpert J, et al.: Major depressive disorder with anger attacks and cardiovascular risk factors. *Int J Psychiatry Med* 2007; 37(1):99-111.

[82]   Rabe-Jablonska J and Poprawska I: Levels of serum total cholesterol and LDL-cholesterol in patients with major depression in acute period and remission. *Medical Science Monitor: international medical journal of experimental and clinical research* 2000; 6(3):539-47.

[83]   Rutledge T, Reis SE, Olson M, Owens J, Kelsey SF, Pepine CJ, et al.: Psychosocial variables are associated with atherosclerosis risk factors among women with chest pain: the WISE study. *Psychosomatic Medicine* 2001; 63(2):282-8.

[84]   Siegman AW, Malkin AR, Boyle S, Vaitkus M, Barko W, and Franco E: Anger, and plasma lipid, lipoprotein, and glucose levels in healthy women: the mediating role of physical fitness. *Journal of behavioral medicine* 2002; 25(1):1-16.

[85]   Jamison RL, Hartigan P, Kaufman JS, Goldfarb DS, Warren SR, Guarino PD, et al.: Effect of homocysteine lowering on mortality and vascular disease in advanced chronic kidney disease and end-stage renal disease: a randomized controlled trial. *Jama* 2007; 298(10):1163-70.

[86]   Fraguas R, Jr., Papakostas GI, Mischoulon D, Bottiglieri T, Alpert J, and Fava M: Anger attacks in major depressive disorder and serum levels of homocysteine. *Biol Psychiatry* 2006; 60(3):270-4.

[87]   Werstuck GH, Lentz SR, Dayal S, Hossain GS, Sood SK, Shi YY, et al.: Homocysteine-induced endoplasmic reticulum stress causes dysregulation of the cholesterol and triglyceride biosynthetic pathways. *J Clin Invest* 2001; 107(10):1263-73.

[88]   Brummett BH, Babyak MA, Siegler IC, Mark DB, Williams RB, and Barefoot JC: Effect of smoking and sedentary behavior on the association between depressive symptoms and mortality from coronary heart disease. *The American journal of cardiology* 2003; 92(5):529-32.

[89]   Iosifescu DV, Clementi-Craven N, Fraguas R, Papakostas GI, Petersen T, Alpert JE, et al.: Cardiovascular risk factors may moderate pharmacological treatment effects in major depressive disorder. *Psychosomatic Medicine* 2005; 67(5):703-6.

[90]   Kubzansky LD, Kawachi I, Spiro A, 3rd, Weiss ST, Vokonas PS, and Sparrow D: Is worrying bad for your heart? A prospective study of worry and coronary heart disease in the Normative Aging Study. *Circulation* 1997; 95(4):818-24.

[91]   Kawachi I, Sparrow D, Vokonas PS, and Weiss ST: Symptoms of anxiety and risk of coronary heart disease. The Normative Aging Study. *Circulation* 1994; 90(5):2225-9.

[92]   Coryell W, Noyes R, and Clancy J: Excess mortality in panic disorder. A comparison with primary unipolar depression. *Arch Gen Psychiatry* 1982; 39(6):701-3.

[93]   Fraguas R, Jr., Iosifescu DV, Alpert J, Wisniewski SR, Barkin JL, Trivedi MH, et al.: Major depressive disorder and comorbid cardiac disease: is there a depressive subtype with greater cardiovascular morbidity? Results from the STAR*D study. *Psychosomatics* 2007; 48(5):418-25.

[94]   Carney RM, Blumenthal JA, Stein PK, Watkins L, Catellier D, Berkman LF, et al.: Depression, heart rate variability, and acute myocardial infarction. *Circulation* 2001; 104(17):2024-8.

[95]   Kamarck TW, Everson SA, Kaplan GA, Manuck SB, Jennings JR, Salonen R, et al.: Exaggerated blood pressure responses during mental stress are associated with enhanced carotid atherosclerosis in middle-aged Finnish men: findings from the Kuopio Ischemic Heart Disease Study. *Circulation* 1997; 96(11):3842-8.

[96]   Schwartz SW, Cornoni-Huntley J, Cole SR, Hays JC, Blazer DG, and Schocken DD: Are sleep complaints an independent risk factor for myocardial infarction? *Ann Epidemiol* 1998; 8(6):384-92.

[97]   Mallon L, Broman JE, and Hetta J: Sleep complaints predict coronary artery disease mortality in males: a 12-year follow-up study of a middle-aged Swedish population. *J Intern Med* 2002; 251(3):207-16.

[98]   Maes M, Meltzer HY, Suy E, Minner B, Calabrese J, and Cosyns P: Sleep disorders and anxiety as symptom profiles of sympathoadrenal system hyperactivity in major depression. *J Affect Disord* 1993; 27(3):197-207.

[99]   Coupland NJ, Wilson SJ, Potokar JP, Bell C, and Nutt DJ: Increased sympathetic response to standing in panic disorder. *Psychiatry Res* 2003; 118(1):69-79.

[100]   Carney RM: Psychological risk factors for cardiac events: could there be just one? *Circulation* 1998; 97(2):128-9.

[101]   Frasure-Smith N and Lesperance F: Depression and other psychological risks following myocardial infarction. *Arch Gen Psychiatry* 2003; 60(6):627-36.

In: Psychological Factors and Cardiovascular Disorders   ISBN: 978-1-60456-871-4
Editor: Leo Sher   © 2008 Nova Science Publishers, Inc.

Chapter VIII

DEPRESSION IN CHRONIC HEART FAILURE: EPIDEMIOLOGY, PATHOPHYSIOLOGY AND DIAGNOSTIC TOOLS

John T. Parissis, Maria Nikolaou, Konstadinos Tsitlakidis, Gerasimos Filippatos and Dimitrios Kremastinos

Heart Failure Unit and Second Cardiology Department, University of Athens and Attikon General Hospital, Athens, Greece.

ABSTRACT

Depression is a frequent non-cardiac comorbidity in chronic heart failure (CHF) contributing to the syndrome progression, as well as an independent risk factor for several adverse outcomes in CHF patients, including decreased compliance with treatment recommendations, increases in healthcare costs, hospital admissions and mortality rates. Hypothalamic axis dysregulation, autonomic system dysfunction, rhythm disturbances, pro-inflammatory cytokine activation, endothelial dysfunction and platelet activation are the main pathophysiologic mechanisms linking depression with increased morbidity and mortality in coronary artery disease and CHF. Diagnosis and effective treatment of this disorder may be essential strategies in order to improve the quality of life and prognosis of CHF patients, and require the close cooperation of clinical cardiologists with psychiatrists, especially in outpatient heart failure clinics. However, large clinical trials are needed in order to identify the ideal clinical strategies for the management of CHF patients with depression.

INTRODUCTION

Chronic heart failure is a progressive syndrome characterized by cardiac and vascular dysfunction, impaired exercise capacity, reduced quality of life, and dismal prognosis. Heart failure also carries major clinical and societal consequences. It is the leading cause of hospitalization in the elderly and the most costly cardiovascular disorder in western world [1-7]. Moreover, there is an increased (6 to 9 times) risk of mortality in patients with CHF in comparison to general population [4]. On the other hand, depression is the most prevalent psychiatric condition in general population and is closely associated with the existence of chronic disorders such as malignancies, inflammatory diseases and CHF. This condition seems to be a frequent co-morbidity in CHF patients and an independent risk factor for readmission to the hospital, functional decline, and mortality. This point indicates that early diagnosis of depression in CHF patients is of great importance in order to avoid the detrimental effects of this condition on CHF progression. Clinical depression in CHF is a syndromal diagnosis based on patient history, the report of signs and symptoms (psychomotor retardation, agitation, social withdrawal, loss of appetite, or insomnia) and the exclusion of competing diagnoses. However, there are many difficulties in real clinical practise in order to detect and treat early this condition in CHF patients as the overlapping of depressive symptoms with the somatic features of CHF makes the diagnosis confused. This chapter summarizes the current knowledge about the prevalence, prognostic importance and pathophysiologic mechanisms that link depression and CHF and lead to patient clinical worsening. Finally, this article describes the recommended strategies (derived by clinical trials and personal clinical experience) for recognizing and diagnosing depression in CHF.

EPIDEMIOLOGY AND PROGNOSTIC IMPORTANCE OF DEPRESSION IN CHRONIC HEART FAILURE

Prevalence

The prevalence of full clinical picture of depression in CHF can be detected in 14-26%, while single depressive symptoms exist in 24-85% of CHF patients [8]. This wide range of prevalence rates can be explained by the different assessment instruments sample sizes and selection criteria of the studied patients [8]. In the recent meta-analysis of 36 clinical trials [9], clinically significant depression was present in 21.5% of CHF patients and varied by the use of questionnaires versus diagnostic interview (33.6% and 19.3%, respectively).

Depression may be more common in women than men. Reported prevalence rates range from 11% to 67% for women and 7 to 63% for men. There is also evidence that depressive symptoms are more common in white men than black men with CHF [10]. There is a strong relationship between major depression and New York Heart Association (NYHA) class [9]. Higher prevalence rates of depression are associated with worse NYHA functional class. The rate of depression in patients with NYHA class III is nearly double than that of patients with functional class II. In the recent meta-analytic review [9], the prevalence of depressive symptoms in NYHA class I patients was 11%, while NYHA class IV patients exhibited depressive symptoms in a percentage of 42%. In contrast, no significant relation of major depression with left ventricular ejection fraction or prior hospitalization for CHF was found [9].

Several other characteristics also affect prevalence rates. Major depression is more common in patients who are disabled, who have a history of depression, or who have comorbid chronic obstructive pulmonary disease (COPD) or sleep apnoea syndrome [8]. COPD and sleep apnoea were associated with major depression in univariate analyses but were not retained as independent correlates.

In contrast, analyses based on geographic location showed nearly identical point of estimates of prevalence of depression rates in CHF patients in the USA and Canada (20.3%) and Europe (21%) [10]. Four independent social factors of developing depression in CHF patients have also been identified: living alone, alcohol abuse, financial burden from medical care, and a worse baseline CHF-specific health status [11].

Prognostic Importance

Depression may contribute to the development of CHF in susceptible populations to a greater degree than it does in otherwise healthy populations. Recently, it has been reported that depression is independently associated with a substantial increase in the risk of CHF among older patients with isolated systolic hypertension [12]. There is also strong evidence that the presence of depression is independently associated with a decline in health status and an increase in the risk of hospitalization and death for patients with existing CHF, regardless of its aetiology [13,14,15]. For example, a large retrospective epidemiologic study [14] showed that the existence of depression in CHF patients is associated with greater than 2-fold increased risk of mortality as well as a 3-fold increased risk of readmission in the first year after index admission, controlling for age, NYHA class and left ventricular ejection fraction. Recent meta-analysis [9] also demonstrated higher rates of death and secondary events (risk ratio=2.1, confidence interval 1.7 to 2.6), trends towards increased health care use, and higher rates of hospitalization and emergency department visits among depressed CHF patients. Finally, depressive symptoms [estimated by Zung self-rated depression scale (SDS)] in CHF are correlated well with plasma b type natriuretic peptide (BNP) concentrations and provide additive value to this established prognostic marker in predicting adverse clinical outcomes [16].

PROPOSED PATHOPHYSIOLOGIC MECHANISMS OF ADVERSE OUTCOMES

The potential pathophysiologic pathways underlying the linkage between depression and CHF outcomes can be summarized in Table 1. There are at least six major mechanisms that have been postulated to play a pivotal role in the development and progression of CHF in depressed patients:

Table 1. Depression-induced pathophysiologic mechanisms that lead to the worsening of heart failure syndrome

A) **Biologic mechanisms**
   - Common genetic predisposition
   - Autonomic system dysfunction (increased sympathetic activity)
   - Hypothalamic axis over-reactivity
   - Increased pro-coagulant activity
   - Endothelial dysfunction
   - Increased activity of serotonin
   - Excessive pro-inflammatory cytokine activation
   - Reduced levels of omega-3-fatty acids
   - Stress-induced ischemia
   - Toxic effects of anti-depressant drugs (e.g tricyclic)

B) **Psychosocial factors**
   - Reduced compliance to medical treatment and diet restrictions
   - De-conditioning
   - Impaired social support

Increased Pro-Coagulant Activity

Disturbances in platelet activation and aggregation may lead to hypercoagulability, thrombosis predisposition into vasculature, and acute ischemic events [8]. The extent of the increased platelet activity, the quantity of functional GPIIb/IIIa receptors and platelet de-granulation (as reflected by increased platelet factor 4 or plasma concentrations of b-thromboglobulin) in depressed CHF patients appear to be greater than those of depressed patients without CHF or atherosclerotic disease [17,18]. Finally, patients with depressive symptoms had higher levels of fibrinogen and increased risk for thrombotic cardiovascular events than those without this condition [19,20].

Hyperactivity of the Hypothalamic-Pituitary-Adrenal Axis

This condition is characterized by hypercortisolemia, elevated corticotropin-releasing factor in cerebrospinal fluid, blunting of the adrenocorticotropic hormone response to corticotropin-releasing factor challenge, non-suppression of cortisol secretion in response to dexamethasone, prolactin hyper-secretion, pituitary and adrenal gland enlargement, and sympathetic hyperactivity, as evidenced by hyper-secretion of norepinephrine, elevated plasma norepinephrine concentration and elevated urinary concentrations of norepinephrine and its metabolites [8,20].

Autonomic Nervous System Dysfunction

This abnormal condition is associated with reduced heart rate variability and therefore less parasympathetic protection from fatal arrhythmias [20,21]. Also QT variability was found to be significantly higher in depressed than non-depressed patients with coronary artery disease. This may reflect a greater increased risk for arrhythmias and sudden death for depressed patients [20,21]. Many indicators of cardiovascular autonomic dysregulation including elevated resting and 24-hour heart rates, increased heart rate responses to physical stressors, reduced heart rate variability and baroreceptor sensitivity, and high variability in ventricular repolarization, have been associated with increased mortality and cardiac morbidity, especially in vulnerable populations of heart disease such as post-myocardial infarction (MI) and CHF patients [20-23].

Excessive Inflammatory Activation

This process is characterized by increased circulating pro-inflammatory cytokines and decreased anti-inflammatory cytokines. Figure 1 describes pathophysiological events associated with a dysregulated neurohormonal–hypothalamic axis and immune activation, which lead to the development of depression in CHF. Heart failure is a multisystem disorder that affects not only the cardiovascular system but also the musculoskeletal, renal, hematopoietic, neuroendocrine and immune systems [24]. Several experimental and clinical observations suggest that CHF represents a state of chronic inflammation with increased levels of pro-inflammatory cytokines (tumor necrosis factor-alpha, interleukin 1, 2 and 6) [24,25]. Although the origin of elevated levels of these substances is not yet clear, they may contribute largely to the progression of the disease and deterioration of the clinical status of CHF patients [26,27]. Moreover, it has been recently reported that emotional distress, central monoamine abnormalities and hypothalamic-pituitary-adrenal axis activation observed in depression are associated with abnormal peripheral immune responses and over-expression of circulating pro-inflammatory cytokines [28,29,30]. The coexistence of CHF with depression seems to lead to an excessive activation of pro-inflammatory mediators causing vicious cycles of further clinical deterioration in these conditions [30-33]. Although pro-inflammatory cytokines are large hydrophilic molecules that are unlikely to cross the blood-brain barrier, however there are some proposed mechanisms by which peripherally released cytokines communicate with the brain, such as the conversion of cytokine signal into secondary signals mediated by nitric oxide or prostaglandin production by endothelium of brain blood vessels, the active transport of these molecules across the blood-brain barrier, and, finally, the transmission of cytokine signals through specific receptors which activate catecholaminergic pathways into specific brain regions [28,29,30]. The effects of cytokines on the nervous and endocrine systems close the loop between the brain and immune system, which indicates that neural-immune interactions are bi-directional [34].

The current literature has not yet addressed the definite role of cytokines as therapeutic targets in comorbid depression and CHF. As there is only indirect evidence that reduction of pro-inflammatory mediators may beneficially modulate depressive personality, additional research and large-scale clinical trials are required to clarify the effect of any kind of immunomodulatory treatment on depression in patients with CHF and excessive immune activation.

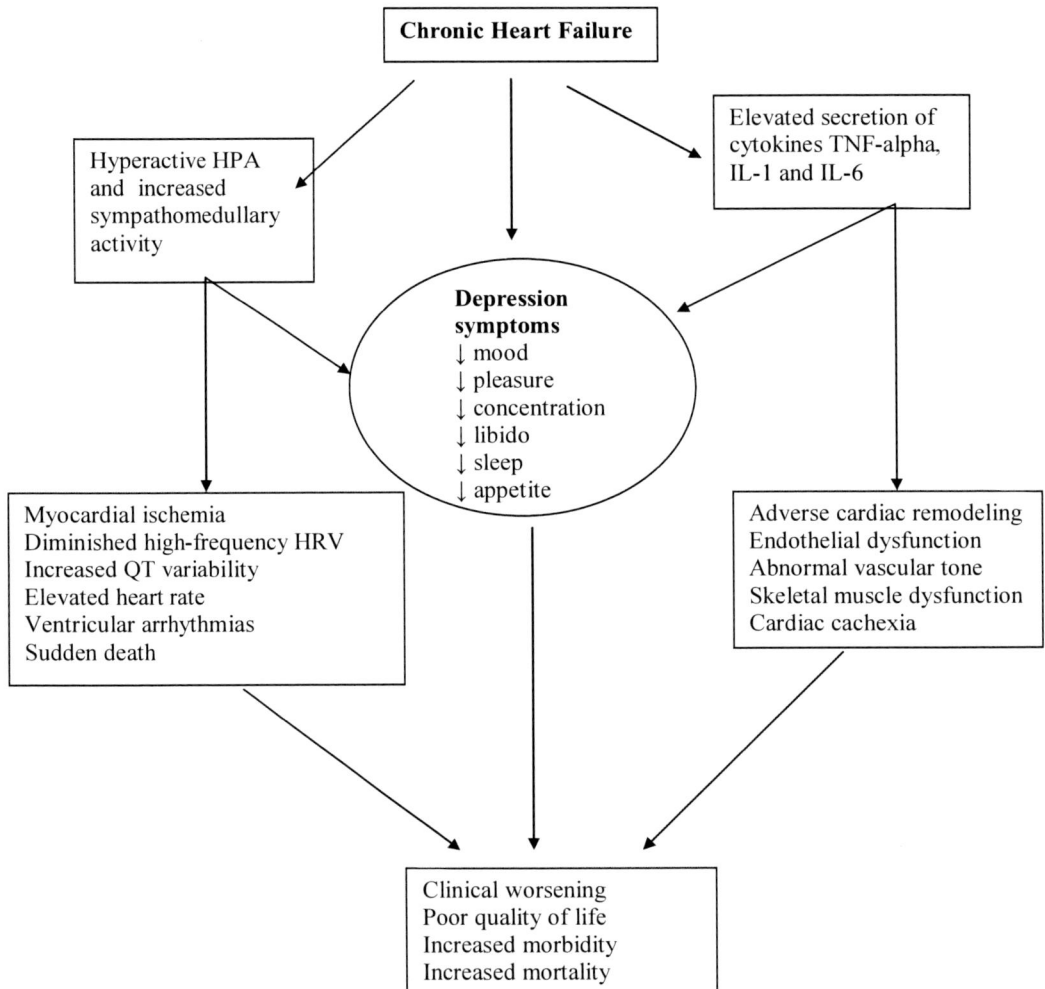

Figure 1. Schematic representation of the pathophysiological role of the dysregulated neurohormonal-hypothalamic axis and immune activation in depression of CHF patients. (HPA: hypothalamic axis, TNF: tumor necrosis factor, IL: interleukin, HRV: heart rate variability) (Modified for reference 30).

Endothelial Dysfunction

Abnormal endothelial function and impaired vasorelaxation may be also common disorders in CHF and depression [30,35]. Rajagopalan et al. [36] found that untreated young patients with major depression without known traditional cardiovascular risk factors had significantly lower brachial arterial response to reactive hyperemia than age- and sex-matched comparison subjects. Depressed patients had also higher levels of endothelial activation substances such as soluble adhesion molecules sICAM-1 and E-selectin, and the chemokine monocyte chemoattractant protein-1. Finally, there is increasing evidence that depression may be associated with alterations of nitric oxide pathways, which affect adversely vascular tone, and promote exercise intolerance and worsening of somatic symptoms in CHF patients [30,37].

Impaired Compliance to Treatment and Life Style Recommendations

The presence of depression may lead to decrease adherence of CHF patients to appropriate medical therapy [8,22]. Depressive patients with CHF are also less likely to embrace healthy lifestyle behaviours and dietary restrictions [8,22]. Ziegelstein et al. [38] evaluated 144 post-MI patients and found that patients with depressive symptoms had poorer adherence to diet, exercise, smoking cessation, stress reduction and regular socializing. In another study [39], depressive patients with CHF had more frequently sodium retention and volume overload as a cause of acute decompensation and hospital admission than patients without depressive symptoms. A meta-analysis by Matteo et al. [40] examining depression as a risk factor for non-adherence with medical treatment in a wide range of patients with medical illness (end-stage renal disease, cancer, CHF) found that depressives were three times more likely than non-depressives to be no-adherent to any medical advice by their health care provider. Furthermore, other investigators [41] looking at psychosocial variables and compliance, specifically in CHF patients, found that higher mental health was predictive of overall compliance behaviour. Thus, depressive CHF patients may be at a higher risk of non-receiving optimum medical treatment. These observations suggest that depression-induced non-adherence to medical treatment and life style modifications may be an additional risk factor for adverse outcomes among CHF patients as well as an important (reversible) cause of syndrome clinical and hemodynamic deterioration [8,22].

DIAGNOSTIC EVALUATION OF DEPRESSIVE DISORDER IN CHRONIC HEART FAILURE

Depression is an important contributor to CHF progression that needs special attention and early diagnosis, as it is associated with increased morbidity and mortality, poorer health related quality of life, reduced adherence to medication and secondary prevention life style changes. Psychiatric diagnosis of a depressive episode or major depression relies on the International Classification of Diseases 10th revision (ICD-10) [42] or on the Diagnostic and Statistical Manual for Mental Disorders, 4th Edition (DSM-IV) criteria [43] for main and additional symptoms. According to ICD-10, minor depression is diagnosed with 2 main and 2 additional symptoms, with or without somatic component, while major depression needs 3 main and 4 additional ones, with or without somatic component (Table 2). According to DSM-IV criteria, the presence of 5 or more symptoms, with at least one main, for a minimum of 2 weeks, is compatible with the diagnosis of major depression, while the presence of 2-4 symptoms, with at least one main, identifies minor depression (Table 2). Since presentation, severity and course of depression vary, a continuous spectrum of dysthymia, minor depression, subsyndromal depression and atypical depression must also be considered.

In general practice, almost half of the depressed patients remain undiagnosed and as a result untreated [44]. Assessing depressive symptomatology in heart failure patients may be even more confounding due to the overlap between the somatic manifestations of depression, such as fatigue, loss of energy, changes in sleep and appetite and CHF symptoms or normal psychological reactions to hospitalizations. On the other hand, CHF patients often present with the unusual *hidden depressive signs*: Instead of the usual sadness with insufficiency, low self-esteem, feelings of guilt or other more emotional expressions of depressed mood, they often experience affective irritability (emotional instability with anger, hostility, sudden crying or rage, hypersensitivity to acoustic stimuli or negative criticism) as well as anxiety, chronic worrying, multiple organic or hypochondriac problems [9].

Table 2. Classification criteria for depressive disorder

Depressive episode according to ICD-10	Depressive disorder, single episode according to DSM-IV
In typical mild, moderate or severe depressive episodes, depending on the number and severity of the symptoms, the patient suffers for at least two weeks from: A. Main symptoms • Worsened mood • Reduced capacity for enjoyment and loss of interest • Reduced energy and decresed activity, with marked tiredness B. Additional symptoms • Reduced capacity for concentration • Reduced self esteem and self-confidence • Ideas of guilt or worthlessness • Negative-pesimistic perspectives of future • Thoughts of self harm or suicide • Disturbed sleep • Decreased appetite C. Somatic symptoms (at least 4) • Loss of interest and pleasurable feelings • Waking in the morning several hours before the usual time • Depression is worse in the morning • Marked psychomotor retardation, agitation • Loss of appetite • Weight loss (5% during last month) • Loss of libido	A. Five or more of the following symptoms were present during the same 2-week period and represent a change from earlier functioning. There must be at least one main symptom: Main symptoms • Depressed mood • Loss of interest or pleasure Additional symptoms • Fatigue or loss of energy • Decreased ability to think or concentrate, indecisiveness • Insomnia or hypersomnia • Feelings of worthlessness or guilt • Recurrent thoughts of death or suicidal ideation • Psychomotor agitation or retardation • Significant weight loss or gain B. The symptoms do not meet the criteria for a mixed episode C. The symptoms cause clinically significant distress or impairment in social, occupational or other important areas D. The symptoms are not due to the direct physiological effects of a substance (e.g. drug or medication abuse) or a general medical condition (e.g. hypothyroidism) E. The symptoms are not better accounted for by bereavement (e.g. after the loss of a loved one), they persist for more than 2 months or are characterized by marked functional impairment, morbid preoccupation with worthlessness, suicidal ideation, psychotic symptoms or psychomotor retardation.

Since the identification of depressed patients, although crucial, is often not obvious, many questionnaires have been developed for routine assessment by the clinicians. These case-finding instruments are self-rated, require about 5 minutes to complete, include questions assessing depressed mood and anhedonia and according to a recent systematic review, may identify major depression with a median sensitivity of 85% and a median specificity of 74% in general population [45]. It seems that operating characteristics of various instruments are similar and the selection of a particular instrument should depend on issues such as feasibility, administration and scoring times, and the instruments' ability to serve additional purposes, such as monitoring severity or response to therapy [45].

The most frequently used instruments among CHF patients are listed in Table 3. The BDI is a 21-item instrument measuring clinical manifestations of depression that correspond to the DSM-IV criteria. Patients are asked to select the statement that best describes how they felt in the past 2 weeks. A sum score is used to indicate the severity of depressive symptomatology. It has been suggested that assessment of depression in medical ill patients may be confounded by elevated somatic symptoms as a result of their illness and BDI subscales scores may be warranted to avoid misinterpretations of overlapping symptomatology. Nevertheless, its ease of use and ample documentation of its reliability and validity make it a feasible tool for depression screening [46].

Table 3. Characteristics of various depression screening instruments used in heart failure populations

Instrument [Ref]	Items n	Answer format	Score range	Cut-off levels
BDI [46]	21,13,7	4 statements of symptoms severity per item	0-63	10-18 mild 19-29 moderate ≥30 severe
CES-D [48]	20,10	4 frequency ratings	0-60	≥16
MOS-D [45]	8	Frequence ratings	0-1 (log reg)	≥0.06
GDS [52]	30,15	Yes or no	0-30	≥11
HADS [47]	14	4 statements of symptoms severity per item	0-21	≥11
PRIME-MD [45]	2	Yes or no	0-2	≥1
PRIME-MD (PHQ) [8]	9	4 frequency ratings	0-9 for diagnosis 0-27 for response	5-9 minor 10-14 moderate 15-19 major 20-27 severe
SDS [49]	20	4 frequency ratings	20-80	40-48 minor 49-56 moderate 57-80 severe
2 QUESTIONS [53]	2	Yes or no	0-2	2
HAM-D [50]	17, 22	Multiple choice		10–17 mild 17 moderate >17 severe

BDI: Beck Depression Inventory, GDS: Geriatric Depression Scale, HADS: Hospital Anxiety Depression Scale, MOS-D: Medical Outcomes Study Depression Scale, PRIME-MD: Primary Care Evaluation of Mental Disorders, PRIME-MD (PHQ): Patient Health Questionnaire, SDS: Zung Self-Assessment Depression Scale, HAM-D: Hamilton Rating scale for depression.

The HADS is a 14-item self-report measure designed for use with medical patients. It consists of 2 subscales with 7 items assessing depression and 7 items measuring anxiety on 4 point rating scales ranging from 0 (complete lack of endorsement) to 3 (complete endorsement). The scores may be interpreted as normal, mild, moderate or severe ranges of depression or anxiety [47].

The CES-D is a brief 20-item self-report instrument designed to measure depressive symptomatology in the general and psychiatric populations which correspond to the DSM-IV criteria. It appears to be more sensitive to mild presentations of depressive symptoms and is a useful screening tool rather than establishing the diagnosis of severe depression [48]. The Medical Outcomes Study Depression Screen (MOSD) is a depression specific instrument, which was developed by combining two questions from the Diagnostic Interview Schedule with six questions from the CESD. A calculator is needed to apply the logistic regression scoring method [45].

Zung SDS has been designed to provide a quantitative assessment of the subjective experience of depression. It contains 20 items covering affective, psychological and somatic features of depression. Non-depressed individuals typically score less than 40, while 40 to 80 cover various grades of depressive symptomatology [49]

The Hamilton Rating Scale for Depression is an observer rating scale, not a self-report test and is considered as the gold standard among other depression rating scales. It contains a relatively large number of somatic symptoms and relatively few cognitive or affective ones [50].

However, the validity and reliability of most scales as screening instruments for depressive disorder have been established in depressed patients without somatic comorbidity. These questionnaires may have a different sensitivity in identifying patients with depression and heart failure, because some aspects of their cardiovascular disease may disturb psychometric abilities of depression rating scales, leading to an overrepresentation of somatic symptoms and to false-positive test results. It has been suggested that optimum cut-off levels in coronary artery disease may differ from the generally accepted values [51]. However there is no evidence for heart failure patients yet, so further studies are needed in order to modify the scoring system in specific populations.

Thus, given the limited existing data about depression assessment in heart failure units, a reasonable strategy could be to screen initially all patients with two self-rated case-finding instruments. Since all instruments have proven to be of equal predictive value in primary care, one should choose those he considers as more "user friendly". If both instruments are negative for depressive symptomatology, the clinician may repeat assessment in 3-6 months. If scoring is borderline the clinician should optimize CHF treatment and repeat assessment in next visit. If one or both instruments are positive, the patient should refer to a psychiatrist for a personalised interview, in order to diagnose and treat if needed, depression. Correct management always includes a basic workup of potential organic factors contributing to depressive symptomatology which may require specific treatment (e.g., diabetes, thyroid dysfunction, anaemia, malignant tumours, Parkinson's disease, dementia).

REFERENCES

[1]   Ho KK, Pinsky JL, Kannel WB, Levy D. The epidemiology of heart failure: the Framingham Study. *J AmColl Cardiol* 1993;22:6A-13A.

[2]   McMurray JJ, Svebak S. Epidemiology, aetiology, and prognosis of heart failure. *Heart* 2000;83:596–602.

[3]   Senni M, Tribouilloy CM, Rodeheffer RJ, et al. Congestive heart failure in the community: trends in incidence and survival in a 10-year period. *Arch Intern Med* 1999;159:29–34.

[4]   Levy D, Kenchaiah S, Larson M. Long-term trends in the incidence of and survival with heart failure. N Engl J Med. 2002;347:1397-1402

[5]   American Heart Association. *Heart disease and stroke statistics*-2003 update. Dallas (TX): American Heart Association; 2003

[6]   Jiang W, Alexander J, Christopher E, et al. Relationship of depression to increased risk of mortality and rehospitalization in patients with congestive heart failure. *Arch Intern Med.* 2001;161:1849-56.

[7]   Thom T, Haase N, Rosamond W, et al. Heart disease and stroke statistics 2006 update: a report from the American Heart Association Statistics Committee and Stroke Statistics Subcommittee. *Circulation* 2006;113:e85-e151.

[8]   Norra C, Skobel EC, Arndt M, Schauerte P. High impact of depression in heart failure: early diagnosis and treatment options. *Int J Cardiol* 2008;125(2):220-31.

[9]   Rutledge T, Reis VA, Linke SV, Greenberg BH, Mills PJ. Depression in Heart Failure: A Meta-Analytic Review of Prevalence, Intervention Effects, and Associations With Clinical Outcomes. *J Am Coll Cardiol* 2006;48;1527-37.

[10]   Evans DL, Charney DS, Lewis L, et al. Mood disorders in the medically ill: scientific review and recommendations. *Biol Psych* 2005;58:175– 89.

[11]   Havranek E, Spertus J, Masoudi F, Jones P, Rumsfeld J. Predictors of the onset of depressive symptoms in patients with heart failure. *J Am Coll Cardiol* 2004;44:2333-38.

[12]   Abramson J, Berger A, Krumholz HM, Vaccarino V. Depression and risk of heart failure among older persons with isolated systolic hypertension. *Arch Intern Med* 2001;161:1725–30.

[13]   Vaccarino V, Kasl S, Abramson J, Krumholz HM. Depressive symptoms and risk of functional decline and death in patients with heart failure. *J Am Coll Cardiol* 2001;38:199 –205.

[14]   Rumsfeld JS, Havranek EP, Masoudi F, et al. Depressive symptoms are the strongest predictors of short-term declines in health status in patients with heart failure. *J Am Coll Cardiol* 2003;42:1811–1817.

[15]   Koenig HG. Depression in hospitalized older patients with congestive heart failure. *Gen Hosp Psychiatry* 1998;20:29–43.

[16]   Parissis J, Nikolaou M, Farmakis D, et al. Clinical and prognostic implications of self-rating depression scales and plasma B-type natriuretic peptide in hospitalised patients with chronic heart failure. *Heart* 2008;94(5):585-9.

[17]   Laghrissi-Thode F, Wagner WR, Pollock BG, Johnson PC, Finkel MS. Elevated platelet factor 4 and b-thromboglobulin plasma levels in depressed patients with ischemic heart disease. *Biol Psychiatry* 1997;42: 290–5.

[18]   Whyte EM, Pollock BG, Wagner WR, et al. Influence of serotonin-transporter-linked promoter region polymorphism on platelet activation in geriatric depression. *Am J Psychiatry* 2001;158:2074–6.

[19] Von Kanel R Mills PJ, Fainman C, Dimsdale JE. Effects of psychological stress and psychiatric disorders on blood coagulation and fibrinolysis: a biobehavioral pathway to coronary artery disease? *Pshychosom Med* 2001;63:531-44.

[20] Joynt KE, Whellan DJ, O' Connor CM. Why is depression bad for the failing heart? A review of the mechanistic relationship between depression and heart failure. *J Card Fail* 2004; 10(3):258-70.

[21] Konstam V, Moser D, De Jong M. Depression and anxiety in heart failure. *J Card Fail* 2005;11:455-62.

[22] Gorman JM, Sloan RP. Heart rate variability in depressive and anxiety disorders. *Am Heart J* 2000;140 (Suppl. 4):77-83.

[23] Carney RM, Blumenthal JA, Stein PK, et al. Depression, heart rate variability, and acute myocardial infarction. *Circulation* 2001; 104:2024-8.

[24] Mann DL. Mechanisms and models in heart failure: a combinatorial approach. *Circulation* 1999;100:999-1008

[25] Blum A, Miller A. Pathophysiological role of cytokines in congestive heart failure. *Annu Rev Med* 2001;52:15–27.

[26] Adamopoulos S, Parissis J, Kremastinos D. A glossary of circulating cytokines in chronic heart failure. *Eur J Heart Fail* 2001;3:517-26.

[27] Anker SD, Von Haehling S. Inflammatory mediators in chronic heart failure: an overview. *Heart* 2004;90:464-470.

[28] Maes M. Major depression and activation of the inflammatory response system. *Adv. Exp. Med. Biol.* 1999;461:25-46.

[29] Pasic J, Levy WC, Sullivan MD. Cytokines in depression and heart failure. *Psychosom. Med.* 2003;65:181-193.

[30] Parissis J, Fountoulaki K, Paraskevaidis I, Kremastinos D. Depression in chronic heart failure: novel pathophysiological mechanisms and therapeutic approaches. *Expert Opin Investig Drugs* 2005;14:567-77.

[31] Parissis J, Adamopoulos S, Rigas A, et al. Comparison of circulating pro-inflammatory cytokines and soluble apoptosis mediators in patients with chronic heart failure with versus without symptoms of depression. *Am J Cardiol* 2004;94:1326-8.

[32] Ferketich A.K, Ferguson J.P, Binkley P.F. Depressive symptoms and inflammation among heart failure patients. *Am Heart J* 2005;150:132-6.

[33] Moorman A, Mozaffarian D, Wilkinson C, et al. In patients with heart failure elevated soluble TNF-receptor 1 is associated with higher risk of depression. *J Card Fail* 2007;13:738-43.

[34] Watkins LR, Maier SF, Goehler LE. Cytokine-to-brain communication: a review and analysis of alternative mechanisms. *Life Sci.* 1995;57:1011-1026.

[35] Adamopoulos S, Parissis J, Kremastinos D. Endothelial dysfunction in chronic heart failure. *Eur J intern Med* 2002;13:233-39.

[36] Rajagopalan S, Brook R, Rubenfire M, et al. Abnormalbrachial artery flow-mediated vasodilation in young adults with major depression. *Am J Cardiol* 2001; 88:196–98.

[37] Parissis J, Fountoulaki K, Filippatos G, Adamopoulos S, Praskevaidis I, Kremastinos D. Depression in coronary artery disease: novel pathophysiologic mechanisms and therapeutic implications. *Int J Cardiol* 2007;116:153-60.

[38]   Ziegelstin RC, Bush DE, Fauerbach JA. Depression, adherence behavior and coronary disease outcomes. *Arch. Intern. Med.* 1998;158:808-14.

[39]   Moser DK, Worster PL. Effect of psychosocial factors on physiologic outcomes in patients with heart failure. *J. Cardiovasc. Nurs.* 2000;14:106-15.

[40]   DiMatteo MR, Lepper HS, Croghan TW. Depression is a risk factor for non-compliance with medical treatment: meta-analysis of the effects of anxiety and depression on patient adherence. *Arch. Intern. Med.* 2000;160:2101-07.

[41]   Evangelista LS, Berg J, Dracup K. Relationship between psychosocial variables and compliance in patients with heat failure. *Heat Lung* 2001;30:294-301.

[42]   World Health Organization. Tenth Revision of the International Classification of Diseases, Chapter (V): mental and behavioural disorders (including disorders of psychological development). *Clinical Descriptions and Diagnostic Guidelines.* WHO, 1991.

[43]   American Psychiatric Association. Diagnostic and Statistical Manual of Mental Disorders. DSM-IV-TR 5th edition. Washington DC: American Psychiatric Press; 2000.

[44]   Kessler RC, Berglund P, Demler O, et al. The epidemiology of major depressive disorder: results from the national comorbidity survey replication (NCS-R). *JAMA* 2003;289:3095-105.

[45]   Williams JW, Pignone M, Ramirez G, Stellato CP. Identifying depression in primary care: a literature synthesis of case-finding instruments. *General Hospital Psychiatry* 2002;24:225–237.

[46]   Beck AT, Ward CH, Mendelson M, Mock J, Erbaugh J. An inventory for measuring depression. *Arch Gen Psychiatry* 1961;4:561–71.

[47]   Shen BJ, Wachowiak PS, Brooks LG. Psychosocial factors and assessment in cardiac rehabilitation. *Eur Med Phys* 2005;41:75-91.

[48]   Radloff LS. The CES-D scale: a self report depression scale for research in the general population. *Appl Psychol Meas* 1977;1:385–401.

[49]   Zung WWK, Richards CB, Short MJ. Self-rating depression scale in an outpatient clinic. *Arch Gen Psychiatry* 1965;13:508-15.

[50]   Hamilton M. A rating scale for depression. *J Neurol Neurosurg Psychiatry* 1960;23:56–62.

[51]   51.J Strik, A Honig, Lousberg R, Denollet J. Sensitivity and Specificity of Observer and Self-Report Questionnaires in Major and Minor Depression Following Myocardial Infarction. *Psychosomatics* 2001;42:423-28.

[52]   Yesavage JA, Brink TL, Rose TL et al. Development and validation of a geriatric depression screening scale: a preliminary report. *J Psychiatr Res* 1982–83;17:37-49.

[53]   Mc Manus D, Pipkin SS, Whooley MA. Screening for depression in patients with coronary heart disease. *Am J Cardiol* 2005;96:1076-81.

In: Psychological Factors and Cardiovascular Disorders   ISBN: 978-1-60456-871-4
Editor: Leo Sher   © 2008 Nova Science Publishers, Inc.

Chapter IX

DIAGNOSING DEPRESSION AND QUALITY OF LIFE IN PATIENTS WITH CHRONIC HEART FAILURE

Nicole Holzapfel, Thomas Müller-Tasch, Wolfgang Herzog and Beate Wild

Department of Psychosomatic and General Internal Medicine, Medical Hospital, University of Heidelberg, Germany.

ABSTRACT

Chronic heart failure (CHF) is a common and disabling disease with high mortality and poor prognosis. Many patients with CHF suffer additionally from a severely reduced quality of life and depression. Despite the high prevalence rates and the significance of depression for the course of physical illness, depression often goes unrecognized and untreated in clinical practice, especially among CHF patients. There is an increasing need to diagnose and treat depressive co-morbidity and reduced quality of life in clinical routine in CHF.

The poor recognition rates of depression in CHF patients might be explained by several factors related to patients, physicians and the health care system. However, a crucial reason for difficulties in diagnosing depression may be found in the symptom overlap between the two disorders: Symptoms like fatigue, difficulties in concentrating, general indisposition or insomnia can occur in both depression and heart failure.

Specific risk factors for depression in CHF patients, such as higher NYHA functional class or younger age can help to identify CHF patients with depression. A standard screening, which identifies depression and psychosocial strains without being too complex or time-consuming and which leads to clearly defined treatment consequences, can amend the diagnostic process.

INTRODUCTION

Chronic heart failure (CHF) is a common and disabling disease with poor prognosis, high mortality, increasing incidence and prevalence [1]. Its typical symptom trias is dyspnea, limited physical functioning, and peripheral edema. CHF is the most common reason for hospitalization in older patients [2] and CHF patients have the highest hospitalization rates among all patients groups [3]. The lifetime risk for CHF is estimated 1 out of 5 for both men and woman [3].

Compliance to a strict and complex healthcare regimen is essential to prevent further deterioration of CHF symptoms and to allow the patients to lead an acceptable life. According to current guidelines, CHF patients are required to regularly take various medications and follow specific behavioural patterns such as daily weighing, limited fluid and sodium intake, moderate exercise, a ban on smoking and limited alcohol consumption [4]. Coping with these strict requirements, functional impairments and physical symptoms is difficult and exhaustive for any length of time [5]. Many patients with CHF suffer from a severely reduced quality of life [6,7] and comorbid depressive disorders are common: While 4 to 10% of the general population in the United States and Europe meet diagnostic criteria for depressive disorders (12-month prevalence rates) [8,9], 11 to 25% of CHF outpatients and 35 to 70% of CHF inpatients are estimated to suffer from depressive disorders [10]. Rutledge et al. [11] concluded in their meta-analytic review that a clinically significant depression is present in at least 1 out of 5 patients. As an important symptom of depressive disorders, suicide risk is also increased in patients with CHF [12].

A number of studies have examined the importance of depression and reduced quality of life on the course of illness and prognosis: Jiang et al. [13], for example, found that the diagnosis of major depression was associated with increased mortality after three months and one year in patients with CHF. Rumsfeld et al. [14] showed that depressive symptoms are a strong predictor of a short-term worsening of heart failure specific symptoms. Jünger et al. [15] concluded that depression is a strong predictor of increased mortality in CHF patients.

A reduced quality of life seems also to be predictive for unscheduled readmissions and mortality [7,16,17]. However, the prognostic value of the patient's quality of life may reflect confounding with comorbid depression and severity of the disease [18].

Despite the obvious negative effects of depression and a reduced quality of life on the course of CHF, these factors often go unrecognized and untreated in clinical practice [19,20]. Koenig [21] concluded that persistent depression was not recognized in 40% of older CHF inpatients. Only 5-7 % of the CHF patients take an antidepressant [22,23].

The present chapter addresses the question as to how this discrepancy can be explained and possibly overcome.

Difficulties in Diagnosing Depression and Reduced Quality of Life in Clinical Practise

The poor recognition rates of depression in general and in CHF patients in particular [19,20,21] might be explained by several factors related to patients, physicians, and the health care system [24]: Patients may not want to disclose emotional distress to their physicians, being afraid of getting the label of a mental disorder or a psychiatric diagnosis. Some patients may also interpret their feelings and thoughts as being part of their medical illness instead of presume a depressive disorder. In primary care settings the prevalent disorders reported by depressive patients are sleep disturbances, fatigue or pain and not emotional symptoms [24]. From the physicians and the health care aspect time is often too limited to be able to question the patient about problems and worries.

Then again some physicians may also not have been trained to recognize typical and atypical depressive symptoms [10] or they may only focus on somatic rather than psychological complaints.

However, another crucial reason for difficulties in diagnosing depression may be found in the symptom overlap between the two disorders: Core symptoms of a depressive disorder are a depressed mood and loss of interest or pleasure in every day activities. Important secondary symptoms are feelings of worthlessness or guilt, sleep disturbance, loss of energy, fatigue, changes in appetite, weak concentration, suicide ideations and psychomotor agitation/retardation. Symptoms such as fatigue, concentration deficits, general indisposition or insomnia can - especially in the older population- occur in both depression and heart failure. This symptom overlap may make the diagnosis and monitoring of depression symptoms during the CHF treatment process more difficult. Given the high co-morbidity rate of depression in CHF and the reported difficulties in diagnosing depression there is an increasing need not only to individually optimize heart failure treatment, but also to optimize the diagnosis and to discuss treatment options of depressive symptoms in CHF patients [10,19,21,25]. However, as O'Connor and Joynt [10] have pointed out, it is important that clinicians and patients realize that CHF is not necessarily accompanied by depression.

Depression Profile in Patients with and Without Chronic Heart Failure

In order to improve the diagnosis of depression in CHF patients, an awareness of the specific symptom profile of depression as presented in CHF patients is necessary. In the past a number of studies have compared depressive symptom patterns in patients with and without somatic comorbidity [26], or in patients recruited in medical and psychiatric settings [27]. So far the findings have remained ambiguous: While an earlier study concluded that there is no clinically relevant difference in the depression symptom profile in medical and non-medical populations [28], another study demonstrated that the features discriminating depressed patients with and without comorbid physical illness were cognitive symptoms such as hopelessness, suicidal ideation and feelings of guilt [27]. In a recent study, Simon and von Korff [26] found only modest differences in the severity of somatic depression symptoms in depressed patients with and without medical co-morbidity - they concluded that the DSM-IV diagnostic criteria do not require modification for patients with medical co-morbidity.

A comparison between depressed patients with and without CHF with respect to severity of individual DSM-IV depressive symptoms (measured with the PHQ-9) revealed significant differences in the depression profile: Depressed patients with CHF reported significantly lower levels of depressed mood and worthlessness / guilt than depressed patients without

CHF. In contrast, no significant group differences were found for any of the other depression symptoms [29].

Increasing evidence may now be found that the diagnostic features discriminating between depressed patients with and without CHF seem to be the cognitive-emotional symptoms of depression, not the somatic symptoms. A possible explanation for this finding is that 38% of depressed medical patients understand their emotional problems as a consequence of their physical illness [30] – thus patients with medical conditions may attribute their depression to their physical illness as an external, non-controllable factor. Perhaps this external attribution of depression prevents self-reproaches, feelings of worthlessness and guilt.

These findings may partially explain the low recognition rate of depression in patients with CHF: Given their specific depression profile, CHF patients might report less often feelings of hopelessness, worthlessness, and guilt in their medical history, so that clinicians might not consider the presence of a depressive comorbidity. Due to the substantial overlap of somatic symptoms between depressive disorders and CHF, depression may often be dismissed as the somatic symptom burden of heart failure. To improve this situation, medical training should address the fact that depressive disorders may appear in different forms in patients with and without CHF.

HOW A STANDARD SCREENING CAN AMEND THE DIAGNOSTIC PROCESS

Specific risk factors for depression in CHF patients, i.e. higher NYHA functional class [11,23] and younger age [31] can help to identify CHF patients with depression. In addition a standard screening, which identifies depression and psychosocial strains without being too complex or time-consuming and leads to clearly defined treatment consequences for CHF patients, can amend the diagnostic process. A short and easy to handle instrument is the nine-item depression module from the Patient Health Questionnaire (PHQ-9) [32,33,34]. The PHQ was particular designed for use in primary care and diagnoses depressive disorders using criteria from the Diagnostic and Statistical Manual of Mental Disorders, Fourth Edition (DSM-IV) (American Psychiatric Association, 35). The sensitivity (98%) and specificity (80%) of the PHQ-9 has proven to be excellent [36]. Each of the nine items ranges from 0 to 3 points. The recommended cut-off point for detecting a depressive disorder is a sum-score of 9 points; the cut-off for a major depressive disorder is 11 points. As an alternative, the applied categorical evaluation of the PHQ as suggested by Spitzer et al. [37] might be used. Spitzer et al. found that if patients confirm at least two symptoms in the depression scale with "more than half the days" within the last two weeks, and one of these items is item 1 or 2 (affective symptoms) a "depressive syndrome" may be diagnosed. A major depression is diagnosed if patients agree to five of the nine depression items with at least "more than half the days". In addition, the last item of the questionnaire asks for suicidal ideations, this enables high-risk patients to be quickly identified. For a very short screening, the two-item Patient Health Questionnaire (PHQ-2) can be used. This has also proven to be valid and reliable [38]. Other long-established screening instruments are for example the HADS

[39,40], the Beck Depression Inventory [41], or the Symptom Checklist [42]. Studies have shown that depression questionnaires for diagnosing and monitoring depression are on the whole comparable [38,43,44].

The patient's self-assessment of health related quality of life can be measured by the thirty six-item short form health survey (SF-36) [45]. This questionnaire is a generic multidimensional instrument consisting of eight subscales (physical functioning, role functioning physical, bodily pain, general health perceptions, vitality, social functioning, role functioning emotional and mental health) and a physical and mental health summary measure. SF-36 scores are converted to a scale of 0 to 100, a higher score indicating a better quality of life.

Although on first sight, such a screening process may increase the work load for the physician and the team, the increased efficiency in screening for depression and quality of life may further improve prognosis and well-being in CHF patients.

CONCLUSION

The presence of physical symptoms in patients with CHF is almost normal and can of course be the result of heart disease. If a patient, however, does not only describe but complains about his symptom burden, if there is a discrepancy between the objective measures of heart failure severity (left ventricular ejection fraction, natriuretic peptides, etc.), and the symptom complaint, if heart failure remains stable but the symptom complaint increases; or if, on the contrary, the patient does not complain about anything or even hardly talks any more – all of that can be a sign that the patient simply is not well. So, the primary means of diagnosing depressive disorders in CHF patients is to be aware of the possibility and to encourage the patient to report on his subjective well-being, keeping the symptom overlap between both disorders and the specific features of depression in CHF in mind. Considering the limited time in clinical routine, the application of short and easy to handle screening instruments may help to successfully complete this important task. Evidence about the effect of specific psychosocial interventions in depressive heart failure patients is still lacking [46]. So, when a depressive co-morbidity has been diagnosed, an individual and pragmatic approach with regard to psychotherapeutic support and/or antidepressive medication can be recommended, taking the patients motivation and preferences into consideration.

REFERENCES

[1] Muntwyler J, Abetel G, Gruner C, Follath F. One-year mortality among unselected outpatients with heart failure. *Eur Heart J* 2002; 23: 1861-1866.

[2] Graves EJ. Detailed diagnosis and procedures: National Hospital Discharge Survey, 1990. *Vital Health Statistics* 1992; 13 (113): 1-224, DHHS Pub. 92-1774.

[3] Lloyd-Jones DM, Larson MG, Leip EP, Beiser A, D'Agostino RB, Kannel WB, Murabito JM, Vasan RS, Benjamin EJ, Levy D. Lifetime risk for developing congestive heart failure: the Framingham Heart Study. *Circulation* 2002; 106: 3068-3072.

[4] Swedberg K, Cleland J, Dargie H, Drexler H, Follath F, Komajda M, Tavazzi L, Smiseth OA, Gavazzi A, Haverich A, Hoes A, Jaarsma T, Korewicki J, Levy S, Linde C, Lopez-Sendon JL, Nieminen MS, Pierard L, Remme WJ; Task Force for the Diagnosis and Treatment of Chronic Heart Failure of the European Society of Cardiology. Guidelines for the diagnosis and treatment of chronic heart failure: Executive summary (update 2005): The Task Force for the Diagnosis and Treatment of Chronic Heart Failure of the European Society of Cardiology. *Eur Heart J* 2005; 26 (11): 1115-1140.

[5] Koenig HG, Vandermeer J, Chambers A, Burr-Crutchfield L, Johnson JL. Comparison of major and minor depression in older medical inpatients with chronic heart and pulmonary disease. *Psychosomatics* 2006; 47 (4): 296-303.

[6] Jünger J, Schellberg D, Krämer S, Haunstetter A, Zugck C, Herzog W, Haass M. Health related quality of life in patients with congestive heart failure: comparison with other chronic diseases and relation to functional variables. *Heart* 2002; 87: 235-241.

[7] Konstam V, Salem D, Pouleur H, Kostis J, Gorkin L, Shumaker S, Mottard I, Woods P, Konstam MA, Yusuf S. Baseline quality of life as a predictor of mortality and hospitalization in 5,025 patients with congestive heart failure. SOLVD Investigations. Studies of Left Ventriculare Dysfunction Investigators. *Am J Cardiol* 1996; 78(8): 890-5.

[8] Demyttenaere K, Bruffaerts R, Posada-Villa J, Gasquet I, Kovess V, Lepine JP, Angermeyer MC, Bernert S, de Girolamo G, Morosini P, Polidori G, Kikkawa T, Kawakami N, Ono Y, Takeshima T, Uda H, Karam EG, Fayyad JA, Karam AN, Mneimneh ZN, Medina-Mora ME, Borges G, Lara C, de Graaf R, Ormel J, Gureje O, Shen Y, Huang Y, Zhang M, Alonso J, Haro JM, Vilagut G, Bromet EJ, Gluzman S, Webb C, Kessler RC, Merikangas KR, Anthony JC, von Korff MR, Wang PS, Brugha TS, Aguilar-Gaxiola S, Lee S, Heeringa S, Pennell BE, Zaslavsky AM, Ustun TB, Chatterji S. Prevalence, severity, and unmet need for treatment of mental disorders in the World Health Organization World Mental Health Surveys. *JAMA* 2004; 291: 2581-2590.

[9] Kessler RC, Berglund P, Demler O, Jin R, Koretz D, Merikangas KR, Rush AJ, Walters EE, Wang PS. The epidemiology of major depressive disorder: results from the National Comorbidity Survey Replication (NCS-R). *JAMA* 2003; 289: 3095-3105.

[10] O' Connor CM, Joynt KE. Depression: are we ignoring an important comorbidity in heart failure? *J Am Coll Cardiol* 2004; 43 (9): 1550-1552.

[11] Rutledge T, Reis VA, Linke SE, Greenberg BH, Mills PJ. Depression in heart failure. *J Am Coll Cardiol* 2006; 48 (8): 27-1537.

[12] Juurlink DN, Herrmann N, Szalai JP, Kopp A, Redelmeier DA. Medical illness and the risk of suicide in the elderly. *Arch Intern Med* 2004 164 (11): 1179-1184.

[13] Jiang W, Alexander J, Christopher E, Kuchibhatla M, Gaulden LH, Cuffe MS, Blazing MA, Davenport C, Califf RM, Krishnan RR, O'Connor M. Relationship of depression to increased risk of mortality and rehospitalization in patients with congestive heart failure. *Arch Intern Med* 2001; 161(15): 1849-56.

[14] Rumsfeld JS, Havranek E, Masoudi FA, Peterson ED, Jones P, Tooley J, Krumhoolz HM, Spertus JA, for the Cardiovascular Outcomes Research Consortium (CORC).

Depressive symptoms are the strongest predictors of short-term declines in health status in patients with heart failure. *J Am Coll Cardiol* 2003; 42 (10): 1811-7.

[15] Juenger J, Schellberg D, Müller-Tasch TH, Raupp G, Zugck CH, Haunstetter A, Zipfel ST, Herzog W, Haass M. Depression increasingly predicts mortality in the course of congestive heart failure. *Eur J Heart Fail* 2005; 7: 261-267.

[16] Bouvy ML, Heerdink ER, Laufkens HG, Hoes AW. Predicting mortality in patients with heart failure: a pragmatic approach. *Heart* 2003; 89: 605- 9.

[17] Jaagosild P, Dawson NV, Thomas C, Wenger NS, Tsevat J, Knaus WA, Califf RM, Goldman L, Vidaillet H, Connors AFJr. Outcomes of acute exacerbation of severe congestive heart failure: quality of life, resource use, and survival. SUPPORT Investigators. The Study to Understand Prognosis and Preferences of Outcomes and Risks of Treatments. *Arch Intern Med* 1998; 158 (10): 1081-9.

[18] Faller H, Strök S, Schowalter M, Steinbüchel T, Wollner V, Ertl G, Angermann CE. Is health-related quality of life an independent predictor of survival in patients with chronic heart failure? *J Psychosom Res* 2007; 63 (5): 533-538.

[19] Davidson JR, Meltzer-Brody SE. The underrecognition and undertreatment of depression: what is the breadth and depth of the problem? *J Clin Psychiatry* 1999; 60 Suppl 7: 4-9.

[20] Alexopoulos GS, Borson S, Cuthbert BN, Devanand DP, Mulsant BH, Olin JT, Oslin DW. Assessment of late life depression. *Biol Psychiatry* 2002; 52 (3): 164-174.

[21] Koenig GK. Recognition of depression in medical patients with heart failure. *Psychosomatics* 2007; 48:338-347.

[22] Gottlieb SS, Khatta M, Friedmann E, Einbinder L, Katzen S, Baker B, Marshall J, Minshall S, Robinson S, Fisher ML, Potenza M, Sigler B, Baldwin C, Thomas SA. The influence of age, gender, and race on the prevalence of depression in heart failure patients. *J Am Coll Cardiol* 2004; 43 (9): 1542-1549.

[23] Holzapfel N, Zugck C, Müller-Tasch T, Löwe B, Wild B, Schellberg D, Nelles M, Remppis A, Katus H, Herzog W, Jünger J. Routine screening for depression and quality of life in outpatients with congestive heart failure. *Psychosomatics* 2007; 48: 112-116.

[24] Goldman LS, Nielsen NH, Champion HC, for the Council on Scientific Affairs, American Medical Association. Awareness, diagnosis, and treatment of depression. *J Gen Intern Med* 1999; 14: 569-580.

[25] Boyd CM, Darer J, Boult C, Fried LP, Boult L, Wu AW. Clinical practise guidelines and quality of care for older patients with multiple comorbid diseases. *JAMA* 2005; 294: 716-724

[26] Simon GE, von Korff M. Medical co-morbidity and validity of DSM-IV depression criteria. *Psychol Med* 2006; 36: 27-36.

[27] Clark DA, Cook A, Snow D. Depressive symptom differences in hospitalized, medically ill, depressed psychiatric inpatients and nonmedical controls. *J Abnorm Psychol* 1998; 107: 38-48.

[28] Coulehan JL, Schulberg HC, Block MR, Zettler-Segal M. Symptom patterns of depression in ambulatory medical and psychiatric patients. *J Nerv Ment* 1988; Dis 176: 284-288.

[29] Holzapfel N, Müller-Tasch T, Wild B, Jünger J, Zugck C, Remppis A, Herzog W, Löwe B. Depression profile in patients with and without chronic heart failure. *J Affect Disord* 2008; 105/1-3: 53-62.

[30] Löwe B, Schulz U, Gräfe K, Wilke S. Medical patients' attitudes toward emotional problems and their treatment. What do they really want? *J Gen Intern Med* 2006; 21: 39-45.

[31] Freedland KE, Rich MW, Skala JA, Carney RM, Davila-Roman VG, Jaffe, A. S., 2003. Prevalence of depression in hospitalized patients with congestive heart failure. *Psychosom. Med. 65*, 119-128.

[32] Spitzer RL, Kroenke K, Williams JB, Patient Health Questionnaire Primary Care Study Group. Validation and utility of a self-report version of PRIME-MD: the PHQ primary care study. *JAMA* 1999; 282: 1737-1744.

[33] Kroenke K, Spitzer RL, Williams JB. The PHQ-9. Validity of a brief depression severity measure. *J Gen Intern Med* 2001; 16: 606-613.

[34] Löwe B, Kroenke K, Herzog W, Gräfe K. Measuring depression outcome with a brief self report instrument: sensitivity to change of the Patient Health Questionnaire (PHQ-9). *J Affect Disord* 2004; 81: 61-66.

[35] American Psychiatric Association 2000. Diagnostic and Statistical Manual of Mental Disorders DSM-IV-TR. 4th edition. Text revision edition. *American Psychiatric Association*, Washington DC.

[36] Löwe B, Spitzer RL, Gräfe K, Kroenke K, Quenter A, Zipfel S, Buchholz C, Witte S, Herzog W. Comparative validity of three screening questionnaires for DSM-IV depressive disorders and physicians' diagnoses. *J Affect Disord* 2004; 78: 131-140.

[37] Spitzer RL, Kroenke K, Williams JB. Patient health questionnaire primary care study group. Validation and utility of a self-report version of PRIME-MD: The PHQ primary care study. *JAMA* 1999 282:1734-1744

[38] Löwe B, Kroenke K, Gräfe K. Detecting and monitoring depression with a two-item questionnaire (PHQ-2). *J Psychosom Res* 2005 58: 163-171

[39] Herrmann C. International experiences with the Hospital Anxiety and Depression Scale - a review of validation data and clinical results. *J Psychosom Res* 1997; 42: 17-41.

[40] Zigmond AS, Snaith RP. The hospital anxiety and depression scale. *Acta Psychiatr Scand* 1983; 67: 361-370.

[41] Beck AT, Beck RW. Screening depressed patients in family practice: a rapid technic. *Postgrad Med* 1972; 52: 81-85.

[42] Derogatis LR. The SCL-90-R. Baltimore, Md: *Clinical Psychometrics Research*: 1975.

[43] Mulrow CD, Williams JW, Gerety MB, Ramirez G, Montiel OM, Kernber C. Case-finding instruments for depression in primary care settings. *Ann Intern Med* 1995 122: 913-921.

[44] Whooley MA, Avins AL, Miranda J, Browner WS. Case-finding instruments for depression. Two questions are as good as many. *J Gen Intern Med* 1997 12: 439-445.

[45] Ware JE, Sherbourne CD. The MOS 36-item short-form health survey (SF-36). I. Conceptual framework and item selection. *Med Care* 1992; 30 (6): 473-483.

[46] Lane DA, Chong AY, Lip GYH. Psychological interventions for depression in heart failure. *Cochrane Database Syst Rev 1*: CD 003329.

In: Psychological Factors and Cardiovascular Disorders   ISBN: 978-1-60456-871-4
Editor: Leo Sher   © 2008 Nova Science Publishers, Inc.

Chapter X

HEART FAILURE: THE MANIFESTATIONS AND IMPACT OF NEGATIVE EMOTIONS

Doris S.F. Yu

The Nethersole School of Nursing, The Chinese University of Hong Kong,
SAR Hong Kong, PRC.

ABSTRACT

Heart failure is an important public health problem worldwide. The fatal, progressively deteriorating nature of this disease, together with its debilitating symptoms, lead to poor psychosocial adjustment among the sufferers. High level of negative emotions has been reported by this vulnerable group of patients, and resulted in multiple deleterious effects on their health outcomes. A body of knowledge in psychosomatic medicine has indicated the effects of stress management techniques on clinical and health outcomes of cardiovascular patients, more attention need to be given to its application to heart failure management.

INTRODUCTION

Heart failure (HF) is a pervasive cardiac syndrome that exposes patients to the distressing symptoms of fatigue and dyspnea, limited functional ability, restricted lifestyle, frequent attacks of disease exacerbation and repeated hospital admissions. As a result, this disease is not only physically debilitating, but it also arouses high levels of negative emotions to the patients. This chapter will give a brief overview of the worldwide epidemiology of heart failure. The transactional model of stress [1] is then elaborated to provide the framework for understanding the way negative emotions, particularly anxiety and depression, in relation to ineffective coping in HF patients has been manifested. In addition, the direct psycho-physiological pathway and the indirect behavioral pathway are outlined to explain the detrimental effects of negative emotions on HF patients' overall well-being. Empirical evidence about the roles of negative emotional in affecting the health outcomes of heart failure patients are summarized. Stress management techniques are recommended as a crucial component in enhancing the disease management for patients with heart failure.

EPIDEMIOLOGY OF HEART FAILURE

Heart failure (HF) is an important public problem that affects people in both developed and developing countries [2-3]. Instead of a disease, HF is defined as "a complex clinical syndrome that can result from any structural or functional cardiac disorder that impairs the ability of the ventricle to fill with or eject blood" [4]. This definition provides the explanation for HF frequently occurring as a clinical endpoint of many cardiovascular disorders, especially those that impair cardiac function or strain the cardiac workload [5]. It also explains the epidemiological trend of HF to proceed in an opposite direction to the improvement in medical technology for extending the life expectancies of various cardiovascular pathologies.

HF has high prevalence worldwide. The estimated crude annual incidence of HF in the general population of developed countries ranges from one to five per 1000, with the crude annual prevalence reported as 20 per 1,000 [6]. In Western countries, HF affects approximately 1% of the population in the United Kingdom [7]. There are also about five million HF patients in the United States of America, and the newly diagnosed cases are reported as being 500,000 per annum [4]. The figure remains high in Canada and HF affects more than 400,000 Canadians, with over 50,000 new cases occurring annually [8]. Indeed, Morgan, et al [9] reported that up to 10% of elderly people in Europe were diagnosed as having ventricular systolic dysfunction when they were assessed with echocardiogram. More recent study also indicated that the lifetime risk of developing HF in Western countries is very alarming and reported as high as 20% [10]. The incidence and prevalence of HF are also found to be age-dependent, with a 5-fold to 10-fold increase for each decade of age [11-13]. In the United Kingdom, the prevalence of HF rises from <1% in those aged < 65 to > 5% among those aged 65 - 79 and 10 - 12% among those of over 80 years of age [13]. The situation is even worse in the southwestern European, with the prevalence of HF shoot up drastically from 4.36% in the overall population to 7.63% in the 60-69 years old group, and 12.7% in the 70-79 years old group [14].

THE MANIFESTATION OF HEART FAILURE

HF is a debilitating and progressively deteriorating disorder [4]. Ineffective myocardial pumping that leading to lack of adequate tissue perfusion causes the cardinal signs and symptoms of fatigue, dyspnea, activity intolerance, venous congestion, peripheral and pulmonary congestion to the patients. The compromised myocardium contractility also initiates compensatory mechanisms which further deteriorate the disease progression. These mechanisms involve a series of activations of neuro-hormonal systems, including the rennin-angiotensin-aldosterone system, sympathetic nervous system, the vasopressin system and the cardiac activation of cytokines [15]. Patients with HF are therefore characterized by an elevation of circulating or tissue levels of epinephrine, angiotensin II, aldosterone, endotheline, renin and cytokines. Such physiological changes further stress the myocardial workload though increasing sodium and fluid retention and inducing vasoconstriction. These detrimental changes may also exert a direct toxic effect on cardiac cells and stimulate myocardial fibrosis. Both the myocardial function and structure are therefore threatened, resulting in further disease deterioration [16].

PREVALENCE OF NEGATIVE EMOTIONS IN HEART FAILURE

Negative emotions commonly occur as a result of a maladaptive reaction to chronic illness. The pervasive impact of HF puts the patients at especially high risk of developing sustained emotional problems. Mood disturbances, especially in the form of anxiety and depression, have been widely documented for this vulnerable group. Lainscak and Keber [17] identified that more than 50% of HF patients complained the psychological symptoms of anxiety and depression. Riedinger, et al [18] and Yu, et al [19] also detected the high levels of such negative emotions experienced by either the Cauasian or non-Cauasian HF patients. They found that mood disturbance was a far more prominent problem in affecting HF patients when compared with a group of normative population. Similar findings have been reported in earlier studies [20-21]. They even found the levels of anxiety and depression reported by HF patients was far higher than those reported by the patients of coronary artery disease (CAD) or those undergone cardiac surgery.

In particular, depression appears to be the most prevalent psychological problem that affects patients with HF. The manifestation of this psychological problem takes different forms including depressed mood, minor depression or even major depression. Murberg, et al [22] found that as many as 39% of HF patients ($N = 119$) reported depressive symptoms and among them, almost 40% were categorized as having moderate to severe depression. Vaccarino, et al [23] recruited a larger sample of HF patients ($N = 426$) revealed a similar situation, that 33.5% and 9% of HF patients were respectively rated as having moderate and high level of depressive symptoms on the Geriatric Depression Scale. Indeed, it is also common for the negative emotion of depression to manifest as a psychiatric morbidity among the hospitalized HF patients. In the recent survey done by Freedland, et al [24], they found that 20% of hospitalized HF patients ($N = 682$) met the Diagnostic and Statistical Manual (4th ed.) [25] for a current major depression and 16% of them also met the criteria for minor depression. In addition, more than half of the sample (51%) was also identified as probably depressed by the Beck Depression Inventory. Koenig [26] reported even worse situation. They found that 36.5% ($N = 107$) of hospitalized HF patients met the criteria for major depression and 21.5% for minor depression. This prevalence rate was significantly higher than that of the non-HF cardiac patients (17%, $p < .002$). Indeed, major depression also presented as a persistent psychiatric problem, as almost 40% of these patients failed to have a remission after one year following their discharge.

THE TRANSACTIONAL MODEL OF STRESS

The high prevalence of negative emotions in HF patients can be explained by the transactional model of stress. This model is a very promising framework for explaining the emotional manifestation of chronic illness, as it not only takes into account the characteristics of illness in contributing to chronic illness, but also gives consideration to the impact of personal attributes and the person's immediate environment to the consequences of illness.

The transactional model of stress is proposed by Lazarus and Folkman [1]. In this model, stress is defined as "a particular relationship between the person and the environment that is appraised by the person as taxing or exceeding his or her resources and endangering his or her well-being." [1, p.19]. According to this definition, stress is regarded as an encounter between the person and the environment, which arouses his or her awareness, and brings about cognitive appraisal of the event, by that individual. Lazarus [27] described cognitive appraisal as a series of repeated evaluations of the impact of the encountered stimulus in relation to oneself. The process is depicted as consisting of two steps: primary and secondary appraisal. In the primary appraisal, the individual makes a judgment about the possible impact of a stimulus that he or she encounters in the environment. There are three kinds of stimulus that would be perceived as stressful. They include those that cause harm or cause loss; those that threaten and those that impose a challenge to the individual. Upon perceiving a stimulus as stressful, secondary appraisal takes place. This is another process in the cognitive evaluation, during which the individual considers the availability, controllability and effectiveness of their coping options, as well as their future expectation of how the stimulus will change as it progresses. The whole process of cognitive appraisal is individualized, as it depends on the influence of the physiological, psychological, social and developmental factors of the individual concerned [28]. The individual appraises the stressors from the standpoint of his or her own motives and beliefs, acquired through the whole course of lives [27]. The socio-demographic and developmental characteristics of the individual, such as their psychodynamic equilibrium, ego structure and past experience, also influence the appraisal outcome [29]. The role of social support in the secondary appraisal is also prominent. It affects the coping ability of the individual in responding to a stressful stimulus, and gives rise to different interpretations of the stimulus [30].

Apart from the cognitive response to stress, affective, physiological and behavioral responses also take place and are described as "by-products of cognition" [31, p.11]. In fact, affective response usually accompanies each cognitive response. Primary appraisal of stressful stimuli usually gives rise to a generalized global anxiety reaction. Secondary appraisal, in turn, arouses more specific emotions. Plutchik, et al [32], who developed a systematic model of emotion, indicated that there are four pairs of basic bipolar emotions including a) fear and anger; b) joy and sadness; c) acceptance and distrust and d) expectancy and surprise. The negative emotions are more likely to occur in stressful situations [27]. Such emotions are originally adaptive in function. They not only serve as barometer that offer the individual feedback about themselves and their relationship with the environment, but also act as compelling signal in motivating him/her to cope with the situation in a more effective manner [33]. Negative emotions also initiate a set of physiological activities to support the body for the subsequent adaptive behavior. Such physiological responses are the result of hormonal stimulation and sympathetic activation, with the purpose of preparing the body for its "flight and fight response". The resulting end-organ activities, such as dilation of the coronary vessels, the vasodilatation of voluntary muscles and decreased peristalsis, are all considered the physiological display of stress.

In addition to the physiological response, the behavioral response, which is translated from the affective response, is also displayed. Lazarus [34] identified this response as the initiation of the ego-mechanism to ameliorate the perceived threat or to manage stressful emotions, and he called it "coping behavior". It consists of behavioral and cognitive efforts that serve to either manage or alter the source of stress, or to regulate the emotional response [35-36]. The effort which serves the former function is called "problem-focused coping" while the effort that serves the second function is called "emotional-focused coping" [1]. As implied in the functions of coping behavior, effective coping does not necessarily mean mastery of the stressful stimuli, but learning to "tolerate, minimize, accept or ignore the irresolvable stimuli" [1, p. 140] and, as such, is also an effective alternative.

Lazarus [27] considered a constellation of coping responses, including all those in the affective, physiological and behavioral dimensions, as being strategies that ultimately bring about changes in the situation. Any changes, which happen during the stressful situation as a result of coping, would then feedback to the individual and act as precursors to the cognitive reappraisal of the situation [34]. This would engender another set of affective, physiological and behavioral responses. This process of appraisal, coping and reappraisal of the stressful stimuli, takes place in a continuous manner until adaptation occurs. The constantly changing relationships between a person and his/ her environment are, therefore, reflected in the word "transaction" of the model. Adaptation refers to a situation in which there is a balance between the demands of the situation and the coping ability of the individual and results in the restoration of equilibrium and preservation of integrity [36]. On the other hand, when the impact of the stressful stimuli is very devastating, and repeated coping attempts fail to meet the demands of the situation, maladaptation results. In such a situation, the prolonged affective response, which evolves during the continuous process of coping, will convert into a negative mood state, and will result in arousing more detrimental physiological and maladaptive behavior.

THE MANIFESTATION OF NEGATIVE EMOTIONS IN HF PATIENTS

The chronic, debilitating and progressively deteriorating nature of heart failure poses great challenges to almost every aspects of the patients' everyday life. Previous studies have examined the ways that this vulnerable group conceived their life situation [37-43]. The results indicated that the course of HF disease was consistently conceived as arousing irresolvable stress to the patients. Negative conceptions of their life situation were dominant and could be categorized by three prominent negative views. They included 1) ambiguity in making sense of the illness experience; 2) feelings of incapacitation in coping with symptom of fatigue; and 3) feelings of dysfunction of their whole being. By the transactional model of stress, the high prevalence of negative emotions in patients with heart failure occurs as a result of ineffective coping and concomitant negative appraisals of their own situation.

Ambiguity in Making Sense of the Illness Experience

Effective adaptation to a chronic illness requires the patients to define the meaning of their life in living with the limitations and constraints imposed by the course of the disease [30]. The process of searching for new meaning commonly occurs through the steps of cognitive appraisal and reappraisal as described in the transactional model of stress [1], during which an individual attempts to interpret and cope with the impact of the disease on their overall being. HF is a syndrome that imposes multi-faceted debilitating effects on the life situation of the patients. Previous studies examining the adaptation process of HF patients consistently revealed their ambiguity in making sense of this disease. Their inability to search for new meaning in their own situations eventually triggered various maladaptive emotional responses.

Stull, et al [43] adopted a qualitative approach in examining the process of adaptation of HF patients. They found that the patients perceived the initial manifestation of the disease as a crisis event that placed them in a new and uncertain life situation. They experienced great difficulty in making sense of the cause of HF and the associated impact of the disease on the various aspects of their lives. The process of searching for new meaning was mainly hindered by fluctuations in their debilitating symptoms, the concomitant hospital admissions, the disruption to their usual role in life and identity, and the limited treatment options. Winters [44] also identified the high levels of uncertainty in HF patients. In addition to the above-mentioned causes, she found that feelings of uncertainty were related to the frequent change in the treatment regime, waiting for the diagnostic results, a lack of orientation about the treatment outcome and their future. Stull, et al [43] reported patients' concomitant emotional responses as feeling "scared", "worried" and "nervous". Some patients also conjured up the image of being near death.

Mahoney [37] examined the patients' experience in adapting to HF in a similar manner and used the words "disruption" and "incoherence" to illustrate the way the patients conceived their illness experience. In her study, the HF patients described their own situation as very burdensome. The impact of HF on the physical, emotional, social, economic and spiritual aspects of their lives greatly disrupted the usual order of patients' existence. The distressing symptoms and progressively deteriorating nature of the disease added difficulty to the patients in making sense out of the illness experience. The narrative findings such as "my (the patient) heart is the tug of war" (p. 432) and "this (the disease) doesn't get better" (p.432) reflected the patients' strong feeling of anxiety, struggling, uncertainty and loss of control in responding to the illness. Other studies also found that the HF patients described themselves or their own situation as "nowhere to turn to", "don't feel any harmony within myself" [39] and "if the machine (patient himself) is finish, …you've to accept it." [38, p. 583]. All of these narratives, indeed, indicated their internal sense of lacking harmony in living with HF. They also conceived the illness experience as imposing a hopeless and uncontrollable situation for them to cope with.

The results of the above-mentioned studies indicate that HF imposes a very distressing experience on the patients. They cognitively constructed this condition as not merely a disease that should be eliminated, but also as an illness experience that exerted an extraordinary demand on them. Their reported feelings of uncertainty, powerlessness, hopelessness and despair also implied the disease had challenged and exhausted their resources and ability to cope. Indeed, the loss of ability to control their situation was identified as one of the significant determinants of anxiety and depression in chronically ill patients [45]. Patients, who internalized a fatalistic view of their condition and future, were also at a high risk of developing depression, especially when the condition persists [46]. Other studies also identified the significant relationship between a high level of uncertainty and emotional distress, mood disturbance and anxiety among HF patients [21,47].

Feeling of Incapacitation in Coping with the Symptom of Fatigue

Fatigue is a common symptom that affects patients with various chronic illnesses. This symptom is also integral to HF [48-50], as a result of the underperfusion of skeletal muscle and other bodily tissues [51]. Although previous studies only identified sleep disturbance, physical symptoms and functional capacity as significantly relating factors [48,50], HF patients not only conceived this symptom as a physical condition, but also a psychological barrier, inhibiting them from participating in a fuller life. Studies examining their conception revealed that a prominent feeling of incapacitation resulted from this symptom.

Schaefer and Shober Potylycki [41] interviewed a group of HF patients (N = 38) and found that fatigue was a very prominent problem, affecting more than 70% of the sample. The patients described this symptom as not only a kind of physical tiredness, but a mental tiredness as well. They used the term "an undercurrent" to illustrate the effect of this symptom in compromising their ability. Their conceptions of fatigue including "tired muscle", being "done for", being "listless and unable to care for themselves" (p. 264) also conveyed their internal feelings of helplessness and decreased self-worthiness. They felt that they had lost their power and motivation to continue with their physical and social activities. They were annoyed and had lost any ambition for their future. Some of them were even afraid that fatigue would overcome them completely and that they would no longer be able to function. Martensson, et al [38] reported similar findings when using a phenomenological approach to examine the life experience of HF patients (N = 12). The patients described this symptom as not only a physically loss of power, but also a lack of mental motivation to initiate intended activities. Symptoms of fatigue as manifested in HF patients, therefore, not only exhausted their physical energy, but also depleted their mental will and power to assume a fuller way of life. Feelings of not being in control of their own lives were the dominant ones to emerge from findings of these two studies.

In fact, the feeling of incapacitation that resulted from their fatigue might be related to the adoption of the ineffective coping strategy of 'behavioral disengagement'. This is one of the avoidance strategies commonly used by chronically ill patients to overcome the symptom of fatigue, and is characterized by physical inactivity and withdrawal from daily life [52]. The reason for patients using this maladaptive illness behavior is commonly based on their belief that limiting activity and minimizing stress will help them to avoid a relapse and hasten their recovery [53-54]. In fact, this coping mechanism will actually further reduce the patients' tolerance of exertion. A vicious circle would be initiated and resulted in more fatigability and disability, and eventually leading to more negative emotions [55], frustration and even demoralization [56].

Fatigue is therefore perceived as an "overwhelming" feeling by HF patients, which wear out their entire well-being. The associated feelings of restriction in both their physical capacity and role, and in their social functioning, not only give rise to a strong sense of powerlessness over their own situation, but also devalue their entire existence. These negative views of themselves, their experience and their future have been identified as prominent factors in precipitating the negative emotion of depression in HF patients [57]. Indeed, Friedman and King [50] demonstrated the significant correlation between fatigue, as manifested in HF patients, and their perceived stress ($r = .43$, $p < .01$) and a lower level of life satisfaction ($r = -.36$, $p < .01$). Yu, et al [58] also identified fatigue as a significant factor among a wide range of socio-demographic and clinical variables associated with anxiety and depression in this vulnerable group.

Feeling of Dysfunction of Their Whole Being

The manifestation of HF results in very debilitating consequences for the patients. Distressing symptoms of fatigue and dyspnea, a compromised activity tolerance level, a complex self-care regime, their treatment-related lifestyle restriction, the relapse of cardiac event and the frequent hospital readmission, not only greatly diminish their physical independency, but also impose great challenges on them when it comes to continuing with their social participation and role fulfillment. Previous studies, which examined the ways HF patients conceived their life experience, found that the disease greatly threatened the self-system of the patients, and induced a strong feeling of dysfunction in their whole being [28-40,42].

Martensson, et al [38,39] found that HF patients had greater difficulty in adapting to their loss of role function and physical independency, and this resulted in a higher level of psychological distress. The patients reported a sense of worthlessness and restriction, as the symptoms limited their ability to continue with their usual role. They perceived themselves as being a burden to the people around them, with their own self-identity being greatly threatened. Feelings of anxiety were most prominent and gave rise to a sense of insecurity. The narrated feeling of "big cut-backs everywhere" [39, p.1220] was the best way the HF patients had of illustrating their internal sense of the lack of harmony within themselves.

Another study reported similar findings and revealed the physical and social losses as leading to high levels of psychological symptoms in HF patients [40]. Stanley [42] also found that anxiety was especially dominant in HF patients whose social role had been disturbed, and such feelings mainly stemmed from the fear of becoming a burden to their children. He commented that patients with acquired functional disabilities would inevitably encounter additional losses, such as loss of function, role and body image. Such experience of loss and the concomitant feeling of their own diminished integrity, precipitate the negative emotions of depression and anxiety [45,57]. Nickel, et al [59] also found that disablement in conducting usual activities was a significant predictor for anxiety (relative risk (RR) = 3.1, p = .001) and depression (RR = 3.8, p = 2.9) in patients with chronic cardiac disease. Indeed, Murberg, Bru, Aarsland, and colleagues (1998) identified perceived limitation in performing daily activities and leisure pursuits as a significant factor in contributing to the great variance in the depression score among HF patients (β = .69, p< .01). Tsay and Chao [60] also reported similar results in Chinese HF patients and identified a significant negative relationship between functional status and depressive symptoms (r = -.33, p < .001).

In summary, previous studies examining the life conception of HF patients revealed their prominent problems of adaptation. The three negative conceptions included ambiguity in making sense of the illness experience, the feeling of incapacitation in coping with the symptom of fatigue, and their feelings of dysfunction in their whole being, were dominant among this vulnerable group. According to the transactional model of stress [1], the persistence of such negative cognitive conception greatly hindered effective adaptation to the disease, and resulted in the configuration of the negative emotions including both anxiety and depression.

IMPACTS OF NEGATIVE EMOTIONS: A THEORETICAL EXPLANATION

The persistent manifestation of such negative emotions is not only detrimental to patients' psychological integrity, but also arouses harmful physiological responses and maladaptive behavior in the individual. The ultimate effect is especially deleterious to their cardiovascular health and the disease progression. In fact, the ways in which negative emotions impact so detrimentally on health have been widely described, and labeled as the direct psycho-physiological and indirect behavioral pathways [61-65].

The Direct Psycho-physiological Pathway

The direct psycho-physiological pathway delineates the direct detrimental effect of negative emotions on cardiovascular health. According to the transactional model of stress [1], manifestation of negative emotions is followed by the initiation of a physiological response in order to enhance the coping of an individual. However, when negative emotions are experienced continually in a persistent manner, the associated physiological arousal will be intensified, and will result in excessive activation of the sympathetic-adrenal-medullary (SAM) system and the hypothalamic-pituitary-adrenocortical (HPA) axis [66-68]. The direct psycho-physiological pathway describes the relationship between excessive negative emotional arousal and the subsequent pathological changes in cardiovascular system.

Detrimental Activation of the SAM System in HF Patients

The detrimental effect of persistent activation of the SAM is related to the altered ratio of sympathetic and parasympathetic activities, in which sympathetic activity becomes more predominant [64]. This is because the change in autonomic response brings about a series of physiological changes including increased blood pressure, heart rate, circulatory levels of epinephrine and nonepinephrine and constriction of peripheral of blood vessels. Several studies have demonstrated increased sympathetic activity in cardiac patients who have high levels of psychological distress [69-70]. All of these physiological responses have been implicated in the development of cardiovascular diseases, such as coronary artery disease (CAD) [71] and HT [72]. Indeed, the physiological responses associated with prolonged SAM activation are especially deleterious to HF patients who are already characterized by a greatly increased sympathetic outflow. Such responses have been found to precipitate two pathological conditions of myocardial ischemia and cardiac arrhythmia in this vulnerable group.

For the condition of myocardial ischemia, excessive SAM activation increases the rate and force of myocardial contraction as well as the vascular tone, resulting in a greater myocardial workload. On the other hand, the myocardial blood supply is compromised as excessive SAM activation a) increases the coronary artery spasm especially in those who have a coronary endothelium injury [73,74]; b) decreases coronary vasodilatation in response to stress [74], c) promotes platelet aggregation [76] which precipitates a coronary thrombobtic event [77], lowers the threshold for myocardial ischemia [78] and produces atherogenesis [78]; d) evokes an intra-lumenal haemodynamic shearing force which promotes the formation of atherosclerosis by inducing endothelial damage [79] and e) stimulates immunological reaction within blood vessel walls which accelerates the formation of plague [80]. SAM activation therefore alters the condition of the myocardial blood supply and demand factors, and precipitates the condition of myocardial ischemia.

As far as the development of cardiac arrhythmia is concerned, two mechanisms have been suggested as attributing to the effect. Firstly, SAM activation increases the circulating level of epinephrine and nonepinephrine. Both of these hormones reduce the repetitive extra systole threshold of the heart and thereby decrease electrical stability of the myocardium [81]. This condition would be worse if the patients already presented with myocardial ischemia [82]. Secondly, the SAM activation also reduces the heart rate variability through an alteration of the autonomic nervous regulation [83]. The reduced heart rate variability is, in fact, an important triggering factor for cardiac arrhythmia [84]. Previous studies have also shown that reduced heart rate variability is an important risk factor for mortality among patients with HF [85,86].

Detrimental Activation of the HPA Axis in HF Patients

HPA hyperactivity is detrimental to the condition of HF, as it further compromises the myocardial blood supply. The excessive activation of the HPA axis increases the circulating level of corticotropin-releasing hormone, adrenocorticotropic hormone and cortisol [66]. These three hormones would affect fat metabolism and blood pressure regulation, and cause the pathological conditions of hypercholesterolemia, hypertriglyceridemia and HT [64]. High levels of cortisol also cause damage to the vascular endothelial cell and intima and delay normal healing of blood vessels [87]. All of these pathological conditions would precipitate the development of atherosclerosis and further decrease the coronary blood flow. The nourishment of myocardium is further reduced, and aggravating the manifestation of symptoms in HF. Previous study has also demonstrated the effect of HPA activity in developing atherosclerosis [88].

The Indirect Behavioral Pathway

The indirect behavioral pathway focuses the discussion on the behavioral changes that occur in response to high levels of negative emotions and places people at risk of disease onset and of increased severity [62,89]. The impact of negative emotions in hindering an individual from performing effective self-care and maintaining the quality and quantity of social relationships are suggested as being responsible for poor health outcomes in patients with cardiac diseases. As effective self-care management is an essential element in the successful control of HF, and social support also serves as an important resource to buffer stress associated with chronic illness, the behavioral changes associated with persistent negative emotions would cause further detrimental impact on the health outcomes of HF patients.

The relationship between negative emotions and poor self-care management is suggested as being the cause of poor motivation and morale in patients who are following a treatment regime [90]. High levels of psychological stress impair the cognitive function of chronically ill patients and can prevent them from making sound decision about monitoring and managing their own physical condition and seeking health care [91]. There is abundant empirical evidence to suggest that the effect of high levels of psychological distress on the effective management of the treatment regimen of cardiac patients. Romanelli, et al [92] found that older patients with myocardial infarction and a higher level of psychological distress were less likely to be adhering to the dietary modification, medication and exercise regimen 4 months after hospitalization. Other studies revealed similar findings and showed that depressed cardiac patients were less adherent to their cardiac medication regimen [93], lifestyle risk factor interventions and cardiac rehabilitation programs [94]. A high level of negative emotions therefore compromises effective self-care management in HF patients, and aggravates poor health outcomes.

Previous studies also demonstrated the suggestion of the indirect behavioral pathway concerning the influence of negative emotion on the patient's interaction with their social system. They found that high levels of psychological distress interfered with the enactment of normative social roles, participation in necessary social interactions and the quality of interaction with their social network [95,96]. Moreover, having to offer continuing support to persons who are psychologically distressed may also exhaust and disintegrate their social network [66]. All of these behavioral changes reduce the network size and interfere with its function of promoting positive health practice, enhancing psychosocial care and providing resources for facing the stressful situation [97]. Indeed, previous studies have demonstrated the increased risk of HF patients, who have higher levels of psychological distress, in developing social isolation and loneliness [98]. Social support has been consistently identified as an important factor in relating and predicting positive health outcomes in cardiac patients [99-101], so the social behavioral changes that are associated with high levels of negative emotions in HF patients, further hinder effective adaptation. Figure 1 outlines the manifestation of negative emotions as a result of ineffective coping in patients with heart failure and the mechanisms for the negative emotions to exhibit its detrimental impact on their health outcomes.

IMPACTS OF NEGATIVE EMOTIONS: AN UPDATE OF EVIDENCE

The impact of negative emotions on the health outcomes of patients with general cardiac disease or HF has been extensively investigated. The accumulated evidence concurs with the theoretical propositions of the direct psycho-physiological pathway and the indirect behavioral pathway. Negative emotions have proved to be a very powerful factor in compromising almost every dimension of the HRQL. There is empirical evidence suggesting their detrimental effect in aggravating cardiac symptoms, decreasing functional status, reducing HRQL, increasing cardiac events and even in increasing hospital readmissions and mortality rates.

Spertus, et al [102] determined the influence of depression on disease specific symptoms, functional status and HRQL in 1,282 outpatients with CAD. By using the Mental Health Inventory, they found that there were marked differences between depressed and non-depressed patients in all of these parameters, with the latter group demonstrating more favorable outcomes. When conducting the follow-up reassessment (n = 1025) three months later, the disease-specific functional status was found to have deteriorated in patients who remained depressed or whose depression had increased, but not in their non-depressed counterparts. The authors therefore concluded that there was a synchrony of change between depression and functional status in this disease group.

Indeed, similar findings were reported in 344 patients with myocardial infarction (MI). [103]. By comparing the longitudinal health outcomes of probable cases with the non-cases of anxiety and depression as categorized by the Hospital Anxiety and Depression Scale (HADS), anxiety and depression were identified as the significant predictors for poor physical, psychological and social outcomes, when measured by the Short Form-36 HRQL scale at both 3 months and 6 months endpoints. In addition, the distressed patients demonstrated more functional deficits across a range of important activities of daily living (p = .0008), leisure (p = .006) and social (p = .0001) activities, and reported statistically non-significant a greater number of physical symptoms including chest pain and breathlessness. They were also more frequent users of primary care visits (p < .05) and home visits by their general practitioner for routine or emergency care (p < .05).

Numerous studies reported consistent findings in demonstrating the prominent effect of negative emotions in worsening the various dimensions of HRQL in cardiac patients. Steffens, et al [104] found that the presence of psychological distress was significantly associated with more functional impairment in patients with CAD. The patients had more than doubled the risk of developing deficits in performing self-maintenance (odds ratio (OR): 3.28, 95% CI: 1.35-7.95, p<.001) and instrumental activities of daily living (OR: 2.70, 95% CI: .58-12.56, p<.001). The detrimental effects of psychological distress on the other health

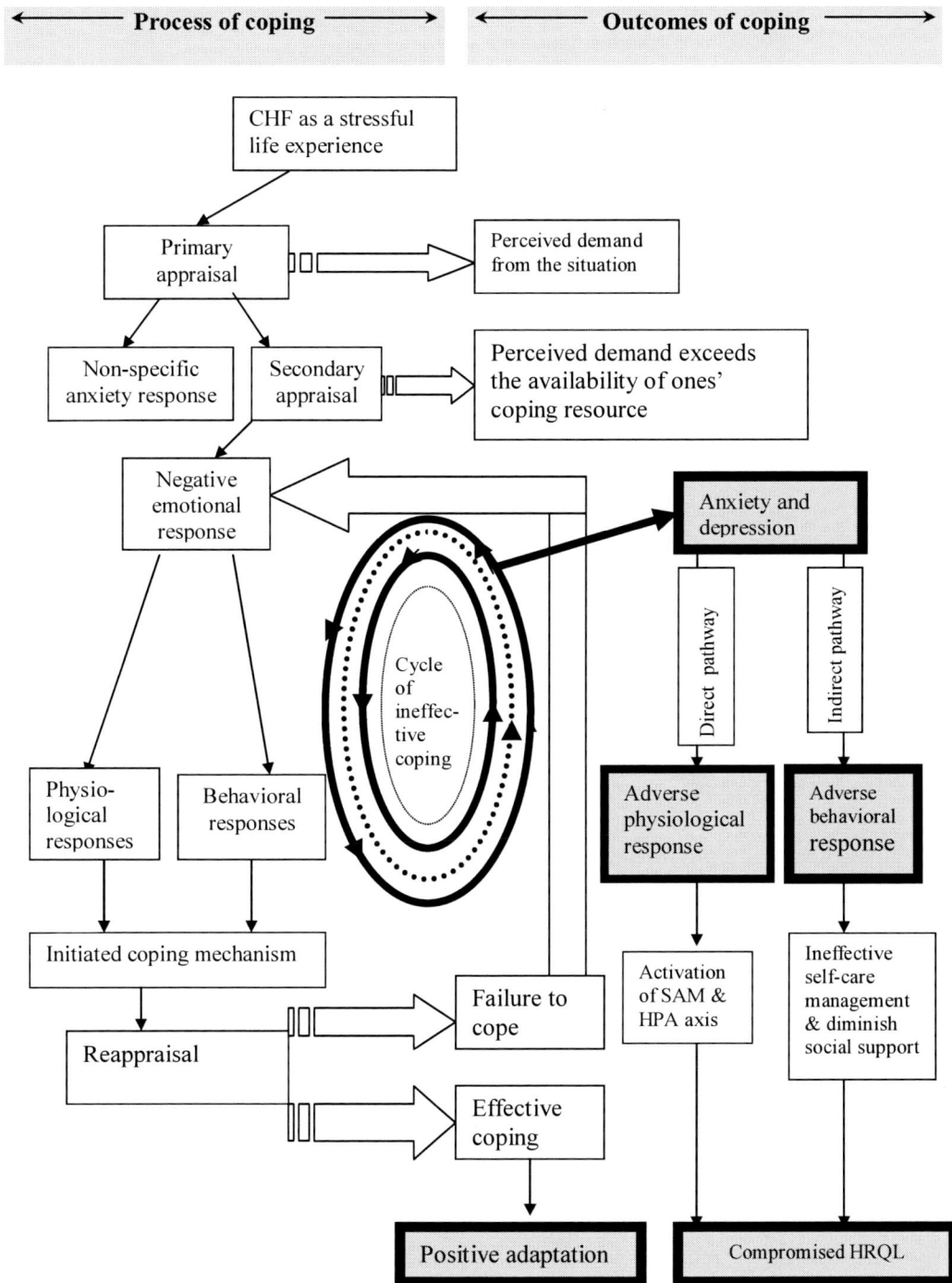

Figure 1. The process and outcomes of coping of heart failure patients. The patients who experience persistent ineffective coping would have mood disturbance and impaired health-related quality of life (HRQL).

outcomes were similar. The depressed CAD patients were twice as likely to develop adverse cardiac symptoms, functional impairments and poorer HRQL, when compared with their non-depressed counterparts who had similar demographic, cardiac and co-morbid characteristics [105]. All of the pervasive prognostic impact of negative emotions on an individual's well-being also affect patients with MI, and manifested in an even longer-term manner. In particular, depression was found to worsen all aspects of the HRQL of MI patients over a period of 1 year [106], and even up to five years [107]. In addition, Denollet and Brutsaert [108] found that patients with MI who experienced anxiety and depression were more likely to have cardiac events in six to ten years, and the odd ratios were reported as 3.4 (95% CI: 1.2 – 9.6) and 4.3 (95% CI: 1.4 – 13.3) respectively. Psychological distress was even found to be a significant predictor of mortality in cardiac patients and the adjusted hazard ratio was reported to be as high as 4.29 (95% CI: 3.14-5.44, p = .013) [109].

When applied specifically to patients with HF, negative emotions exerted similar deleterious effects on the HRQL of the sufferers. Clarke, et al [110] conducted a large-scale longitudinal study to examine the predictive power of psychological distress on the functional status of 2,922 HF patients. The results indicated that anxiety and depression, as measured by the Profile of Mood States, were significant predictors for the presence of impairment in the intermediate activity of daily living at one year, with RR = 1.83 (95% CI: 1.47-2.27) and RR = 1.96 (95% CI: 1.59-2.42) respectively. A comparable increase in the risk of impaired social activities (OR: 1.39 – 1.72) was also noticed. All of these findings were independent of the influences of baseline functional status, comorbid medical condition and disease progression of HF over the intervening year. This well-designed study therefore provided definite evidence suggesting the detrimental impact of negative emotions on the physical and social functioning of HF patients. Vaccarino, et al [23] reported similar findings, and depression was found to predict greater functional decline in HF patients (OR = 1.10 - 1.82; $p < .004$), after adjusting for the possible influences of the baseline demographic, functional and clinical variables. In addition to affecting their actual functional level in day-to-day life, negative emotions also affected the patients' perceived functional status. Skotzko, et al [111] found that 42% of the depressed HF patients ($N = 33$), as diagnosed by the Center for Epidemiological Studies Depression Scale, tended to under-estimate their functional ability when compared with their non-depressed counterparts, even though both groups had comparable energy expenditure, maximal heart rate and maximal oxygen consumption.

There is other evidence that demonstrates the role of negative emotions in worsening the disease progression and prognosis of HF patients. Murberg, et al [22] examined the relationship between negative emotions and disease symptoms amongst a group of 199 HF patients, who were recruited from an outpatient cardiology practice. They revealed a significant bivariate correlation between depression and the symptoms of dyspnea ($r = .37$, $p < .001$) as well as perceived physical limitation ($r = .64$, $p < .001$). After controlling the effect of disease severity, as measured by the New York Heart Association Classification (NYHA) and the Plasma N-terminal atrial natriuretic factor, depressed mood was also found to be a significant predictor of mortality in this vulnerable group, with a hazard ratio of 1.9 ($p = .002$). In addition, Jiang, et al [112] also identified that the HF patients who were comorbid with major depression, were more than twice as likely as the non-depressed, and mildly depressed patients to be readmitted to hospital within 1 year of discharge, with OR = 2.57

(95% CI: 1.16-5.68, p = .04) and OR = 2.98 (95% CI: 1.17-7.59, p = .03) respectively. These calculated odd ratios were independent of the influence of demographic characteristics, disease severity and etiological factors. A more recent study provided even more alarming findings [113]. When the influence of baseline socio-demographic, functional and clinical conditions was eliminated, the risk of death in clinically depressed HF patients was as high as three times as that of their non-depressed counterparts (hazards ratio: 3.0, 95% CI: 1.4-6.4, p = .004).

The above studies provided strong evidence of the detrimental effects of negative emotions on the various dimensions of HRQL and on the disease progression of HF patients. Indeed, psychological factors were found to override the other clinical and socio-demographic factors in determining their HRQL. Dracup, et al [20] examined the relationship between HRQL and different soico-demogarphic, psychological and clinical factors of HF patients. They identified that depression as the most predominant factor, which independently accounted for a 34% variance in HRQL in this vulnerable group. A more recent study echoes these findings [19]. Among a wide scope of demographic, social and clinical factors, psychological distress, as measured by the HADS, was the most significant predictor of disease-specific HRQL in HF patients (N = 227), and also accounted for 34% of its variance. These studies indicate that negative emotions will be a very significant risk marker for poor health outcomes in HF patients.

RECOMMENDATIONS ON CLINICAL PRACTICE

With the dominance of the biomedical model in the health care context, enormous resources and expertise have been invested in the development of advanced medical treatments for HF patients. However, in relation to the nature and prognosis of the disease, the advances in medical treatment for HF patients do not result in a marked improvement in their morbidity and mortality. The hospital admission and mortality rates for this vulnerable group remain high. As a result, it is critically important to extend the mainstay of treatment for HF from the present advanced medical therapy to those interventions that are targeted at ameliorating the predictors for poor health outcomes. This is especially true when the incidence of HF is expected to rise in the next decade. Moser and Worster [114], indeed, made the same point when discussing the direction of current health care practice for HF patients.

Negative emotions, from both a theoretical and an empirical perspective, have a very detrimental prognostic impact on almost every vital aspect of the well-being of HF patients. Independent of any medical risks, evidence consistently indicates negative emotions significantly predict higher morbidity and mortality in this vulnerable group of patients. Any unrecognized and untreated psychological distress or impaired HRQL would, therefore, be transferred directly into a further rise in the astronomical health care costs for this group of patients. Accordingly, there is a pressing need for health care professionals to target the psychological risk factors for prompt intervention.

Stress management techniques (SMT) have been widely used as a clinical intervention to promote the successful adaptation of patients who are suffering from various chronic illnesses. It covers a range of therapeutic techniques, including progressive muscle relaxation, guided imagery, autogenic training, and breathing exercise, which can be used either individually or in combination. The ultimate purpose of SMT is "to eliminate those stresses that can be eliminated; to master stress that cannot be eliminated; and to develop techniques for recognition and modification of an individual's own response to stress" [115, p. 575]. This specification accords with the transactional model of stress [1], which categorized coping as being either problem-focused or emotional-focused. As applied to HF patients, SMT would be most relevant to be used to promote their emotional coping and, hence, eliminate the emotional etiological factor in the deterioration of cardiac pathology.

The effectiveness of SMT in promoting emotional coping and clinical outcomes in patients with various cardiac pathologies such as hypertension, coronary artery disease (CAD) and myocardial infarction (MI) has been widely documented. Evidence consistently indicated that SMT is effective in alleviating negative emotions, mediating the biological risk factors for the progression of cardiac disease, lessening the symptoms, reducing the recurrence of cardiac condition and mortality [116-118]. There is also increasing evidence to suggest the therapeutic effects of SMT in HF patients. While the beneficial effect of SMT on emotional well-being is most convincing [119-124], some studies also demonstrated its effects in reducing symptom control [119,121,124] as well as lowering excessive sympathetic-related physiologic arousal [119].

Deterring by all these empirical evidence, SMT should be incorporated as an adjunctive non-pharmacological intervention in the context of care for elderly patients with HF. In the last two decades, multi-disciplinary disease management program has emerged as a model of care to enhance the health outcomes of HF patients [125-127]. Such programs can either be launched in hospital setting as a discharge intervention, or be launched in community health care settings such as heart failure clinic, geriatric day care center and integrated community rehabilitation center. However, a review indicated that the integral component of these programs is limited to intensive patient education, exercise training, drug titration, intensive disease surveillance through follow-up telephone call, home visit or clinic visits. Psychological care intervention is found to be almost absent or just limited to non-specific support or counseling [128]. Indeed, the Disease Management Association of America [129] emphasizes the importance of incorporating humanistic outcomes in the evaluation of any disease management program. SMT, which has a particularly positive impact on the psychological status of elderly HF patients, therefore, need to be considered as an integral element of the disease management program, in order to enhance their post-discharge outcomes in a more holistic manner. Indeed, SMT has been found to be an acceptable and feasible intervention for heart failure patients [130]. It can be taught to the patients during their hospital stay or in out-patient setting. Using group-based training is also recommended as it is a means to provide the client with peer support and enhance their adherence behavior to non-pharmacological behavior [131]. Involving the family members or friends, especially for older patients, is also effective, as their support not only serve to reinforce proper techniques, but also motivates patients to practice regularly by promoting the feeling of closeness [132]. Providing self -help materials such as taped instruction and information booklets can facilitate self-directed learning and promote skill development. Patients can, hence, use it more effectively to cope with stress associated with the illness experience.

Effective management of chronic illness, indeed, emphasizes the importance of patients undertaking their own self-care [133], integrating SMT into the care of HF patients as a self-regulatory technique, provides a good opportunity for them to independently and actively participate in their own care.

CONCLUSION

The symptomatic, relapsing and progressively deteriorating nature of heart failure not only causes debilitating physical insults, but also poses enormous psychological burden to the patients. Although research evidence indicated the manifestation and detrimental impact of negative emotions in patients with heart failure, psychological intervention that is specifically designed to assist patients to combat negative emotions, has received least attention. In views of the convincing evidence in suggesting the effects of SMT on not only the psychological but also the physical outcomes of patients with cardiac pathology, including heart failure, this intervention should be incorporated as a crucial component in the heart failure management.

REFERENCES

[1]   Lazarus RS, Folkman S: *Stress, appraisal and coping*. New York: Springer Pub. Co, 1984.

[2]   Levy D, Kenchaiah S, Larson MG, Benjamin EJ, Kupka MJ, Ho KK, Murabito JM. Vasan RS: Long-term trends in the incidence of and survival with heart failure. *New Eng J Med* 2002; 347(18): 1397-402.

[3]   Mendez GF, Cowie MR: The epidemiological features of heart failure in developing countries: a review of the literature. *Int J Cardiol*, 2001; 80(2-3): 213-9.

[4]   Hunt SA, Baker DS, Chin MH, Cinquegrani MP, Feldman AM, Francis GS: ACC/AHA the 1995 Guidelines for the evaluation and management of heart failure, 2001.   Retrieved   Dec   18,   2007   from http://www.americanheart.org/downloadable/heart/   101320118293HFGuideline Final/pdf.

[5]   Ho KK, Pinsky JL, Kannel WB, Levy D: The epidemiology of heart failure: the Framingham study. *J Am Coll Cardiol* 1993; 22(4 Suppl A): 6A-13A.

[6]   Cowie MR, Mosterd A, Wood DA, Deckers JW, Poole-Wilson PA, Sutton G C, Grobbee DE: The epidemiology of heart failure. *Eur Heart J* 1997; 18(2): 208-25.

[7]   Petersen S, Rayner M: Coronary Heart Disease Statistics 2002 Edition. British Heart Foundation Health Promotion Research Group. Oxford: Department of Public Health, University of Oxford, 2002.

[8]   Naylor CD, Slaughter P. (Eds.): *Cardiovascular health and services in Ontario: an ICES atlas* (1st ed.). Toronto: ICES, 1999.

[9]   Morgan S, Smith H, Simpson I, Liddiard GS, Raphael H, Pickering RM, Mant D: Prevalence and clinical characteristics of left ventricular dysfunction among elderly

patients in general practice setting: cross sectional survey. *BMJ* 1999; 318(7180): 368-72.

[10]   Campbell DJ: Heart failure: how we prevent the epidemic? *Med J Aust* 2003; 179(8): 422-5.

[11]   Funk M, Krumholz HM: Epidemiologic and economic impact of advanced heart failure. *J Cardiovas Nurs* 1996; 10(2): 1-10.

[12]   Kannel WB, Belanger AJ: Epidemiology of heart failure. *Am Heart J* 1991; 121: 951-7.

[13]   McDonagh TA, Morrison CE, Lawrence A, Ford I, Tunstall-Pedoe H, McMurray JJ, Dargie HJ: Symptomatic and asymtomatic left-ventricular systolic dysfunction in an urban population. *Lancet* 1997; 350(9081): 823-33.

[14]   Ceia F, Fonseca C, Mota T, Morais H, Matias F, de Sousa A et al: Prevalence of chronic heart failure in Southwestern Europe: the EPICA study. *Eur J Heart Fail* 2002; 4(4): 531-9.

[15]   McMurray JJ, Stewart S: Epidemiology, aetiology, and prognosis of heart failure. *Heart* 2000, 83(5), 596-602.

[16]   Wiseman S, LeJemetek TH, Sonnenblick EH: Congestive heart failure in the elderly. In, DD Tresch, WS Aronow (Eds.), *Cardiovascular disease in the elderly patient* (2nd ed., pp. 467-480). NY: Marcel Dekker, 1999.

[17]   Lainscak M, Keber I: Patient's view of heart failure: from the understanding to the quality of life. *Eur J Cardiovas Nurs* 2003; 2(4): 275-81.

[18]   Riedinger MS, Dracup KA, Brecht ML, Padilla G, Sarna L, Ganz PA: Quality of life in patients with heart failure: do gender differences exist? *Heart Lung* 2001; 30(2): 105-16.

[19]   Yu DSF, Lee TF, Woo, J: Correlates of health-related quality of life in elderly Chinese patients with heart failure. *Res Nurs Health* 2004; 27(4): 332-44.

[20]   Dracup K, Walden JA, Lynne W, Stevenson W, Brecht ML: Quality of life in patients with advanced heart failure. *J Heart Lung Transplant* 1992: 11(2 Pt 1), 273-9.

[21]   Hawthorne MH, Hixon ME: Functional status, mood disturbance and quality of life in patients with heart failure. *Prog Cardiovas Nurs* 1994; 9(1): 22-32.

[22]   Murberg TA, Bru E, Aarsland T, Svebak S: Functional status and depression among men and women with congestive heart failure. *Int J Psychiatry Med* 1998; 28(3): 273-91.

[23]   Vaccarino V, Kasl SV, Abramson J, Krumholz HM. Depressive symptoms and risk of functional decline and death in patients with heart failure. *J Am Coll Cardiol* 2001; 38(1): 199-205.

[24]   Freedland KE, Rich MW, Skala JA., Carney RM, Davila-Roman VG, Jaffe AS: Prevalence of depression in hospitalized patients with congestive heart failure. *Psychosom Med* 2003; 65(1): 119-28.

[25]   American Psychiatric Association Work Group to Revise DSM-III. *Diagnostic and Statistical Manual of Mental Disorders* (4th ed.). Washington, DC: American Psychiatric Association, 1994.

[26]   Koenig HG: Depression in hospitalized older patients with congestive heart failure. *Gen Hosp Psychiatry* 1998; 20(1): 29-43.

[27]   Lazarus RS: Progress on a cognitive-motivational-relational theory of emotion. *Am Psychol* 1991; 46(8): 819-34.

[28]   Molassiotis A: A conceptual model of adaptation to illness and quality of life for cancer patients treated with bone marrow transplants. *J Adv Nurs* 1997; 26(3): 572-9.

[29]   Rodin G, Craven J, Littlefield C: *Depression in the medically ill: an integrated approach.* NY: Brunner/Mazel, 1991.

[30]   Molassiotis A, van den Akker OB, Boughton BJ: Perceived social support, family environment and psychosocial recovery in bone marrow transplant long-term survivors. *Soc Sci Med* 1997; 44(3): 317-25.

[31]   Scott DW, Oberst MT, Dropkin MJ: A stress-coping model. *Adv Nurs Sci* 1980; 3: 9-23.

[32]   Plutchik R, Kellerman H, Conte HR: A structural theory of ego defences and emotions. In C. E. Izard (Ed.), *Emotions in personality and psychopathology* (pp. 227-260). NY: Plenum Press, 1979.

[33]   Stuart GW: Emotional responses and mood disorder. In. G. W. Stuart, & S. J. Sundeen (Eds.), *Principles and practice of psychiatric nursing* (5th ed., pp. 413-451). St Louis: Mosby, 1995.

[34]   Lazarus, R. S: Coping theory and research: past, present, and future. *Psysom Med* 1993; 55(3): 234-47.

[35]   Lazarus RS, Cohen JB, Folkman S, Manner A, Schafer C: Psychological stress and adaptation: some unresolved issues. In H Selye (Ed.), *Seyle's guide to stress research* (pp. 90-117). NY: Van Nostrandt Reinhold, 1980.

[36]   Lazarus RS, DeLongis A, Folkman S, Gruen R: Stress and adaptational outcomes. The problem of confounded measures. *Am Psychol* 1985: 40(7): 770-85.

[37]   Mahoney JS: An ethnographic approach to understanding the illness experiences of patients with congestive heart failure and their family members. *Heart Lung* 2001: 30(6): 429-36.

[38]   Martensson J, Karlsson JE, Fridlund B: Male patients with congestive heart failure and their conception of the life situation. *J Adv Nurs* 1997; 25(3): 579-86.

[39]   Martensson J, Karlsson JE, Fridlund B: Female patients with congestive heart failure: how they conceive their life situation. *J Adv Nurs* 1998; 28(6): 1216-24.

[40]   Rhodes DL, Bowles CL: Heart failure and its impact on older women's lives. *J Adv Nurs* 2002; 39(5): 441-9.

[41]   Schaefer KM, Shober Potylycki MJ: Fatigue associated with congestive heart failure: use of Levine's Conservation Model. *J Adv Nurs* 1993; 18(2): 260-8.

[42]   Stanley M: Congestive heart failure in the elderly. *Geriatric Nurs* 1999; 20(4): 180-5.

[43]   Stull DE, Starling R, Haas G, Young JB: Becoming a patient with heart failure. *Heart Lung* 1999; 28(4): 284-92.

[44]   Winters CA: Heart failure: living with uncertainty. *Prog Cardiovas Nurs* 1999; 14(3): 85-91.

[45]   Pennix BW, Beekman ATF, Ormel J, Kriegsman DMW, Boeke AJP, Van Eijk JT, Deeg DJ: Psychological status among elderly people with chronic disease: Does type of disease play a part? *J Psychosom Res* 1996: 40(5): 521-34.

[46]   Buckwalter KC, Babich KS: Psychologic and physiologic aspects of depression. *Nurs Clin North Am* 1990; 25(4): 945-54.

[47]   Christman NJ, McConnell EA, Pfeiffer C, Webster KK, Schmitt M, Ries J: Uncertainty, coping, and distress following myocardial infarction: transition from hospital to home. *Res Nurs Health* 1988; 11(2):71-82.

[48]   Broström A, Strömberg A, Dahlström U, Fridlund B: Patients with congestive heart failure and their conceptions of their sleep situation. *J Adv Nurs* 2001; 24(4): 520-9.

[49]   Drexler H, Coats AJ: Explaining fatigue in congestive heart failure. *Ann Rev Med* 1996; 4: 241-56.

[50]   Friedman MM, King KB: Correlates of fatigue in older women with heart failure. *Heart Lung* 1995; 24(6): 512-8.

[51]   Wilson JR, Mancini DM, Dunkman WB: Exertional fatigue due to skeletal muscle dysfunction in patients with heart failure. *Circulation* 1993; 87(2): 470-5.

[52]   Ray C, Jefferies S, Weir WR: Coping and other predictors of outcome in chronic fatigue syndrome: a 1-year follow-up. *J Psychosom Res* 1997; 43(4): 405-15.

[53]   Sharpe M, Hawton K, Seagroatt V, Pasvol G: Follow up of patients presenting with fatigue to an infectious diseases clinic. *BMJ* 1992; 305(6846): 147-52.

[54]   Surawy C, Hackmann A, Hawton K, Sharpe M: Chronic fatigue syndrome: a cognitive approach. *Beh Res Ther* 1995; 33(5): 535 –44.

[55]   Janz NK, Janevic MR, Dodge JA, Fingerlin TE, Scork MA, Mosca LJ, Clark NM: Factors influencing quality of life in older women with heart disease. *Med Care* 2001; 39(6): 588-98.

[56]   Deale A, David AS: Chronic fatigue syndrome: evaluation and management. *J Neuropsychiatr Clin Neurosci* 1994; 6(2): 189-94.

[57]   Johnson LH, Roberts SL: A cognitive model for assessing depression and providing nursing interventions in cardiac intensive care. *Intensive & Crit Care Nurs* 1996; 12(3): 138-46.

[58]   Yu DSF, Lee DTF, Woo J, Thompson DR: Correlates of psychological distress in elderly patients with congestive heart failure. *J Psychosom Res* 2004; 57: 573-81.

[59]   Nickel JT, Brown KJ, Smith BA: Depression and anxiety among chronically ill heart patients: age differences in risk and predictors. *Res Nurs Health* 1990; 13(2): 87-97.

[60]   Tsay SL, Chao YF: Effects of perceived self-efficacy and functional status on depression in patients with chronic heart failure. *J Nurs Res* 2002; 10(4): 271-8.

[61]   Carney RM, Freedland KE, Miller GE, Jaffe AS: Depression as a risk factor for cardiac mortality and morbidity: a review of potential mechanism. *J Psychosom Res* 2002; 53(4): 897-902.

[62]   Kubzansky LD, Kawachi I: Going to the heart of the matter: do negative emotions cause coronary heart disease? *J Psychosom Res* 2000; 48(4-5): 323-37.

[63]   Lovallo WR, Gerin W: Psychophysiological reactivity: mechanisms and pathways to cardiovascular disease. *Psychosom Med* 2003; 65(1): 36-45.

[64]   Musselman DL, Evans DL, Nemeroff CB. The relationship of depression to cardiovascular disease: epidemiology, biology, and treatment. *Arch Gen Psychiatr* 1998; 55(7): 580-92.

[65] Rozanski A, Blumenthal JA, Kaplan J: Impact of psychological factors on the pathogenesis of cardiovascular disease and implications for therapy. *Circulation* 1999; 99(16): 2192-217.

[66] Cohen S, Rodriguez MS: Pathway linking affective disturbances and physical disorders. *Health Psychol* 1995; 14(5): 374-80.

[67] Kamarck T, Jennings JR: Biobehavioral factors in sudden cardiac death. *Psychol Bull* 1991; 109(1): 42-75.

[68] Ritchie JC, Nemeroff CB: Stress, the hypothalamic-pituitary-adrenal axis, and depression. In JA McCubbing, PG Kaufmann, CB Nemeroff (Eds.), *Stress, neuropeptides and systemic disease* (pp. 181-197). San Diego, C.A.: Academic Press, 1991.

[69] Roose SP, Dalack GW: Treating the depressed patient with cardiovascular problems. *J Clin Psychiatry* 1992; 53(Suppl): 25-31.

[70] Veith RC, Lewis N, Linares OA, Barnes RF, Raskind MA, Villacres EC, Murburg MM, Ashleigh EA, Castillo S, Peskind ER: Sympathetic nervous system activity in major depression. Basal and desipramine-induced alternations in plasma norepinephrine kinetics. *Arch Gen Psychiatry* 1994; 51(5): 411-22

[71] Manuck SB, Marsland AL, Kaplan JR, Williams JK: The pathogenicity of behavior and its neuroendocrine mediation: an example from coronary artery disease. *Psychosom Med* 1995; 57(3): 257-83.

[72] Krantz DS, Manuck SB: Acute psychophysiologic reactivity and risk of cardiovascular disease: a review and methodologic critique. *Psychol Bull* 1984; 96(3): 435-64.

[73] Boltwood MD, Taylor CB, Burke MB, Grogin H, Giacomini J: Anger report predicts coronary artery vasomotor response to mental stress in atherosclerotic segments. *Am J Cardiol* 1993; 72(8): 1316-65.

[74] Lacy CR, Contrade RJ, Robbins ML, Tannenbaum AK, Moreyra AE, Chelton S, Kostis JB: Coronary vasoconstriction induced by mental stress (simulated public speaking). *Am J Cardiol* 1995; 75(7): 503-05.

[75] Dakak N, Quyyumi AA, Eisenhofer G, Goldstein DS, Cannon RO. III: Sympathetically mediated effects of metal stress on the cardiac microcirculation of patients with coronary artery disease. *Am J Cardiol* 1995; 76: 125-130.

[76] Ardlie NG, McGuiness JA, Garett JJ: Effect on human platelets of catecholamines at levels achieved in the circulation. *Atherosclerosis* 1985; 58(1-3), 251-59.

[77] von Kanel R, Mills PJ, Fainman C, Dimsdale JE: Effects of psychological stress and psychiatric disorders on blood coagulation and fibronolysis: a biobehavioral pathway to coronary artery disease? *Psychosom Med* 2001; 63(4): 531-44.

[78] Markovitz JH, Matthews KA: Platelets and coronary heart disease: Potential psychophysiologic mechanisms. *Psychosom Med* 1991: 53(6): 643-68.

[79] Kawachi I, Sparrow D, Vokonas PS, Weiss ST: Decreased heart rate variability in men with phobic anxiety (data from the Normative Aging Study). *Am J Cardiol* 1995; 75(14): 882-5.

[80]   Kop WJ, Cohen N: Immune system involvement in cardiovascular disease. In R. Ader, D. L. Felten, & N. Cohen (Eds.), *Psychoneuroimmunology* (3rd ed., pp. 525-545). San Diego, CA: Academic, 2000.

[81]   Hohnloser SH, Verrier RL, Lown B: Effects of adrenergic and muscarinic receptor stimulation on serum potassium concentrations and myocardial electrical stability. *Cardiovasc Res* 1986; 20(12): 891-6.

[82]   Kovach JA, Nearing BD, Verrier RL: Angerlike behavioral state potentiates myocardial ischemia-induced T-wave alternans in canines. *J Am Coll Cardiol* 2001; 37(6): 1719-25.

[83]   Stein PK, Carnet RM, Freedland KE, Skala JA, Jaffe AS, Kleiger RE, Rottman JN: Severe depression is associated with markedly reduced heart rate variability in patients with stable coronary heart disease. *J Psychosom Res* 2000; 48(4-5): 493-500.

[84]   Stein PK, Kleiger RE: Insights from the study of heart rate variability. *Ann Rev Med* 1999; 50, 249-61.

[85]   Saul JP, Arai Y, Berger RD, Lilly LS, Colucci WS, Cohen RJ: Assessment of autonomic regulation in chronic congestive heart failure by heart rate spectral analysis. *Am J Cardiol* 1998; 61(15): 1292-9.

[86]   van Ravenswaaij-Arts CM, Kollee LA, Hopman JC, Stoelinga GB, van Geijn HP: Heart rate variability. *Ann Intern Med* 1993; 118(6): 436-47.

[87]   Arbogast BW, Neumann JK, Arbogast LY, Leeper SC, Kostrzewa RM: Transient loss of serum protective activity following short-term stress: a possible biochemical link between stress and atherosclerosis. *J Psychosom Res* 1994; 38(8): 871-84.

[88]   Black PH, Garbutt LD: Stress, inflammation and cardiovascular disease. *J Psychosom Res* 2002; 52(1), 1-23.

[89]   Schneiderman N, Antoni MH, Saab PG, Ironson G: Health psychology: psychosocial and biobehavioral aspects of chronic disease management. *Annu Rev Psychol* 2001; 52, 555-80.

[90]   Littman AB: Review of Psychosomatic aspects of cardiovascular disease. *Psychother Psychosom* 1993; 60(3-4): 148-67.

[91]   Cohen S, Williamson GM: Stress and infectious diseases in humans. Psychol Bull 1991; 109(1): 5-24.

[92]   Romanelli J, Fauerbach JA, Bush DE, Ziegelstein RC: The significance of depression in older patients after myocardial infarction. *J Am Geriatr Soc* 2002; 50(5): 817-22.

[93]   Carney RM, Freedland KE, Eisen SA, Rich MW, Jaffe AS: Major depression and medication adherence in elderly patients with coronary artery disease. *Health Psychol* 1995; 14(1): 88-90.

[94]   Ziegelstein RC, Fauerbach JA, Stevens SS, Romanelli J, Richter DP, Bush DE: Patients with depression are less likely to follow recommendations to reduce cardiac risk during recovery from a myocardial infarction. *Arch Intern Med* 2000; 160(12): 1818-23.

[95]   Krishnan KR, George LK, Pieper CF, Jiang W, Arias R, Look A, O'Connor C: Depression and social support in elderly patients with cardiac disease. *Am Heart J* 1998; 136(3): 491-5.

[96] Murberg TA, Bru E, Miller J, Aarsland T, Svebak S: Social support, social disability and their role as predictors of depression among patients with congestive heart failure. *Scand J Soc Med* 1998; 26(2): 87-95.

[97] Cohen S: Psychosocial models of the role of social support in the etiology of physical disease. *Health Psychol* 1988; 7(3): 269-97.

[98] Carles RA: The association between disease severity, functional status, depression and daily quality of life in congestive heart failure patients. *Qual Life Res* 2004; 13(1): 63-72.

[99] Cuijpers P: Mortality and depressive symptoms in inhabitants of residential homes. *Int J Geriatr Psychiatr* 2001; 16(2): 131-8.

[100] Krumholz HM, Butler J, Miller J, Vaccarino V, Williams CS, Mendes de Leon CF, Seeman TE. Kasl SV. Berkman LF: Prognostic importance of emotional support for elderly patients hospitalized with heart failure. *Circulation*, 1998; 97(10): 958-64.

[101] Shih SN, Shih FJ: Health needs of lone elderly Chinese men with heart disease during their hospitalization. *Nurs Ethics* 1999; 6(1): 58-72.

[102] Spertus JA, McDonell M, Woodman CL, Fihn SD: (2000). Association between depression and worse disease-specific functional status in outpatients with coronary artery disease. *Am Heart J* 2000; 140(1): 105-10.

[103] Mayou RA, Gill D, Thompson DR, Day A, Hicks N, Volmink J et al: Depression and anxiety as predictors of outcome after myocardial infarction. *Psychosom Med* 2000; 62(2): 212-19.

[104] Steffens DC, O'Connor CM, Jiang WJ, Pieper CF, Kuchibhatla MN, Arias RM et al: The effect of major depression on functional status in patients with coronary artery disease. *J Am Geriatr Sco* 1999; 47(3), 319-22.

[105] Rumsfeld JS, Magid DJ, Plomondon ME, Sales AE, Grunwald GK, Every NR, Spertus JA: History of depression, angina, and quality of life after acute coronary syndromes. *Am Heart J* 2003; 145(3): 493-9.

[106] Lane D, Carroll D, Ring C, Beevers DG, Lip GY: Mortality and quality of life 12 months after myocardial infarction: effects of depression and anxiety. *Psychosom Med* 2001; 63(2): 221-30.

[107] Sullivan MD, LaCroix AZ, Spertus JA, Hecht JD: Five-year prospective study of the effects of anxiety and depression in patients with coronary heart disease. *Am J Cardiol* 2000; 86(10): 1135-40.

[108] Denollet J, Brutsaert DL: Personality, disease severity, and the risk of long-term cardiac events in patients with a decreased ejection fraction after myocardial infarction. *Circulation,*1998; 97(2): 167-73.

[109] Frasure-Smith, N. F., Lespérance, F., & Talajic, M. (1995). Depression and 18-month prognosis after myocardial infarction. *Circulation*, 91(4), 999-1005.

[110] Clarke SP, Frasure-Smith N, Lespérance F, Bourassa MG : Psychosocial factors as predictors of functional status at 1 year in patients with left ventricular dysfunction. *Res Nurs Health* 2000; 23(4): 290-300.

[111] Skotzko CE, Krichten C, Zietowski G, Alves L, Freudenberger R, Robinson S, Fisher M. Gottlieb SS: Depression is common and precludes accurate assessment of

functional status in elderly patients with congestive heart failure. *J Card Fail* 2000; 6(4): 300-5.

[112] Jiang W, Alexander J, Christopher E, Kuchibatla M, Gaulden LH, Cuffe MS, Blazing MA. Davenport C. Califf RM. Krishnan RR. O'Connor CM: Relationship of depression to increased risk of mortality and rehospitalization in patients with congestive heart failure. *Arch Intern Med* 2001; 161(15): 1849-56.

[113] Faris R, Purcell H, Henein MY, Coats AJS: Clinical depression is common and significantly associated with reduced survival in patients with non-ischaemic heart failure. *Eur J Heart Fail* 2002; 4(4): 541-51.

[114] Moser DK, Worster PL: Effect of psychosocial factors on physiologic outcomes in patients with heart failure. *J Cardiovas Nurs* 2000; 14(4): 106-15.

[115] Robinette A: Coping with stress in nursing practice. In. PD Barry (Ed.), *Psychosocial Nursing: care of physically ill patients and their families* (3rd ed., pp. 575). Philadelphia: Lippincott, 1996.

[116] Linden W, Stossel C, Maurice J: Psychosocial interventions for patients with coronary artery disease: a meta-analysis. *Arch Intern Med* 1996; 156(7): 745-52.

[117] Blumenthal JA, Jiang W, Babyak MA, Krantz DS, Frid DJ, Coleman RE, Waugh R. Hanson M. Appelbaum M. O'Connor C. Morris JJ: Stress management and exercise training in cardiac patients with myocardial ischemia. Effects on prognosis and evaluation of mechanisms. *Arch Intern Med* 1997; 157(19): 2213-23.

[118] Black JL, Allison TG, Williams DE, Rummans TA, Gau GT : Effect of intervention for psychological distress on rehospitalization rates in cardiac rehabilitation patients. *Psychosom* 1998; 39(2): 134-43.

[119] Kortis JB, Rosen RC, Cosgrove NM, Shindler DM, Wilson AC: Nonpharmacologic therapy improves functional and emotional status in congestive heart failure. *Chest* 1994; 106:996-1001.

[120] Moser DK, Dracup K, Woo MA, Stevenson LW: Voluntary control of vascular tone by using skin-temperature biofeedback-relaxation in patients with advanced heart failure. *Altern Ther Health Med* 1997; 3: 51-9.

[121] Klaus L, Beniaminovitz A, Choi L, Greenfield F, Whitworth GC, Mehmet CO, Mancini DM: Pilot study of guided imagery use in patients with severe heart failure. *Am J Cardiol* 2000; 86: 101-4.

[122] Luskin F, Reitz M, Newell K, Quinn TG, Haskell WA: A controlled pilot study of stress management training of elderly patients with congestive heart failure. *Prev Cardiol* 2002; 168-76.

[123] Chang BH, Hendricks A, Zhao Y, Rothendler JA, LoCastro JS, Slawsky MT: A relaxation response randomized trial on paitnets with chronic heart failure. *J Cardiopulm Rehabil* 2005; 25: 149-57.

[124] Yu DSF, Lee DTF, Woo J: Effects of relaxation therapy on psychological distress and symptom status in older Chinese patients with heart failure. *J Psychosom Res* 2007; 62: 427-37.

[125] Barrella P, Della ME : Managing congestive heart failure at home. *AACN Clinical Issues*, 1998; 9(3), 377-88.

[126] de Loor S, Jaarsma T: Nurse-managed heart failure programmes in the Netherlands. *Eur J Cardivas Nurs* 2002; 1(2): 123-9.

[127] Gorski LA, Johnson K: A disease management program for heart failure: collaboration between a home care agency and a care management organization. *Lippincott's Case Management*, 2003; 8(6): 265-73.

[128] Yu DSF, Thompson DR, Lee DTF: Disease management programmes for older people with heart failure: crucial characteristics which improve post-discharge outcomes. *Eur Heart J* 2006; 27: 596-612.

[129] Disease Management Association of America. Home Page. Retrieved Dec 16, 2007 from http://www.dmaa.org.

[130] Yu DSF, Lee DTF, Woo J: Effects of relaxation therapy on psychologic distress and symptom status in older Chinese patients with heart failure. *J Psychosom Res* 2007; 62: 247-37.

[131] Fraser SN, Spink KS: Examining the role of social support and group cohesion in exercise compliance. *J Behav Med* 2002; 25(3), 233 – 49.

[132] van Dixhoorn JJ: Implementation of relaxation therapy within a cardiac rehabilitation setting. In. DT Kenny, JG Carlson (Eds.), *Stress and health: Research and clinical application* (pp. 355-73). Amsterdam: Harwood Academic, 2000.

[133] Bennett SJ, Cordes DK, Westmoreland G, Castro R, Donnelly E: Self-care strategies for symptom management in patients with chronic heart failure. *Nurs Res* 2000; 49(3): 139-45.

In: Psychological Factors and Cardiovascular Disorders   ISBN: 978-1-60456-871-4
Editor: Leo Sher   © 2008 Nova Science Publishers, Inc.

Chapter XI

SEASONAL MOOD CHANGES AND CORONARY HEART DISEASE

Leo Sher

Department of Psychiatry, Columbia University, and New York State Psychiatric
Institute, New York, NY, USA.

ABSTRACT

Since ancient times people have known about seasonal changes in mood and behavior. Seasonal changes in mood and behavior have been studied extensively over the past two decades. The degree to which seasonal changes affect mood and behavior has been called 'seasonality'. Seasonality of mood and behavior is common in the general population. Coronary heart disease shows a winter peak and summer trough in incidence and mortality. Psychological factors have a considerable impact on the cardiovascular system. Psychological factors may also significantly affect the immune system. Depressive disorders, chronic stress, and bereavement generally have a suppressive effect on parameters of the immune system. There is considerable evidence that coronary heart disease is associated with inflammation and infection. The development of infection and inflammation in the atherosclerotic plaque may be related to the psychological disorders that suppress the immune system. Changes in the immune system may mediate the effect of seasonal depression on the heart and vessels. Seasonal mood changes may contribute to the increased incidence of cardiovascular events in the winter.

SEASONAL MOOD CHANGES

The importance of mind–body relationships is often overlooked and underestimated. Contemporary technomedicine does not pay much attention to the subtle and complex relation between mind and body. However, the influence of psychological factors on the physical and mental condition of healthy and sick people is very considerable.

Since ancient times people have known about the seasonal changes in mood and behavior [1]. The concept of seasonal mood disorders dates back to the dawn of medicine [2,3]. Seasonal depressions were described by the Greek physician Hippocrates circa 400 bc [4]. About 2000 years ago, the Greek philosopher Posidonius wrote that "melancholy occurs in autumn, whereas mania in summer" [5]. In the second century, Greco-Roman physicians were treating depression and lethargy with sunlight directed toward the eyes [6,7]. In 1894, explorer Frederick Cook linked seasonal loss of sunlight to a mood disorder [8]. Cook described a syndrome characterized by a loss of sexual desire and energy, fatigue, and a profoundly depressed mood. The French neurologist Esquirol [9] and the German psychiatrist Kraepelin [10] both described seasonal changes in mood in books published in the years 1845 and 1921, respectively.

Seasonal changes in mood and behavior have been studied extensively over the past two decades [11-16]. The degree to which seasonal changes affect mood and behavior has been called 'seasonality' [11]. Seasonality can manifest to different degrees in different individuals. Seasonality can be viewed in dimensional terms ranging from those who show no seasonal changes to those who show more extreme changes with the seasons. 'Seasonal affective disorder' (SAD), a condition where depressions in fall and winter alternate with non-depressed periods in the spring and summer, is an extreme form of seasonality [12]. It has been suggested that in order for a diagnosis of SAD to be made, the following criteria must be met: a history of a major affective disorder; at least 2 consecutive previous years in which depression developed during fall or winter and remitted by the following spring and summer; absence of any other Axis I psychiatric disorder; and absence of any clear-cut, seasonally changing psychosocial variables that would account for the seasonal variability in mood and behavior [12,15].

Seasonality of mood and behavior is common in the general population [11,16]. A survey in the Washington area in the USA found that approximately 4% of the population have winter SAD and over 10% more have sub-syndromal SAD [11]. Twenty-seven percent of respondents reported that changes with the seasons were a problem for them, 66% reported seasonal changes in energy level, 64% reported some seasonal changes in mood, and 49% reported seasonal changes in weight. Another survey, in New York City, indicated approximately 6% with potential clinical severity, 18% reporting milder symptoms that are bothersome, and 35% noting symptoms but without complaint [16].

SEASONAL VARIATIONS IN CORONARY HEART DISEASE

Coronary heart disease shows a winter peak and summer trough in incidence and mortality [17,18]. An increase in mortality from acute myocardial infarction in the winter was first reported in 1937 [19,20]. Since these initial observations, many researchers reported an increased mortality from coronary heart disease in the winter months [17,18]. An observational study suggests that there is a seasonal occurrence of acute myocardial infarction that is characterized by a marked peak of cases in the winter months and a nadir in the summer months [18]. This pattern was observed in all subgroups analyzed as well as in different geographic areas.

MOOD AND CARDIOVASCULAR ILLNESS

Psychological factors have a very considerable impact on the cardiovascular system [21-26]. Studies of psychiatric patients, community samples and patients with known heart disease show that depression is associated with increased incidence, morbidity, and mortality of cardiovascular disease. Depressive disorders play an important role in the pathogenesis of hypertension, angina, myocardial infarction, and sudden cardiac death. A number of research studies have replicated a consistently strong association between depressed symptoms and risk for coronary heart disease across different population groups and male/female gender [21]. Many studies documented increased cardiovascular morbidity and mortality in cardiac patients with depressive symptoms or major depression, thereby implicating depression as an independent risk factor in the pathophysiologic progression of cardiovascular disease [22]. For example, Frasure-Smith et al. found that depression was associated with a more than four-fold increased risk of mortality during the first 6 months following acute myocardial infarction after adjusting for relevant covariates including left ventricular dysfunction [23]. Moreover, its prognostic significance was equivalent to that of left ventricular dysfunction and previous history of myocardial infarction. In a study of patients undergoing diagnostic cardiac catheterization and arteriography, concomitant major depression was the best predictor of cardiac events during a 1-year follow-up [24]. In patients with congestive heart failure, depressive symptoms are a stronger predictor of New York Heart Association functional class than is left ventricular ejection fraction [25]. Depression, stress, anger, anxiety, and social isolation have been shown to substantially increase risk for myocardial infarction in coronary artery disease patients [23-26].

MOOD, THE IMMUNE SYSTEM AND INFLAMMATION

Psychological factors may significantly affect the immune system [27-29]. Solomon [27] suggests that both the central nervous system and the immune system 'relate the organism to the outside world, both serve functions of defense and adaptation, both result in illness when operating inappropriately or overdefensively, and both have the property of memory and learning from the experience.' It is not surprising that altered immune function can be associated with depression. Depressive disorders, chronic stress, and bereavement generally have a suppressive effect on parameters of the immune system [27,29]. Research data suggest that patients with depression have lower percentages of helper T lymphocytes, fewer suppressor and total T lymphocytes, and a poorer T-cell response to mitogen stimulation than nondepressed controls [29].

Repeated episodes of acute psychological stress, or chronic psychological stress, may induce a chronic inflammatory process culminating in atherosclerosis [30]. These inflammatory events, caused by stress, may account for the approximately 40% of atherosclerotic patients with no other known risk factors. Stress, by activating the sympathetic nervous system, the hypothalamic-pituitary axis, and the renin-angiotensin system, causes the release of various stress hormones such as catecholamines, corticosteroids, glucagon, growth hormone, and renin, and elevated levels of homocysteine, which induce a heightened state of cardiovascular activity, injured endothelium, and induction of adhesion molecules on endothelial cells to which recruited inflammatory cells adhere and translocate to the arterial wall.

CARDIOVASCULAR DISORDERS AND INFECTION

There is considerable evidence that coronary heart disease is associated with inflammation and infection [31-34]. Microbial agents may have a direct effect on the endothelium or smooth muscle of the arterial wall, or have an indirect effect on plague progression or rupture through changes in cross-reactive antibodies, lipid levels, or coagulation factors. Studies done in many laboratories around the world over the past several years have shown an association between inflammation and coronary atherosclerosis with an exacerbation of the inflammatory process during acute myocardial ischemia. Infection with very common organisms (e.g., Helicobacter pylorii and

Chlamydia pneumoniae) may lead to a localized infectious process and a chronic inflammatory reaction in the atherosclerotic plaque. It has been suggested that inflammation in the atherosclerotic plaque may be a causative mechanism for coronary heart disease. Anti-inflammatory agents (e.g., aspirin) and antibiotics may have substantial therapeutic effects in coronary artery disease. Based on the observations that some psychological factors promote the development of disorders of the cardiovascular system, that the same psychological factors decrease immunity and promote infection, and that there is evidence that the infectious process is involved in the pathogenesis of coronary heart disease, I have proposed that the development of infection and inflammation in the atherosclerotic plaque is related to the psychological disorders that suppress the immune system [35-37].

COLD TEMPERATURES AND INFECTION

Both coronary heart disease and respiratory infections exhibit a winter peak [17]. Cold temperatures increase the risk of respiratory infection through the suppression of immune responses and a direct effect on the respiratory system [38-40]. Experimental studies demonstrated that the acute effect of severe chilling is a suppression of several cellular and humoral components of the immune response, including a decrease of lymphocyte proliferation, a down-regulation of the immune cascade, a reduction of natural killer cell count, cytolytic activity, activation of complement, and the induction of heat shock proteins [40]. Most likely, cold temperatures contribute to the increase in incidence and mortality of cardiovascular disorders in the winter months.

CONCLUSION

Studies have suggested that the incidence of AMI is increased in the winter months. Seasonality of mood and behavior is common throughout the general population.

Increased cardiovascular morbidity and mortality in patients with depressive disorders have been well documented. Hence, it is reasonable to suggest that seasonal mood changes may contribute to the increased incidence of AMI in the winter.

This hypothesis has practical applications:

- Patients with cardiovascular disorders who suffer from seasonal mood changes should be identified.
- These patients should receive the appropriate treatment (light therapy, etc) for seasonal depressive symptoms, which may improve the quality of life for these individuals and reduce their incidence of acute myocardial infarction.
- The medical management of these patients should be more careful during the winter months.
- Future studies of pathophysiology, clinical features, and treatment of seasonal mood disorders in patients with cardiovascular illness are merited.

REFERENCES

[1]   Wehr T. A. Seasonal affective disorder. A historical overview. In: Rosenthal N. E., Blehar M. C., eds. *Seasonal affective disorder and phototherapy.* New York: Guilford Press, 1989; 11–32.

[2]   Oren DA, Rosenthal NE. Seasonal affective disorders. In: Paykel ES, ed. *Handbook of Affective Disorders.* 2nd ed. New York: Guilford Press; 1992: 551-567.

[3]   Sher L. Seasonal affective disorder and seasonality: a review. *The Jefferson Journal of Psychiatry* 2000; 15(1): 3-11.

[4]   Hippocrates. Aphorisms. In: Jones WHS, trans-ed. *Hippocrates.* Vol. 4. Cambridge, Mass: Harvard University Press; 1931: 128-129.

[5]   Roccatagliata G. *A History of Ancient Psychiatry.* New York: Greenwood Press; 1986.

[6]   Aretaeus. *The Extant Works of Aretaeus, the Cappadocian.* Adams F, trans-ed. London: Sydenham Society; 1856.

[7]   Aurelianus C. *On Acute Diseases and On Chronic Diseases.* Drabkin IE, trans-ed. Chicago: University of Chicago Press; 1950.

[8]   Cook FA. Gynecology and obstetrics among the Eskimo. *Brooklyn Med J.* 1894; 8: 154-169.

[9]   Esquirol JE. *Mental Maladies. A Treatise on Insanity.* Hunt EK, ed. Philadelphia: Lea and Blanchard; 1845.

[10]   Kraepelin E. *Manic-Depressive Illness and Paranoia.* Barklay RM, trans, Robertson GM, Livingstone E, Livingstone M, eds. Edinburgh: E&S Livingstone; 1921.

[11]   Kasper S, Wehr TA, Bartko J J, Gaist P, Rosenthal NE. Epidemiological findings of seasonal changes in mood and behavior. *Arch Gen Psychiatry* 1989; 46: 823–833.

[12] Rosenthal N E, Sack DA, Gillin JC, Lewy AJ, Goodwin FK, Davenport Y, Mueller P S, Newsome DA, Wehr TA. Seasonal affective disorder: a description of the syndrome and preliminary findings with light therapy. *Arch Gen Psychiatry* 1984; 41: 72–80.

[13] Sher L, Goldman D, Ozaki N, Rosenthal NE. The role of genetic factors in the etiology of seasonal affective disorder and seasonality. *J Affect Disord* 1999; 53: 203–210.

[14] Sher L., Rosenthal N.E., Wehr T.A. Free thyroxine and thyroid-stimulating hormone levels in patients with seasonal affective disorder and matched controls. *J Affect Disord* 1999; 56(2-3): 195-199.

[15] Sher L. Cortisol and seasonal changes in mood and behavior. *Psychiatric Times* 2006; 23(11): 22,24-25.

[16] Terman M. On the question of mechanism in phototherapy for seasonal affective disorder: considerations of clinical efficacy and epidemiology. *J Biol Rhythms* 1988; 3: 155–172.

[17] Pell J. P., Cobbe S. M. Seasonal variation in coronary heart disease. *QJM* 1999; 92: 689–696.

[18] Spencer F. A., Goldberg R. J., Becker R. C., Gore J. M. Seasonal distribution of acute myocardial infarction in the second National Registry of Myocardial Infarction. *J Am Coll Cardiol* 1998; 31: 1226–1233.

[19] Rosahn P. D. Incidence of coronary artery thrombosis. *JAMA* 1937; 109: 1294–1299.

[20] Masters A. M., Dack S., Jaffe H. L. Factors and events associated with onset of coronary artery trombosis. *JAMA* 1937; 109: 546–549.

[21] Barrick C. B. Sad, glad, or mad hearts? epidemiological evidence for a casual relationship between mood disorders and coronary artery disease. *J Affect Disord* 1999; 53: 193–201.

[22] Musselman D. L., Evans D. L., Nemeroff C. B. The relationship of depression to cardiovascular disease. *Arch Gen Psychiatry* 1998; 55: 580–592.

[23] Frasure-Smith N., Lesperance F., Talajic M. Depression following myocardial infarction: impact on 6-month survival. *JAMA* 1993; 270: 1819–1861.

[24] Carney RM, Rich MW, Tevelde A, Saini J, Clark K, Jaffe AS. Major depressive disorder predicts cardiac events in patients with coronary artery disease. *Psychosom Med* 1988; 50: 627–633.

[25] Skala J. A., Freedland K. E., Carney R. M. Depressive symptoms and functional status in patients with congestive heart failure. *Ann Behavior Med* 1995; 17: S130.

[26] Denollet J, Vaes J, Brutsaert DL. Inadequate response to treatment in coronary heart disease: adverse effects of type D personality and younger age on 5-year prognosis and quality of life. *Circulation* 1998; 97(2): 167-173.

[27] Solomon G. F. Immunologic abnormalities in mental illness. In: Ader R. (ed.) *Psychoneuroimmunology*. Orlando: Academic Press, 1981: 259–278.

[28] Olff M. Stress, depression and immunity: the role of defense and coping styles. *Psychiatry Res* 1999; 85: 7–15.

[29] Kiecolt-Glaser J. K., Glaser R. Stress and immune function in humans. In: Ader R., Felten D. L., Cohen N. (eds) *Psychoneuroimmunology*, 2nd edn. San Diego: Academic Press, 1991; 847–867.

[30] Black PH, Garbutt LD. Stress, inflammation and cardiovascular disease. *J Psychosom Res* 2002; 52(1): 1-23.

[31] Gurfinkel E, Bozovich G, Daroca A, Beck E, Mautner B, for the ROXIS Study Group. Randomised trial of roxithromycin in non- Q-wave coronary syndromes: ROXIS pilot study. *Lancet*1997; 350: 404–407.

[32] Danesh J, Collins R, Peto R. Chronic infection and coronary heart disease: is there a link? *Lancet* 1997; 350: 430–436.

[33] Mehta JL, Saldeen TGR, Rand K. Interactive role of infection, inflammation and traditional risk factors in atherosclerosis and coronary artery disease. *J Am Coll Cardiol* 1998; 31: 1217–1225.

[34] Rana JS, Nieuwdorp M, Jukema JW, Kastelein JJ. Cardiovascular metabolic syndrome - an interplay of, obesity, inflammation, diabetes and coronary heart disease. *Diabetes Obes Metab.* 2007; 9(3): 218-32.

[35] Sher L. Depression and cardiovascular disorders. *J Psychiatry Neurosci* 1998; 23: 180–181.

[36] Sher L. The role of the immune system and infection in the effects of psychological factors on the cardiovascular system. *Can J Psychiatry* 1998; 43: 954–955.

[37] Sher L. Effects of psychological factors on the development of cardiovascular pathology: role of the immune system and infection. *Med Hypotheses*1999; 53: 112–113.

[38] Ophir D., Elad Y. Effects of steam inhalation on nasal patency and nasal symptoms in patients with the common cold. *Am J Otolaryngol* 1987; 3: 149–153.

[39] Tyrrell D., Barrow I, Arthur J. Local hyperthermia benefits natural and experimental common colds. *Br Med J* 1989; 298: 1280–1283.

[40] Shephard R. J., Shek P. N. Cold exposure and immune function. *Can J Physiol Pharmacol* 1998; 76: 828–836.

In: Psychological Factors and Cardiovascular Disorders   ISBN: 978-1-60456-871-4
Editor: Leo Sher   © 2008 Nova Science Publishers, Inc.

Chapter XII

THE ROLE OF POSTTRAUMATIC STRESS DISORDER IN CORONARY ARTERY DISEASE: EPIDEMIOLOGY, RISK FACTORS, AND POTENTIAL MECHANISMS

Helle Spindler, Susanne S. Pedersen and Ask Elklit
Department of Psychology, University of Aarhus, Aarhus, Denmark;
CoRPS – Center of Research on Psychology in Somatic diseases,
Tilburg University, Tilburg, The Netherlands.

ABSTRACT

The psychological impact of coronary artery disease (CAD) has mainly been studied in the realm of depression; however, the experience of a cardiac event may also result in the development of posttraumatic stress disorder (PTSD). PTSD in cardiac patients has been associated with non-adherence to medication, increased emotional distress, impaired health-related quality of life, and adverse prognosis, suggesting a potential role for PTSD as a risk factor in CAD. To evaluate the impact of PTSD on CAD prognosis current research on the prevalence of PTSD, the associated risk factors, and the potential mechanisms linking CAD and PTSD are reviewed in order to examine the current status of PTSD as a potential risk factor in CAD.

INTRODUCTION

Coronary artery disease (CAD) is the most prominent cause of death in the Western world today, and due to improvement in treatment options, the number of patients who survive a myocardial infarction has increased substantially. Combined with an ageing population, the burden of CAD is expected to increase significantly in the future posing a major challenge to the health care system [1]. Despite advances in diagnosis and treatment of CAD, patients who survive an initial cardiac event may subsequently experience significant morbidity, and in consequence not benefit optimally from treatment efforts, hence increasing the risk of impaired health-related quality of life, recurrent cardiac events, and mortality [2-6]. Identifying factors that may influence the progression of heart disease is therefore important for secondary prevention.

Cardiac psychology is a multidisciplinary effort that attempts to prevent or minimize serious medical and psychological complications, with the aim of optimizing patients' medical and psychosocial outcomes [7]. In this line of research, posttraumatic stress disorder (PTSD) has been identified as a factor influencing both the onset [8-12] and progression of CAD [13] as well as comprising a possible consequence of CAD [14-19]. In other words, when humans are exposed to a life-threatening, traumatic event, this increases the cardiovascular risk as well as the risk of PTSD [12,17]. PTSD was first introduced into the diagnostic system in 1980 [20], but it was not until 1994 that medical illness was added explicitly as an event qualifying for PTSD in the DSM-IV [21], thereby recognizing medical illness, including CAD, as a sufficient stressor leading to PTSD.

In this chapter, current evidence on the prevalence of PTSD following CAD, knowledge of risk factors for developing PTSD, as well as potential mechanisms linking PTSD to cardiac prognosis, will be presented with the aim of answering the following questions: How prevalent is PTSD in CAD patients? Does PTSD influence cardiac prognosis? The answers to these questions are important, in that they may help determine the importance of addressing PTSD in future CAD research with the same laboriousness as has been the case for depression [22-25], and in turn, whether PTSD in future should be incorporated as a risk factor in clinical cardiology practice on par with traditional biomedical risk factors.

THE NATURE OF POSTTRAUMATIC STRESS DISORDER

The stressor criteria for PTSD in the DSM-IV stipulate that the preceding traumatic event must involve threatened death or serious injury to oneself, and that the subjective response must involve fear, helplessness, or horror. Additional criteria comprise experiencing intrusive and avoidant symptoms, as well as hyperarousal for more than one month. Acute PTSD refers to symptom duration of less than 3 months, whereas chronic PTSD refers to symptom duration of 3 months or more [21]. Evidently, acute cardiac events, such as acute myocardial infarction (MI), fulfill the stressor criteria, however, chronic cardiac events, such as congestive heart failure (CHF), may also qualify as traumatic. In contrast to acute events, CHF is the endstage of most heart diseases incurring a *continuous* risk of sudden death, thereby constituting a *chronic* stressor. Chronic stressors, by nature, recurrently threaten the patient's survival. In the general psychotraumatology literature, ongoing trauma, such as combat, civil war, sexual and physical child abuse, and stalking are considered to be especially traumatogenic, as it is difficult to find a safe haven, as would be possible after a single trauma, such as a car accident.

PTSD shares 80% comorbidity with depression [26]. The impact of depression on prognosis in patients with established CAD has been studied extensively, with depression being associated with a 2-fold increased risk of mortality [22,23], although there is still some debate regarding depression as an independent risk factor in CAD [25]. The question is whether this comorbidity renders the studying of PTSD in its own right obsolete? However, results from pathophysiological studies suggest that although both depression and PTSD have been associated with increased secretion of corticotropin-releasing factor, in PTSD, contrary to the pathophysiology in depression, this increased secretion is associated with hypocortisolaemia, indicating that the pathophysiology of the two disorders may in fact be distinct [27]. In addition, depression and PTSD require different treatment options, as conventional treatment of depression is not aimed at the core symptoms of PTSD, although treatment of PTSD may alleviate depressive symptomatology [28]. Hence, ignoring PTSD while treating depression may result in adverse consequences for cardiac patients [13], especially as intervention studies focusing on depression have shown to have little effect on hard medical outcomes [29-33]. By contrast, preliminary evidence suggests that treatment of PTSD may improve cardiovascular risk factors, e.g. smoking and cholesterol levels [28]. On a final note, risk factors may act in synergy, and adequate attention to all relevant factors seems to be the only way forward towards optimizing secondary prevention in patients with CAD [34,35].

EPIDEMIOLOGY

The occurrence of PTSD in CAD has mainly been studied in patients following MI. The prevalence rate of PTSD in these studies varies from 0% [36] to 35% [37] (see Table 1). While some studies used only patients with a first MI, other studies also included patients with multiple MIs. In patients with a first MI, the prevalence rate varies from 0% [36] to 22% [38], whereas in patients with multiple MIs the prevalence rate ranges from 7.7% [39] to 32% [40]. One study presented data concerning the temporal onset of PTSD and found that only 8% of their PTSD-cases had delayed onset after 12 months [41]. Two studies also examined the PTSD prevalence prospectively, and their results therefore have some bearing on the remission rate of PTSD following MI. In one study the prevalence rate dropped from 24% at 1 month to 14% 9 months post-MI. In another study, the prevalence rate was 23.8% at 6 weeks and 11.8% at 12 weeks post-MI [37]. A related study addressed the prevalence of PTSD in patients with acute coronary syndrome (ACS), a patient group, which also encompasses MI, and found a prevalence of 14.8% 3 months after the index event [42] (see Table 1).

In other groups of cardiac patients, there are far less studies focusing on PTSD as a possible consequence of CAD. Only four studies address the prevalence of PTSD in survivors of sudden cardiac arrest (SCA) (see Table 1). In these studies, the prevalence rate varies from 5% [43] to 38% [44]; the small prevalence rate of 5% was found in a case-control study, which could not support the notion of SCA as a risk factor for the development of PTSD. However, although the main study population was large, the subgroup of SCA patients was small (n = 39) [43]. In the remaining 3 studies, the smallest prevalence rate of 19% was found when assessing PTSD relatively shortly after the index event (mean 9.6 months (range 3-18 months)) [45], whereas studies evaluating the prevalence of PTSD >22 months after the index event found rates of 27% [46] and 38% [44]. Late-onset, additional adverse clinical events, and other accumulating adversities may be possible explanatory factors for this increase in PTSD prevalence over time. Unless studies adjust for previous trauma and trauma during follow-up, it is difficult to tease out the extent to which cardiac disease leads to PTSD or it is due to other life events, in turn making it difficult to ascertain the true prevalence.

Four studies have examined the prevalence of PTSD following cardiac surgery (CS; i.e. coronary artery bypass grafting (CABG), aortic valve replacement (AVR), and cardiac valve replacement (CVR)) (see Table 1). Of these, one study focused on children aged 5-12, who were scheduled for CS due to congenital heart disease, finding a prevalence of PTSD of 12% [47]. In the remaining studies, the prevalence rate varies from 8% [48] to 18% [49]. In all four studies, PTSD-caseness was assessed relatively soon following CS (range 1-12 months). Heart transplantation (HT) is considered in a category of itself, despite HT being a form of CS, since its nature is quite different from the remaining types of CS. Only 2 studies looking at the prevalence of PTSD in relation to HT could be identified (see Table 1). One study did not find any patients with PTSD, however, about 25% of spouses of HT patients displayed symptom levels equivalent to a PTSD diagnosis [50,51]. The only other study in HT patients, prospectively evaluated the prevalence of PTSD at several time points [52-55], and found the prevalence rate to vary from 10.8% [56] to 15.8% [53] dependent on time of assessment. The cumulative prevalence rates at 7, 12, and 36 months post HT were 9.6%, 15.6%, and 17%, respectively [55]. Of note, only one new case of PTSD was identified after 12 months, suggesting that the occurrence of late onset is rare in this population.

In CHF patients, the only study found was the case-control study mentioned above, which also examined the risk of PTSD associated with SCA (see Table 1). However, the CHF subgroup was remarkably larger than the SCA group, and the study found that there was a PTSD prevalence of 7% and that CHF was associated with a 49% increase in the risk of developing PTSD [43]. However, for both cardiac subgroups the generalizability of the results is limited because the study was conducted in a veteran population. To date, there are no studies of PTSD in patients with an implantable cardioverter defibrillator (ICD), however, case studies suggest that the risk of PTSD in ICD patients, especially those patients experiencing shocks, may be imminent [57-59]. In addition, Ladwig and colleagues have shown that ICD patients with high levels of PTSD are at increased risk of mortality [60]. It therefore seems timely, if not overdue, to address the issue of PTSD in ICD patients.

FACTORS ASSOCIATED WITH INCREASED RISK OF PTSD

Besides establishing the risk of PTSD associated with various types of heart disease, it is important to identify factors that may incur an increased risk of PTSD following heart disease in order to enhance secondary prevention (for an overview of risk factors, see Table 1, right). In 1994, Kutz and colleagues [41] were the first to identify factors, such as previous MI or traumatization, as well as the subjective expectation of incapacitation and ethnic origin as risk factors for the development of PTSD in the aftermath of MI. No studies have corroborated previous MI or traumatization as risk factors in MI patients, however, in patients admitted for ACS prior depression [42] was identified as a risk factor, whereas in a study of HT patients prior psychiatric illness in general was a risk factor, although this was for any psychiatric disorder following HT and not just for PTSD [55].

Several studies have focused on factors related to the cardiac event, showing length of hospitalization in HT patients [55], time spent in the ICU for children undergoing CS [47], lack of sedation during resuscitation in SCA patients [44], and subjective intensity of acute pain, and emotional distress in patients admitted for ACS [42] to be risk factors for PTSD. Focusing on MI patients exclusively, perceived threat and severity of the MI [61], awareness of the event as being an MI [62], less perceived control and duration of MI [39], feeling terrified at the time of MI [63], and illness perceptions [37] as well as subjective reactions to MI, i.e. emotional distress [63], dissociation [42,63,64], ASD [65], and intrusion and avoidance symptoms [42,64] have all been identified as risk factors for PTSD.

Other subsequent studies have turned their interest towards more stable factors, such as personality, showing that the distressed (Type D) personality [66], repressive coping [65], neuroticism or negative affect [38,42,67], and alexithymia [62] increased the risk of PTSD following MI. Generally, lack of social support has been associated with an increased risk of PTSD [68,69], and this finding is corroborated both in MI patients [64,70], and in HT patients [55]. Additionally, younger age has been identified as increasing the risk of PTSD both in MI patients [62] and in SCA patients [46], whereas female gender, a well-known risk factor in general PTSD research, has only been identified as increasing the risk of PTSD in HT patients [55].

Given that many different risk factors for PTSD have been identified, there is a need to combine these findings in future research in order to gain a better understanding of the current puzzle of risk factors and their possible interaction.

POTENTIAL PATHWAYS LINKING PTSD AND ADVERSE CAD PROGNOSIS

Recognizing the potential risk of PTSD associated with various types of heart disease is important, because PTSD may have detrimental consequences for the health of cardiac patients. So far, PTSD has been associated with impairments in social functioning, vitality, physical health [61], increased psychological distress [65], impaired quality of life [39], increased anxiety, depression, social dysfunction, and somatic problems [71], and adverse prognosis, including mortality [13,39,53,60,72]. As these findings relate PTSD to an increased risk of impairment or adverse health outcomes, they all corroborate the understanding of PTSD as a potential CAD risk factor. However, in order to consolidate the status of PTSD as a risk factor, it is necessary to elucidate the potential mechanisms through which PTSD exerts its cardio-toxic effects.

Few studies have addressed the issue of mechanisms linking PTSD and adverse cardiac prognosis [13], resulting in the general PTSD literature being used to infer possible mechanisms [17]. A review of the general psychotraumatology literature may serve to generate a theoretical understanding of what may serve as potential mechanisms linking PTSD to adverse cardiac prognosis; however, there is still a paucity of empirical studies of these mechanisms within CAD populations. In several studies, Shemesh and colleagues have shown PTSD to be associated with non-adherence to medication, which in turn increases the risk of adverse clinical events [13,28,72]. The authors suggest that non-adherence to medication may reflect avoidance behavior associated with PTSD, in that ingestion of medication may serve as a reminder of the traumatic cardiac event [13]. In addition, one of these studies also showed PTSD to be associated with increased cardiovascular re-admissions post-MI [13], a finding, which was corroborated in a study by Doerfler and colleagues who found increasing PTSD scores related to more cardiac readmissions [39]. In a later study, Shemesh and colleagues also found that smoking was significantly more common among MI survivors with PTSD than MI survivors without PTSD [28]. Smoking is a well-established cardiovascular risk factor [73]. In sum, behavioral factors associated with PTSD may comprise one of the links between PTSD and adverse cardiac prognosis.

A recent review of PTSD in MI patients focused on possible atherosclerotic mechanisms, suggesting autonomic dysfunction, reduced heart rate variability, decreased cortisol, and a pro-inflammatory state in PTSD as factors exacerbating the atherosclerotic process [17]. Further support for a pro-inflammatory state as a pathophysiological mechanism was found in a recent study showing low-grade systemic pro-inflammatory activity in PTSD patients as compared to controls without PTSD [10]. Another line of research focuses on cardiovascular reactivity to stress. A recent review on cardiovascular effects of acute mental stress suggests that increased heart rate, blood pressure, arrhythmias, coagulation abnormalities, endothelial dysfunction, and platelet activation may serve as potential pathways [12]. Of note, however, acute mental stress cannot substitute the enduring nature of PTSD symptomatology, and therefore results from studies using this research paradigm must be interpreted with caution. The association between mental stress and arrhythmia has been the subject of several studies in ICD patients consistently showing acute mental stress to be associated with an increased rate of arrhythmia [74-76]. Both animal and ICD patient studies suggest that beta-blockade may counter this effect, supporting the hypothesis that symphathetic activation could be one of the underlying mechanisms producing arrhythmia [12]. However, no studies have looked at the effect of PTSD on arrhythmia in ICD patients. Early studies in patients with established CAD has also identified an association between mental stress and silent ischemia [77,78], which has been corroborated in more recent studies [79-81], but again these findings should be replicated in studies of CAD patients with PTSD. The effect of mental stress has also been examined in relation to coagulation and platelet activation [82-84], with one of these studies being conducted in CAD patients [84].

Taken together, these studies show mental stress to be associated with abnormal coagulation, but the effect was short-lived [84]. Recently, however, it was shown that blood coagulation in otherwise healthy individuals with PTSD was associated with a hypercoagulable state compared to a matched sample of trauma-exposed controls without PTSD [11]. This last study expands on earlier research by showing coagulation abnormalities in patients with enduring stress responses as compared to the acute mental stress reported on in earlier studies. The logical next step in this line of research would be to examine coagulation abnormalities in CAD patients with PTSD in comparison with CAD patients without PTSD. On a similar note, Kario and colleagues addressed some of the above mentioned factors in a study of hypertensive outpatients living in an earthquake area and found an increase in blood pressure, blood viscosity determinants, and fibrin turnover, as well as prolonged endothelial cell stimulation in the aftermath of a major earthquake [85]. Although this study incorporated outpatients with hypertension rather than patients with established CAD, hypertension is a risk factor for incident CAD.

In sum, pathophysiological studies consistently seem to identify symphathetic over-activity and reduced parasympathetic cardiac control as a hall-mark in PTSD as well as being a risk factor in CAD [17,86], thus linking PTSD to atherosclerotic progression. This understanding is very much in line with the "allostatic load model" that regards PTSD as challenging the balance of the allostatic systems that usually assist in helping the body adapt to life circumstances [87]. Chronic stress, ie. PTSD, exerts substantial psychobiological demands, in a way that forces the body to find new steady states in which to maintain its vital functions [88]. These new states represent the body's adaptation to stress, but at the same time they require a sustained activity that places the allostatic systems under an excessive load due to chronic over- or underactivity, ie. sympathetic over-activity and reduced parasymphathetic cardiac control. Over time, pathophysiological changes may occur that lead to an increased risk of medical illness [87,88]. The evidence presented so far linking PTSD to atherosclerotic mechanisms is very compelling; however, almost all studies are done within the psychotraumatological research paradigm and then subsequently related to CAD progression, because the atherosclerotic mechanisms associated with PTSD are known cardiovascular risk factors. Therefore, future studies should address whether the proposed atherosclerotic mechanisms exert their cardio-toxic influence in CAD patients in the same way as has been shown in the general psychotraumatology literature.

With regard to depression, much of this work has already been carried out, and depression is now the most recognized psychological risk factor in CAD. In consequence, a considerable amount of research into its associated risk, pathophysiological mechanisms, as well as effects of intervention has been published [22-25]. In contrast, studies on PTSD as a psychological risk factor are few, although they show interesting results. Shemesh and colleagues explored the impact of PTSD and depression on MI survivors and found that PTSD, but not depression, was associated with non-adherence to medication and increased re-admission [13]. In a subsequent pilot study, Shemesh and colleagues showed that cognitive behavioral therapy relieved PTSD symptomatology as well as cardiac risk factors [28]. In addition, they found that depressive symptoms improved in the PTSD treatment group, although this was not statistically significant. However, this was a small study (n= 6), and the lack of statistical significance may be due to lack of power, as other studies, using other trauma populations, have shown that treatment of PTSD may also improve depressive symptomatology [89,90].

PTSD may have considerable consequences for the individual patient as indicated by the pathophysiological studies cited above, however, PTSD in relation to heart disease may also have consequences for society in general in terms of an increased number of cardiac-related re-admissions and recurrent cardiac events [13,39], and health-care consumption [9]. However, although PTSD alone or in combination with depression may lead to an increased use of health services, this use need not be of an inappropriate nature [8].

DISCUSSION

Overall, the bulk of research on PTSD in cardiovascular disease has been conducted in MI patients, with these studies offering a tentative conclusion. The best powered prospective studies found a prevalence rate ranging from 10% [72] to 16% [61,91,92] 6-7 months after the index event and a prevalence rate of 24% and 14% in patients with a first MI at 4-6 weeks and 9 months, respectively [38,70]. A previous study has shown late onset to be rare [41]. Taken together, these studies suggest a prevalence rate of about 15% in MI patients after allowing for a period of remission, which is in accordance with the estimated prevalence in two recent reviews [17,19]. In contrast, another well-powered study found a prevalence of 32% about 10 years after the index event [40]. This study examined MI patients in general practice, and the sample selection, the retrospective methodology, as well as MI-related adversities in the intervening years may be some of the factors explaining the high prevalence of PTSD found in this particular study. Studies examining the incidence of PTSD in CS, SCA, ACS, HF, HT, and ICD are too few and inconclusive to reliably estimate an over-all prevalence rate in each patient group.

The methodology of the studies assessing PTSD prevalence rates shows considerable heterogeneity; hence, appropriate attention to methodology in future studies may be important in order to enhance our understanding of PTSD in relation to CAD. When assessing the prevalence rate of PTSD in CAD patients, it is important to consider the time of assessment, the nature of the cardiac event, and the choice of instrument (e.g. diagnostic interview versus self-report) in order to elucidate the incidence and natural course of PTSD in CAD. Future studies should also be prospective, incorporating multiple assessments of PTSD, both in terms of assessment instrument and time point; yet, no assessment should be carried out sooner than 4 weeks after the index event, in adherence with the diagnostic criteria for PTSD [21]. Of note, researchers should take care in using only validated instruments modified to address the index event in question. Additionally, studies should be sufficiently powered, and pooling of cardiac patient groups to obtain sufficient power should be avoided, as prevalence rates may vary considerably across different types of cardiac conditions [19,45]. Moreover, incorporating a healthy matched control group in order to determine the relative magnitude of the problem may enhance our understanding of the impact of PTSD on CAD patients in comparison to the general population. Future studies adhering to such stringent methodology may be pivotal in bringing this line of research one step further in determining whether PTSD comprises another risk factor in cardiovascular disease.

Despite the preliminary evidence on PTSD in the context of CAD presented in this chapter, studies generally support the relevance of studying PTSD in CAD, especially given the first evidence that PTSD may lead to non-adherence to medication and increased cardiac re-admissions [13,72], and that treatment of PTSD may improve cardiovascular risk factors [28]. So far, no conclusive evidence regarding the risk of mortality associated with PTSD in CAD can be identified. Existing studies are conducted in veteran populations, and findings are inconsistent, with the most recent study showing only PTSD co-morbid with depression to be associated with increased risk of mortality [93-96]. However, this association disappeared when adjusting for health behaviors, which may not be all that surprising given that both depression and PTSD are associated with maladaptive health behaviors, such as smoking [28]. Besides prevalence rates, many studies have also examined risk factors for PTSD and shown that prior history, personality, aspects of the cardiac event, dissociative symptoms, ASD, social support and socio-demographic factors all may influence the development of PTSD. However, this abundance of risk factors has been examined in an unsystematic fashion, and in order to improve our understanding of the association between PTSD and CAD, future studies need to address such possible risk factors in a more systematic and methodologically sound fashion. That is, it is necessary to consider as many as these factors as possible conjointly (e.g. demographic, social, clinical or aspects related to the event) and use the same definition, in order to assess their relative importance as possible risk factors for PTSD. Such a strategy will also be informative regarding an additive or a synergistic effect of risk factors [34]. Additionally, an issue that has been neglected in current research is the impact of clinical risk factors, including disease severity and previous (multiple) cardiac events, as they may serve as confounders for the development of PTSD. This issue is also important for future studies focusing on determining the risk of recurrent cardiovascular events and mortality associated with PTSD in CAD patients. Although some have called for the recognition of depression as an independent cardiovascular risk factor [97], this issue is still under debate, with some evidence suggesting that the association between depression and CAD progression may be confounded by disease severity, rather than there being an independent impact of depression on cardiac prognosis [24,25].

In addition, it must be stressed that focusing on PTSD symptomatology may be of equal importance to focusing on PTSD caseness, especially since subclinical symptoms of PTSD may also result in significant distress. Subclinical PTSD is not uncommon in MI [65,72] and HT patients [52], and distress has been associated with adverse health-related quality of life and prognosis in cardiac patients [3,98,99]. In that respect, examining whether the cardiovascular risk associated with PTSD may also pertain to subclinical PTSD is another aim for future CAD research.

Finally, more pathophysiological studies addressing PTSD in CAD patients are needed. Although the existing body of research suggests that sympathetic over-activity and parasympathetic under-activity may be the major pathophysiological mechanisms [17], most of this evidence is inferred from general stress studies or otherwise healthy populations with PTSD; hence, future studies should address these issues in actual CAD populations. Such a line of research may in turn help provide the grounds for evaluating whether the existing evidence regarding pathophysiological mechanisms has sufficient bearing in CAD populations, or whether CAD pathophysiology changes the way in which PTSD pathophysiology may impact on the progression of the underlying cardiac disease.

CONCLUSION

There has been an increasing interest in PTSD as a risk factor in CAD. Nevertheless, we are still far from seeing PTSD as an accepted risk factor on par with traditional risk factors, such as hypertension and smoking, etc. Current evidence suggests that CAD patients are at increased risk of PTSD, with the prevalence of PTSD in MI patients being around 15%.

However, given the paucity of studies in other cardiac patient groups, it is rather difficult to give an estimate of the prevalence in these groups. In general, there is an urgent need for sufficiently powered studies on PTSD in CAD patients, using systematic and sound methodology to accurately evaluate the prevalence rate of PTSD, to establish the clinical course of PTSD, as well as the prognostic consequences of PTSD across CAD patient groups. There is not yet a clear understanding of which risk factors may lead to the development of PTSD, which factors sustain the condition, and their relative impact, just as little is known about the pathogenic pathways linking PTSD and CAD. Such information is important and would, in turn, contribute to better risk stratification in both research and clinical practice. In the interim, PTSD as a sequel of CAD should not be forgotten in clinical practice given its associated negative health consequences and preliminary evidence suggesting that treatment of PTSD may have a beneficial influence on cardiovascular risk factors.

Table 1. Studies evaluating the prevalence of PTSD in various cardiac populations

Study	Design Time since index event	PTSD measure	Population	PTSD Prevalence	Risk factors
Acute Coronary Syndrome					
Whitehead et al (2006)	Prospective 3 months	PSS-SR	135	14.8%	Subjective intensity of acute pain; prior depression; dissociation, emotional distress during the event, experience of intrusions; negative affectivity; hostility
Myocardial Infarction					
Doerfler et al (1994)	Cross-sectional 6-12 months	IES	27 MI 23 CABG	8 %	-
Kutz et al (1994)	Retrospective 6-18 months	PTSD Inventory	100	25%; (16% *chronic*)	Ethnic origin; prior MI or cardiac hospitalization; prior PTSD; subjective expectation of incapacitation
Van Driel et al (1995)	Prospective (1) 1-2 weeks; (2) 22-26 months	SCID-R	23	(1) (4% *subclinical*) (2) 0 %	-
Bennett et al (1999)	Cross-sectional 9.24 (6-12) months	PDS	44	10.75%	Younger age; alexithymia, awareness of the event as an MI
Bennett et al (2001)	Longitudinal 3 months	PDS	70	3%	Negative affect in hospital; feeling terrified at the time of MI; dissociation during MI
Shemesh et al (2001)	Prospective study 6 months	IES	102	9.8%	-

Study	Design Time since index event	PTSD measure	Population	PTSD Prevalence	Risk factors
Myocardial Infarction (continued)					
Bennett et al (2002)	Prospective 3 months	PDS	89	16%	Initial intrusion and avoidance symptoms; negative affect, lack of social support; dissociation during MI
Ginzburg et al (2002, 2003, 2004)	Prospective 7 months	PTSD Inventory	116	16% *(27.6% subclinical)*	Subjective perception of threat; ASD; perceived severity of MI
Pedersen et al (2003; 2004)	Prospective (1) 4-6 weeks; (2) 9 months	PDS	(1) 112 (2) 104	(1) 24% (2) 14%	Lack of social support; depression; neuroticism
O'Reilly et al (2004)	Case-control 9.6 (3-18) months	SCID, PDS, IES	27	7%	-
Shemesh et al (2004)	Prospective 6 months	IES	65	20 %	-
Doerfler et al (2005)	Cross-sectional 3-6 months	PSS	52	7.7%	Less perceived control during MI; readmissions to hospital, duration of MI; hours of experienced pain during MI
Sheldrick et al (2006)	Prospective (1) 6 weeks; (2) 12 weeks	DTS	17	(1) 23.8% (2) 11.8%	Illness perceptions (identity, timeline, consequences, emotional representation)
Shemesh et al (2006)	Prospective 6 months	IES, PDS	65	22%	-
Jones et al (2007) Chung et al. (2006, 2007, 2008)	Cross-sectional Mean of 10 years since 1st MI	PDS	111	32%	Neuroticism, less agreeableness.
Sudden Cardiac Arrest					
Ladwig et al (1999)	Prospective 39 (22-64) months	IES	21	38 %	Lack of sedation during resuscitation
Martz et al., (2001)	Retrospective, case-control	Diagnosis in medical journal	39	5%	-
Gamper et al (2004)	Prospective 45 (24-66) months	DTS	143	27%	Younger age
O'Reilly et al (2004)	Case-control 9.6 (3-18) months	SCID, PDS, IES	27	19 %	-
Heart Failure					
Martz et al., (2001)	Retrospective, case-control	Diagnosis in medical journal	2313	7%	-

Table 1. (Continued)

Study	Design Time since index event	PTSD measure	Population	PTSD Prevalence	Risk factors
Cardiac Surgery					
Doerfler et al (1994)	Cross-sectional 6-12 months	IES	27 MI 23 CABG	8 %	-
Stoll et al (2000) (100)	Cross-sectional 20 weeks	PTSS-10	51 CABG; 29 AVR	15 %	-
Connolly et al (2003)	Prospective (1) presurgery; (2) 4-8 weeks	DISC	43 children	(1) 0% (2)12 %	Spending more than 48 hours in the ICU
Schelling et al (2003)	Prospective (1) presurgery; (2) 6 months	PTSS-10 (modified)	(1) 184 (2) 148	(1) 4.8% (2) 18.2%	-
Heart Tranplantation					
Dew et al (1996; 1999; 2000; 2001) Stukas et al. (1999)	Prospective (1) 7 months; (2) 12 months; (3) 36 months	SCID	145-191	(1) 9.6%[1] (2) 15.6%[1] (3) 17%[1]	Prior psychiatric history; female gender; length of hospitalization; lower social support; poor family cohesion; poor sense of mastery; poor self-esteem[2]
Bunzel et al (2005, 2007)	6-135 months	IES	41	0%	-

ABBREVIATIONS:

POPULATIONS

MI = Myocardial infarction; CABG = Coronary artery bypass grafting; AVR = Aortic valve replacement.

QUESTIONNAIRES

DISC: Diagnostic Interview Schedule for Children; IES: Impact of Event Scale; PDS: Posttraumatic Diagnostic Scale (based on DSM-IV criteria); PTSS-10: Post-Traumatic Stress Syndrome 10-Questions Inventory (based on DSM-III criteria); DTS: Davidson Trauma Scale (based on DSM-IV criteria); SCID: Structured Clinical Interview; RI: Reaction Index ; PSS-SR: PTSD Symptom Scale-self report version.

DIAGNOSES

ASD: Acute Stress Disorder; PTSD: Post-traumatic Stress Disorder

[1] Cumulative risk; [2] Some of these factors relate to psychiatric disorders in general and not specifically to PTSD.

REFERENCES

[1]　Mackay J, Mensah GA. *The atlas of heart disease and stroke.* Geneva, Switzerland, World Health Organization. 2004.

[2]　Januzzi JL,Jr, Stern TA, Pasternak RC, et al. The influence of anxiety and depression on outcomes of patients with coronary artery disease. *Arch Intern Med.* 2000;160:1913-21.

[3]   Blumenthal JA, Lett HS, Babyak MA, et al. Depression as a risk factor for mortality after coronary artery bypass surgery. *Lancet.* 2003;362:604-9.

[4]   Pedersen SS, Lemos PA, van Vooren PR, et al. Type D personality predicts death or myocardial infarction after bare metal stent or sirolimus-eluting stent implantation: A rapamycin-eluting stent evaluated at rotterdam cardiology hospital (RESEARCH) registry substudy. *J Am Coll Cardiol.* 2004;44:997-1001.

[5]   Soto GE, Jones P, Weintraub WS, et al. Prognostic value of health status in patients with heart failure after acute myocardial infarction. *Circulation.* 2004;110:546-51.

[6]   Vaccarino V, Lin ZQ, Kasl SV, et al. Sex differences in health status after coronary artery bypass surgery. *Circulation.* 2003;108:2642-7.

[7]   Fisher J. Is there a need for cardiac psychology? The view of a practicing cardiologist. In: Allan R, Scheidt SS, editors. Heart & mind: *The practice of cardiac psychology.* Washington, DC, US: American Psychological Association; 1996. p. 125-45.

[8]   Deykin EY, Keane TM, Kaloupek D, et al. Posttraumatic stress disorder and the use of health services. *Psychosom Med.* 2001;63:835-41.

[9]   Friedman MJ, Schnurr PP. The relationship between trauma, post-traumatic stress disorder, and physical health. In: Friedman MJ, Charney DS, Deutch AY, editors. *Neurobiological and clinical consequences of stress: From normal adaptation to PTSD.* Philadelphia: Lippincott-Raven Publishers; 1995. p. 507-24.

[10]   von Kanel R, Hepp U, Kraemer B, et al. Evidence for low-grade systemic proinflammatory activity in patients with posttraumatic stress disorder. *J Psychiatr Res.* 2007;41:744-52.

[11]   von Kanel R, Hepp U, Buddeberg C, et al. Altered blood coagulation in patients with posttraumatic stress disorder. *Psychosom Med.* 2006;68:598-604.

[12]   Qureshi EA, Merla V, Steinberg J, et al. Terrorism and the heart: Implications for arrhythmogenesis and coronary artery disease. *Card Electrophysiol Rev.* 2003;7:80-4.

[13]   Shemesh E, Yehuda R, Milo O, et al. Posttraumatic stress, nonadherence, and adverse outcome in survivors of a myocardial infarction. *Psychosom Med.* 2004;66:521-6.

[14]   Owen RL, Koutsakis S, Bennett P. Post-traumatic stress disorder as a sequel of acute myocardial infarction: An overlooked cause of psychosocial disability. *Coronary Health Care.* 2001;5:9-15.

[15]   McFarlane A. Posttraumatic stress disorder: The intersection of epidemiology and individual psychobiological adaptation. *Current Opinion in Psychiatry.* 2003;16:57-63.

[16]   Tedstone JE, Tarrier N. Posttraumatic stress disorder following medical illness and treatment. *Clin Psychol Rev.* 2003;23:409-48.

[17]   Gander ML, von Kanel R. Myocardial infarction and post-traumatic stress disorder: Frequency, outcome, and atherosclerotic mechanisms. *Eur J Cardiovasc Prev Rehabil.* 2006;13:165-72.

[18]   Pedersen SS. Post-traumatic stress disorder in patients with coronary artery disease: A review and evaluation of the risk. *Scand J Psychol.* 2001;42:445-51.

[19]   Spindler H, Pedersen SS. Posttraumatic stress disorder in the wake of heart disease: Prevalence, risk factors, and future research directions. *Psychosom Med.* 2005;67:715-23.

[20]   *APA. Diagnostic and statistical manual of mental disorders*. 3rd edition ed. Washington DC: American Psychiatric Association; 1980.

[21]   *APA. Diagnostic and statistical manual of mental disorders*. 4th ed. ed. Washington DC: American Psychiatric Association; 1994.

[22]   Barth J, Schumacher M, Herrmann-Lingen C. Depression as a risk factor for mortality in patients with coronary heart disease: A meta-analysis. *Psychosom Med*. 2004;66802-13.

[23]   Van Melle JP, De Jonge P, Spijkerman TA, et al. Prognostic association of depression following myocardial infarction with mortality and cardiovascular events: A meta-analysis. *Psychosom Med*. 2004;66:814-22.

[24]   de Jonge P, Ormel J, van den Brink RH, et al. Symptom dimensions of depression following myocardial infarction and their relationship with somatic health status and cardiovascular prognosis. *Am J Psychiatry*. 2006;163:138-44.

[25]   Nicholson A, Kuper H, Hemingway H. Depression as an aetiologic and prognostic factor in coronary heart disease: A meta-analysis of 6362 events among 146 538 participants in 54 observational studies. *Eur Heart J*. 2006;27:2763-74.

[26]   Kessler RC, Sonnega A, Bromet E, et al. Posttraumatic stress disorder in the national comorbidity survey. *Arch Gen Psychiatry*. 1995;52:1048-60.

[27]   Lyons D, McLoughlin DM. Recent advances: Psychiatry. *BMJ*. 2001 24;323:1228-31.

[28]   Shemesh E, Koren-Michowitz M, Yehuda R, et al. Symptoms of posttraumatic stress disorder in patients who have had a myocardial infarction. *Psychosomatics*. 2006;47:231-9.

[29]   Joynt KE, O'Connor CM. Lessons from SADHART, ENRICHD, and other trials. *Psychosom Med*. 2005;67:S63-6.

[30]   Carney RM, Blumenthal JA, Freedland KE, et al. Depression and late mortality after myocardial infarction in the enhancing recovery in coronary heart disease (ENRICHD) study. *Psychosom Med*. 2004;66:466-74.

[31]   Berkman LF, Blumenthal J, Burg M, et al. Effects of treating depression and low perceived social support on clinical events after myocardial infarction: The enhancing recovery in coronary heart disease patients (ENRICHD) randomized trial. *JAMA*. 2003;289:3106-16.

[32]   Lesperance F, Frasure-Smith N, Koszycki D, et al. Effects of citalopram and interpersonal psychotherapy on depression in patients with coronary artery disease: The Canadian cardiac randomized evaluation of antidepressant and psychotherapy efficacy (CREATE) trial. *JAMA*. 2007;297:367-79.

[33]   Honig A, Kuyper AM, Schene AH, et al. Treatment of post-myocardial infarction depressive disorder: A randomized, placebo-controlled trial with mirtazapine. *Psychosom Med*. 2007;69:606-13.

[34]   Alonzo AA. Acute myocardial infarction and posttraumatic stress disorder: The consequences of cumulative adversity. *J Cardiovasc Nurs*. 1999;13:33-45.

[35]   Rozanski A, Blumenthal JA, Davidson KW, et al. The epidemiology, pathophysiology, and management of psychosocial risk factors in cardiac practice: The emerging field of behavioral cardiology. *J Am Coll Cardiol*. 2005;45:637-51.

[36]   van Driel RC, Op den Velde W. Myocardial infarction and post-traumatic stress disorder. *J Trauma Stress*. 1995;8:151-9.

[37]   Sheldrick R, Tarrier N, Berry E, et al. Post-traumatic stress disorder and illness perceptions over time following myocardial infarction and subarachnoid haemorrhage. *Br J Health Psychol*. 2006;11:387-400.

[38]   Pedersen SS, Middel B, Larsen ML. Posttraumatic stress disorder in first-time myocardial infarction patients. *Heart Lung*. 2003;32:300-7.

[39]   Doerfler LA, Paraskos JA, Piniarski L. Relationship of quality of life and perceived control with posttraumatic stress disorder symptoms 3 to 6 months after myocardial infarction. *J Cardiopulm Rehabil*. 2005;25:166-72.

[40]   Jones RC, Chung MC, Berger Z, et al. Prevalence of post-traumatic stress disorder in patients with previous myocardial infarction consulting in general practice. *Br J Gen Pract*. 2007;57:808-10.

[41]   Kutz I, Shabtai H, Solomon Z, et al. Post-traumatic stress disorder in myocardial infarction patients: Prevalence study. *Isr J Psychiatry Relat Sci*. 1994;31:48-56.

[42]   Whitehead DL, Perkins-Porras L, Strike PC, et al. Post-traumatic stress disorder in patients with cardiac disease: Predicting vulnerability from emotional responses during admission for acute coronary syndromes. *Heart*. 2006;92:1225-9.

[43]   Martz E, Cook DW. Physical impairments as risk factors for the development of posttraumatic stress disorder. *Rehabilitation Counselling Bulletin*. 2001;44:217-21.

[44]   Ladwig KH, Schoefinius A, Dammann G, et al. Long-acting psychotraumatic properties of a cardiac arrest experience. *Am J Psychiatry*. 1999;156:912-9.

[45]   O'Reilly SM, Grubb N, O'Carroll RE. Long-term emotional consequences of in-hospital cardiac arrest and myocardial infarction. *Br J Clin Psychol*. 2004;43:83-95.

[46]   Gamper G, Willeit M, Sterz F, et al. Life after death: Posttraumatic stress disorder in survivors of cardiac arrest - prevalence, associated factors, and the influence of sedation and analgesia. *Crit Care Med*. 2004;32:378-83.

[47]   Connolly D, McClowry S, Hayman L, et al. Posttraumatic stress disorder in children after cardiac surgery. *J Pediatr*. 2004;144:480-4.

[48]   Doerfler LA, Pbert L, DeCosimo D. Symptoms of posttraumatic stress disorder following myocardial infarction and coronary artery bypass surgery. *Gen Hosp Psychiatry*. 1994;16:193-9.

[49]   Schelling G, Richter M, Roozendaal B, et al. Exposure to high stress in the intensive care unit may have negative effects on health-related quality-of-life outcomes after cardiac surgery. *Crit Care Med*. 2003;31:1971-80.

[50]   Bunzel B, Laederach-Hofmann K, Wieselthaler GM, et al. Posttraumatic stress disorder after implantation of a mechanical assist device followed by heart transplantation: Evaluation of patients and partners. *Transplant Proc*. 2005;37:1365-8.

[51]   Bunzel B, Laederach-Hofmann K, Wieselthaler G, et al. Mechanical circulatory support as a bridge to heart transplantation: What remains? Long-term emotional sequelae in patients and spouses. *J Heart Lung Transplant*. 2007;26:384-9.

[52]   Dew MA, Roth LH, Schulberg HC, et al. Prevalence and predictors of depression and anxiety-related disorders during the year after heart transplantation. *Gen Hosp Psychiatry*. 1996;18:48S-61S.

[53]   Dew MA, Kormos RL, Roth LH, et al. Early post-transplant medical compliance and mental health predict physical morbidity and mortality one to three years after heart transplantation. *J Heart Lung Transplant*. 1999;18:549-62.

[54]   Dew MA, DiMartini AF, Switzer GE, et al. Patterns and predictors of risk for depressive and anxiety-related disorders during the first three years after heart transplantation. *Psychosomatics*. 2000;41:191-2.

[55]   Dew MA, Kormos RL, DiMartini AF, et al. Prevalence and risk of depression and anxiety-related disorders during the first three years after heart transplantation. *Psychosomatics*. 2001;42:300-13.

[56]   Stukas AA,Jr, Dew MA, Switzer GE, et al. PTSD in heart transplant recipients and their primary family caregivers. *Psychosomatics*. 1999;40:212-21.

[57]   Hamner M, Hunt N, Gee J, et al. PTSD and automatic implantable cardioverter defibrillators. *Psychosomatics*. 1999;40:82-5.

[58]   Maryniak A, Szumowski L, Walczak F, et al. Post-traumatic stress disorder in a patient with recurrent ICD shocks. The role of RF ablation. *Kardiol Pol*. 2006;64:910-2.

[59]   Neel M. Posttraumatic stress symptomatology in patients with automatic implantable cardioverter defibrillators: Nature and intervention. *Int J Emerg Ment Health*. 2000;2:259-63.

[60]   Ladwig KH, Marten-Mittag B, Baumert J, et al. Posttraumatic stress symptoms as predictor for mortality among patients with implantable cardioverter-defibrillators (ICD). results from the prospective LICAD study. Abstract from the 65th Annual Meeting of the *American Psychosomatic Society*. 2007:105.

[61]   Ginzburg K, Solomon Z, Koifman B, et al. Trajectories of posttraumatic stress disorder following myocardial infarction: A prospective study. *J Clin Psychiatry*. 2003;64:1217-23.

[62]   Bennett P, Brooke S. Intrusive memories, post-traumatic stress disorder and myocardial infarction. *Br J Clin Psychol*. 1999;38:411-6.

[63]   Bennett P, Conway M, Clatworthy J, et al. Predicting post-traumatic symptoms in cardiac patients. *Heart Lung*. 2001;30:458-65.

[64]   Bennett P, Owen RL, Koutsakis S, et al. Personality, social context and cognitive predictors of post-traumatic stress disorder in myocardial infarction patients. *Psychol Health*. 2002;17:489-500.

[65]   Ginzburg K, Solomon Z, Bleich A. Repressive coping style, acute stress disorder, and posttraumatic stress disorder after myocardial infarction. *Psychosom Med*. 2002;64:748-57.

[66]   Pedersen SS, Denollet J. Validity of the type D personality construct in Danish post-MI patients and healthy controls. *J Psychosom Res*. 2004;57:265-72.

[67]   Chung MC, Berger Z, Jones R, et al. Posttraumatic stress disorder and general health problems following myocardial infarction (post-MI PTSD) among older patients: The role of personality. *Int J Geriatr Psychiatry*. 2006;21:1163-74.

[68]   Keane TM, Marshall AD, Taft CT. Posttraumatic stress disorder: Etiology, epidemiology, and treatment outcome. *Annu Rev Clin Psychol.* 2006;2:161-97.

[69]   Guay S, Billette V, Marchand A. Exploring the links between posttraumatic stress disorder and social support: Processes and potential research avenues. *J Trauma Stress.* 2006;19:327-38.

[70]   Pedersen SS, Middel B, Larsen ML. The role of personality variables and social support in distress and perceived health in patients following myocardial infarction. *J Psychosom Res.* 2002;53:1171-5.

[71]   Chung MC, Berger Z, Rudd H. Comorbidity and personality traits in patients with different levels of posttraumatic stress disorder following myocardial infarction. *Psychiatry Res.* 2007 30;152:243-52.

[72]   Shemesh E, Rudnick A, Kaluski E, et al. A prospective study of posttraumatic stress symptoms and nonadherence in survivors of a myocardial infarction (MI). *Gen Hosp Psychiatry.* 2001;23:215-22.

[73]   Smith SC,Jr, Blair SN, Bonow RO, et al. AHA/ACC guidelines for preventing heart attack and death in patients with atherosclerotic cardiovascular disease: 2001 update. A statement for healthcare professionals from the American heart association and the American College of Cardiology. *J Am Coll Cardiol.* 2001;38:1581-3.

[74]   Lampert R, Jain D, Burg MM, et al. Destabilizing effects of mental stress on ventricular arrhythmias in patients with implantable cardioverter-defibrillators. *Circulation.* 2000;101:158-64.

[75]   Lampert R, Joska T, Burg MM, et al. Emotional and physical precipitants of ventricular arrhythmia. *Circulation.* 2002;106:1800-5.

[76]   Peters RW, McQuillan S, Resnick SK, et al. Increased monday incidence of life-threatening ventricular arrhythmias. Experience with a third-generation implantable defibrillator. *Circulation.* 1996;94:1346-9.

[77]   Rozanski A, Bairey CN, Krantz DS, et al. Mental stress and the induction of silent myocardial ischemia in patients with coronary artery disease. *N Engl J Med.* 1988;318:1005-12.

[78]   Deanfield JE, Shea M, Kensett M, et al. Silent myocardial ischaemia due to mental stress. *Lancet.* 1984;2:1001-5.

[79]   Goldberg AD, Becker LC, Bonsall R, et al. Ischemic, hemodynamic, and neurohormonal responses to mental and exercise stress. Experience from the psychophysiological investigations of myocardial ischemia study (PIMI). *Circulation.* 1996;94:2402-9.

[80]   Giubbini R, Galli M, Campini R, et al. Effects of mental stress on myocardial perfusion in patients with ischemic heart disease. *Circulation.* 1991;83:II100-7.

[81]   Gottdiener JS, Krantz DS, Howell RH, et al. Induction of silent myocardial ischemia with mental stress testing: Relation to the triggers of ischemia during daily life activities and to ischemic functional severity. *J Am Coll Cardiol.* 1994;24:1645-51.

[82]   Jern C, Eriksson E, Tengborn L, et al. Changes of plasma coagulation and fibrinolysis in response to mental stress. *Thromb Haemost.* 1989;62:767-71.

[83]   Levine SP, Towell BL, Suarez AM, et al. Platelet activation and secretion associated with emotional stress. *Circulation.* 1985;71:1129-34.

[84]   Grignani G, Soffiantino F, Zucchella M, et al. Platelet activation by emotional stress in patients with coronary artery disease. *Circulation.* 1991;83:II128-36.

[85]   Kario K, Matsuo T, Kobayashi H, et al. Earthquake-induced potentiation of acute risk factors in hypertensive elderly patients: Possible triggering of cardiovascular events after a major earthquake. *J Am Coll Cardiol.* 1997;29:926-33.

[86]   Blechert J, Michael T, Grossman P, et al. Autonomic and respiratory characteristics of posttraumatic stress disorder and panic disorder. *Psychosom Med.* 2007;69:935-43.

[87]   McEwen BS. The neurobiology and neuroendocrinology of stress. implications for post-traumatic stress disorder from a basic science perspective. *Psychiatr Clin North Am.* 2002;25:469,94, ix.

[88]   Kario K, McEwen BS, Pickering TG. Disasters and the heart: A review of the effects of earthquake-induced stress on cardiovascular disease. *Hypertens Res.* 2003;26:355-67.

[89]   Foa EB, Rothbaum BO, Riggs DS, et al. Treatment of posttraumatic stress disorder in rape victims: A comparison between cognitive-behavioral procedures and counselling. *J Consult Clin Psychol.* 1991;59:715-23.

[90]   Bryant RA, Moulds ML, Guthrie RM, et al. Imaginal exposure alone and imaginal exposure with cognitive restructuring in treatment of posttraumatic stress disorder. *J Consult Clin Psychol.* 2003;71:706-12.

[91]   Gotzmann L, Schnyder U. Posttraumatic stress disorder (PTSD) after heart transplant: The influence of earlier loss experiences on posttransplant flashbacks. *Am J Psychother.* 2002;56(4):562-7.

[92]   Ginzburg K. PTSD and world assumptions following myocardial infarction: A longitudinal study. *Am J Orthopsychiatry.* 2004;74:286-92.

[93]   Kinder LS, Bradley KA, Katon WJ, et al. Depression, posttraumatic stress disorder, and mortality. *Psychosom Med.* 2008;70:20-6.

[94]   Boscarino JA. Posttraumatic stress disorder and mortality among U.S. army veterans 30 years after military service. *Ann Epidemiol.* 2006;16:248-56.

[95]   Drescher KD, Rosen CS, Burling TA, et al. Causes of death among male veterans who received residential treatment for PTSD. *J Trauma Stress.* 2003;16:535-43.

[96]   Kasprow WJ, Rosenheck R. Mortality among homeless and nonhomeless mentally ill veterans. *J Nerv Ment Dis.* 2000;188:141-7.

[97]   Rumsfeld JS, Ho PM. Depression and cardiovascular disease: A call for recognition. *Circulation.* 2005;111:250-3.

[98]   Denollet J, Vaes J, Brutsaert DL. Inadequate response to treatment in coronary heart disease: Adverse effects of type D personality and younger age on 5-year prognosis and quality of life. *Circulation.* 2000;102:630-5.

[99]   Rumsfeld JS, Havranek E, Masoudi FA, et al. Depressive symptoms are the strongest predictors of short-term declines in health status in patients with heart failure. *J Am Coll Cardiol.* 2003;42:1811-7.

[100]   Stoll C, Schelling G, Goetz AE, et al. Health-related quality of life and post-traumatic stress disorder in patients after cardiac surgery and intensive care treatment. *J Thorac Cardiovasc Surg.* 2000;120:505-12.

In: Psychological Factors and Cardiovascular Disorders   ISBN: 978-1-60456-871-4
Editor: Leo Sher   © 2008 Nova Science Publishers, Inc.

Chapter XIII

SUB-CLINICAL PSYCHOLOGICAL CONDITIONS AFFECTING CARDIOVASCULAR DISORDERS

Chiara Rafanelli

Faculty of Psychology, University of Bologna, Italy.

ABSTRACT

Using DSM criteria in medical settings, a basic question arises, that is whether patients who do not fulfil these criteria do not indeed present psychological problems which may affect the medical symptoms and are worthy of clinical attention. However, psychological symptoms and personality traits that do not satisfy traditional psychiatric criteria are not well defined; moreover, it is difficult to measure these subtypes of distress and there is always the need for a clinical judgement. In recent years psychosomatic research has focused increasing attention on these clinical and methodological issues. Psychosocial variables that were derived from psychosomatic research were then translated into operational tools, such as Diagnostic Criteria for Psychosomatic Research (DCPR). DCPR diagnoses such as demoralization, irritable mood, type A behavior, illness denial, alexithymia and health anxiety are frequently detected in cardiac patients. The joint use of DSM-IV and DCPR criteria allow then to identify psychological factors that seem to affect cardiologic condition. Clinical and therapeutic implications are discussed by the author.

Substantial data support a strong relationship between cardiovascular diseases (coronary heart disease and congestive heart failure) and psychological conditions, such as clinical depression and anxiety detected by diagnostic criteria in the Diagnostic and Statistical Manual of Mental Disorders (DSM-IV-TR) [1]. However, using DSM criteria in medical settings, a basic question arises, that is whether patients who do not fulfil these criteria do not indeed present psychological problems which may affect the medical symptoms and are worthy of clinical attention. This question appears to be reinforced by the high prevalence of subsyndromal affective symptoms in primary care [2]. The terms "psychological subsyndromal symptoms" (for example anxiety or depressive symptoms which do not fulfil the DSM criteria for an Axis I diagnosis, influencing medical condition through the clinical judgement), "personality traits" -such as Type A behavior- or styles (being mild conditions as opposed to Axis II personality disturbances which are clearly pathological) and "risk health behaviors" have never been clearly defined and enumerated [3]; moreover, it is difficult to measure these subtypes of distress and there is always the need for a clinical judgement [4]. In recent years, psychosomatic research has focused increasing attention on these clinical and methodological issues. Psychosocial variables, observed in various medical settings and derived from psychosomatic research, were then translated, by an international group of investigators, into operational tools, such as Diagnostic Criteria for Psychosomatic Research (DCPR) [5] which may entail clinical value. The DCPR interview [6] detects subclinical psychological syndromes, which allows for identification of 12 psychosomatic clusters such as: alexithymia, type A behavior, irritable mood, demoralization, disease phobia, thanatophobia, health anxiety, illness denial, functional somatic symptoms secondary to a psychiatric disorder, persistent somatization, conversion symptoms and anniversary reaction. Data from different studies have shown that the system has good levels of reliability and validity and that the joint application of the DCPR and DSM-IV improved the identification of psychological problems in patients with a variety of medical disorders [7]. While the DSM provides important operational tools for identifying and treating mood and anxiety disorders in cardiac patients, it fails to provide proper identification, prognostic implications and potential therapeutic implications for this kind of patients in medical practice. The DCPR provides a step in this direction.

CORONARY HEART DISEASE

Coronary heart diseases (CHD) are the number one cause of death and disability in the United States and most European countries. By the time that heart problems are detected, the underlying cause (atherosclerosis) is usually quite advanced, having progressed for decades. There is therefore increased emphasis on preventing atherosclerosis by modifying risk factors, such as healthy eating, exercise and avoidance of smoking. The recent INTERHEART study [8] sought to identify modifiable risk factors for acute MI in more than 25000 patients from 52 countries. As expected, the traditional risk factors of dyslipidemia, diabetes, smoking, hypertension and obesity were all predictive factors of acute MI. However, in a multivariable model, psychosocial factors, such as stress and depression, were stronger for incident MI than diabetes, smoking, hypertension and obesity [9]. Rosengren et al. in the cited study showed, in fact, that feeling sad, blue or depressed for 2 weeks or more in a row was associated with MI across different populations and across groups of people with different ethnic origins [9]. On the other hand, a meta-analysis of 11 studies concluded that depression predicts the development of CHD in initially healthy people [10]. Sensitivity analysis showed that clinical depression was a stronger predictor than depressive mood. Contrary to the findings in this meta-analysis, Rosengren et al [9] did not find a so-called dose-response relation, because the risk of a MI was similarly increased irrespective of the number of items in the DSM depression scale.

Table 1. DCPR demoralization

Demoralization
A 1 Do you feel you have failed to meet your expectations or those of other people (concerningyour work, family, social and/or economic status)?   Yes   No
2 Is there an urgent problem you feel unable to cope with?   Yes   No
3 Do you experience feelings of helplessness, hopelessness, and/or giving up?   Yes   No
B Does your state of feeling exceed a month?   Yes   No
C Did this feeling occur before the manifestation of a physical disorder or exacerbate it?   Yes   No
Diagnosis: A (1 and/or 2 and/or 3) = yes + B = yes + C = yes

(From the Interview for the Diagnostic Criteria for Psychosomatic Research (DCPR) by L. Mangelli, C. Rafanelli, P. Porcelli, G.A. Fava, Department of Psychology, University of Bologna, Bologna, Italy, in: Rafanelli C, Roncuzzi R, Finos L, Tossani E, Tomba E, Mangelli L, Urbinati S, Pinelli G, Fava GA: Psychological assessment in cardiac rehabilitation. Psychother Psychosom 2003; 72: 343-349)

Sub-Clinical Psychological Antecedents

Demoralization

In the international literature there is the need to study other psychological variables related to depression. One aspect of depression, hopelessness, has received particular attention. Recently, prospective epidemiological studies have also reported a relationship between symptoms of hopelessness and the development of CHD through carotid atherosclerosis [11,12]. A related phenomenon is "vital exaustion": Appels and Mulder [13] found that this state, characterized by unusual fatigue, increased irritability and demoralized feelings, is associated with an increased risk of AMI. Schmale and Engel [14] have provided a detailed account for demoralization, which they defined as the "giving up-given up complex". Such a subsyndromal state cannot be identified with psychiatric categories [15]. The DCPR criteria for demoralization [6] (Table 1) identify a syndrome characterized by the patient's consciousness of having failed to meet his or her own expectations or those of others or being unable to cope with some pressing problems. The patient experiences feelings of helplessness, or hopelessness or giving up. In the study by Rafanelli et al. [16], DCPR criteria were used to detect demoralization: 20% of patients were identified as suffering from demoralization one year before the first episode of MI or angina. In 12% of patients there was an overlap between major depression and demoralization. Demoralization could not be considered a cardiac risk factor per se, but the addition of this subsyndromal state to major depression could individuate a subgroup of patients at a greater risk of a cardiac morbidity [16]. In the study by Ottolini et al. [17] at least one DCPR diagnosis was found in all patients; 51% of patients reported demoralization. 14.8% was the overlap rate of DCPR demoralization with DSM-IV mood disorders. There is a phenomenological ground whereby demoralization can be differentiated from major depression [18,19]. In fact in the sample of the cited studies [16,17] the subjects who had a mood disorder did not necessarily present demoralization and vice versa. Moreover, demoralization has been proposed as the common element of all conditions that psychotherapy attempts to relieve [20]. The diagnostic criteria for demoralization attempt to capture the state of feeling that Schmale and Engel [14] outlined as a facilitating factor for the onset of disease to which the individual was predisposed. This factor thus likely decrease individual vulnerability to disease. The results of the study by Rafanelli et al. [16] and Ottolini et al. [17] lend support to the importance of assessing both clinical and subclinical symptoms. Using DCPR criteria, the authors outlined a more specific profile which seems to be characteristic of MI patients.

Table 2. DCPR Irritable mood

Irritable Mood
A 1 When you sometimes feel irritable (either brief or prolonged episodes, occasionally or persistent), do you need to make an increased effort to control your temper? <div align="center">Yes   No</div>
2 Or do you have uncontrollable verbal or behavioral outbursts (e.g. shout, slam the door, bang your fists on the table)? <div align="center">Yes   No</div>
B After that, do you still feel bad? <div align="center">Yes   No</div>
C When you are irritable, do you feel your heart beating fast and other symptoms coming on? <div align="center">Yes   No</div>
Diagnosis: A (1 and/or 2) = yes + B = yes + C = yes

(From the Interview for the Diagnostic Criteria for Psychosomatic Research (DCPR) by L. Mangelli, C. Rafanelli, P. Porcelli, G.A. Fava, Department of Psychology, University of Bologna, Bologna, Italy, in : Rafanelli C, Roncuzzi R, Finos L, Tossani E, Tomba E, Mangelli L, Urbinati S, Pinelli G, Fava GA: Psychological assessment in cardiac rehabilitation. Psychother Psychosom 2003; 72: 343-349)

Irritable Mood

The experience of irritability is part of the normal human repertoire. Everyday stresses, such as noise, traffic, a long wait, a rude answer, may elicit irritable mood [21]. A substantial problem of research on irritability lies in the various ways it is defined. Slater and Roth [22] defined irritability as a mode of response to psychological stimuli of a particular kind, such as those in which the individual is threatened in some way, or is frustrated in a purposive course of action. A considerable body of evidence has suggested a pathogenetic role for anger, hostility and irritable mood in physical illness, both of organic and functional nature [23].

The DCPR definition of irritable mood [6)] (Table 2), a feeling state which requires an increased effort of control over temper by the individual or results in irascible verbal or behavioral outbursts, largely is based on the work of Snaith and Taylor [24]. It may be experienced as brief episodes, in particular circumstances, or it may be prolonged and generalized. Irritability can covary but differs from depressed mood. It may be part of the Type A personality associated with hostile cynism (see the following chapter). In the cited study by Ottolini et al. [17], irritable mood was the most frequent DCPR diagnosis (56% of the patients) retrospectively investigated in a sample of 92 patients at first episode of MI. This syndrome was frequently associated with anxiety disorders.

Health Anxiety

A major problem with the DSM classification of hypochondriacal fears and attitudes is that they only define the most severe end of the spectrum (hypochondriasis, characterized by resistance to medical reassurance and multiple fears). There is evidence [25,26] that other worries are worthy of clinical attention, such as health anxiety. DCPR criteria [6] (Table 3) define health anxiety as generic worry about illness, concern about pain and bodily preoccupations (tendency to amplify somatic sensations). Worries and fears are characterized to readily responding to appropriate medical reassurance, even though new worries may ensue after some time. Health anxiety was one of the most frequent diagnositic finding accounted for 41% of the total sample in the cited study by Ottolini et al. [17]. Health anxiety was frequently associated with mood disorders.

Table 3. DCPR Health anxiety

Health Anxiety
A 1 Are you worried that you may have a serious illness?   Yes   No
2 If you are suffering from common symptoms (e.g. bleeding nose, a cold, headache etc.) do you fear (e.g. become alarmed, consult your local doctor, request medical examinations, go to the hospital emergency department, consult a medical book etc.) they may develop into a serious illness?   Yes   No
B If the physician gives you an appropriate medical reassurance explaining that you don't have any illness and you are healthy, do you trust him?   Yes   No
C Have you experienced these fears for the past 6 months?   Yes   No
Diagnosis: A (1 and/or 2) = yes + B = yes + C = yes

(From the Interview for the Diagnostic Criteria for Psychosomatic Research (DCPR) by L. Mangelli, C. Rafanelli, P. Porcelli, G.A. Fava, Department of Psychology, University of Bologna, Bologna, Italy, in : Rafanelli C, Roncuzzi R, Finos L, Tossani E, Tomba E, Mangelli L, Urbinati S, Pinelli G, Fava GA: Psychological assessment in cardiac rehabilitation. Psychother Psychosom 2003; 72: 343-349)

Type A Behavior

The belief that a pattern of aggressive or irascible behavior is associated with coronary heart disease holds a peculiar and persistent fascination for both the lay public and physicians and psychologists [26]. While the history of the idea can be traced back for at least several centuries, the scientific study of the possible behavioral basis of CHD was laid by the pioneering work of Friedman and Rosenman, who, over 30 years ago, described what they termed the Type A or coronary prone behavior pattern [27,28]. This pattern was characterized by hard driving and competitive behavior, ambition, drive for success, a potential for hostility, a subjective sense of time urgency, devotion to work, restlessness, pronounced impatience, and vigorous speech stylistic and abruptness of gesture [26,29]. People relatively lacking those behavioral characteristics have been designed as type B. Type A behavior is exhibited by persons who are constantly engaged in a struggle to achieve, to outdo others, and to meet deadlines. It is not synonymous with life stress, nor does it represent a response to life stress. Rather, it constitutes a habitual behavioral state whose precursors have been observed in children [29]. It seems that type A behavior represents specific manifest features of an interaction between a set of psychological characteristics and specific stimulus situations that provoke them and promote their full expression (the social environment that offers opportunities and rewards for competitive striving and a related value system, the easy access to a diet rich in saturated fats and calories, tobacco and transportation) [29]. Type A behavior was measured using a mildly challenging structured interview and it was determined both from the content of the subject's answers to the interview questions and also from the style in which they responded. A large number of studies have been conducted in the past 3 decades on the pathogenic role of type A behavior [30] in CHD [31]. The search for these characteristics in noncardiac conditions has been neglected. Various methods of assessment have been used and the results have been rather controversial. Among the instruments for measurement of type A behavior and hostility—the Jenkins Activity Scale, the structured interview, the Minnesota multi- phasic personality inventory (MMPI), the Bortner hostility scale—have been subjected to psychometric testing and incorporated into many cardiovascular cohort studies, including some that have not reported results [32]. The most relevant clinical features of DCPR type A behavior pattern [6] (Table 4), such as excessive degree of involvement in work and pervasive sense of time urgency, elicit stress-related physiologic responses that precipitate or exacerbate symptoms of the medical condition. Unlike other psychosocial factors, type A is distinguished by being the subject of numerous intervention trials [33]. On the basis of early positive findings in the Framingham study [34] and the Western Collaborative Group's eight year follow up [35], among other evidence, the National Institutes of Health declared type A an independent risk factor for CHD. However, with the publication of negative findings [36-38] it was proposed that more specific components of type A, namely hostility and time urgency, appeared to be two key components [31], might be aetiological, although there are conflicting studies. None of the five studies that examined type A or hostility in relation to prognosis among patients with coronary heart disease showed an increased risk; indeed, one suggested a protective effect [32]. Some of the differences are, in all likelihood, due to inadequacies of measurement, such as using the cited simple questionnaires rather than the structured interview [26].

In the cited study by Ottolini et al. [17], 40% of the patients presented Type A behavior detected by DCPR criteria. Type A behavior was frequently associated with anxiety disorders. The results indicate that not all cardiac patients present with type A behavior. In those who do, the onset of irritable mood may interact with type A personality characteristics to increase psychosomatic vulnerability. In those who do not present type A features, the clinical development of symptoms may be different.

Table 4. DCPR Type A behavior

Type A Behavior
A 1 Do you often stay at work after your normal shift to finish some activities subject to deadlines, where you feel particularly responsible? Yes   No
2 Do you often have a strong sense of time urgency to finish activities (either at work or not) you have started? Yes   No
3 *Does the patient have a rapid and explosive speech, abrupt body movements, hand gestures, and tensing of facial muscles?* Yes   No
4 When you feel a strong sense of time urgency, do you become aggressive with the people around you? Yes   No
5 Do you often feel irritable? Yes   No
6 Are you inclined to walk, move, act, and gesticulate quite fast? Yes   No
7 Do you feel you have many ideas and thoughts at the same time? Yes   No
8 Do you feel you are very ambitious at work, desiring for achievements and more recognition than other people? Yes   No
9 Do you feel in competition with your colleagues? Yes   No
B Do you have physical symptoms, such as palpitations, sweating, muscular and stomach pains, intestinal disorders, and/or breathing fast? Yes   Nog
Diagnosis: A (at least 5 characteristics) = yes + B = yes

(From the Interview for the Diagnostic Criteria for Psychosomatic Research (DCPR) by L. Mangelli, C. Rafanelli, P. Porcelli, G.A. Fava, Department of Psychology, University of Bologna, Bologna, Italy, in : Rafanelli C, Roncuzzi R, Finos L, Tossani E, Tomba E, Mangelli L, Urbinati S, Pinelli G, Fava GA: Psychological assessment in cardiac rehabilitation. Psychother Psychosom 2003; 72: 343-349)

Sub-Clinical Psychological Aspects

Illness Denial

One of the most common immediate responses to MI is minimization of danger, called also denial. Illness denial is a maladaptive strategy included in the abnormal illness behavior, defined by Pilowsky [39] as the persistence of a maladaptive mode of perceiving, evaluating and responding to one's health status, despite the fact that a doctor has provided a lucid and accurate appraisal of the situation and management to be followed (if any), with opportunities for discussion, negotiation and clarification, based on adequate assessment of all relevant biological, psychological, social and cultural factors. Denial interferes with the decision process to seek immediate help. Prompt medical treatment is crucial to the survival of MI, and denial of cardiac events may be a primary reason for patient delay. However, denial has yet to be definitively linked to patient delay [40]. Further research is needed on this relationship, because if such a link exists, dramatic reductions of patient delay might be possible. Although denial may be an adaptive behavior towards the first three days of recovery from MI [41], there is strong evidence that prolonged denial of the significance of the illness negatively affects MI recovery outcome once removed from the hospital setting [41,42]. As Sirous [43] concluded in his review on denial in CHD, denial likely has a long-term negative effect on cardiovascular health. The extent and importance of that negative effect on cardiovascular health is still quite unknown due to methodological problems concerning the assessment of denial. In fact, even though a number of scales have been created in attempts to accurately assess and quantify denial and have been used in multiple clinical trials [41,44], there is no standard measurement of denial. The DCPR illness-denying category of abnormal illness behavior [6] (Table 5) provides room for various psychosomatic situations occurring in both medical and surgical cardiac settings. Two alternative explanations have been offered for the denial: 1) denial as a defence against death anxiety, coupled with a tendency to rationalize the symptoms as not related to the heart and 2) denial as minimization of the symptoms' significance to avoid the acceptance of the helplessness of being sick and having to depend on others. Patients with a history of a previous myocardial infarction or angina tend to delay calling for help more than do younger persons having their first experience of chest pain or dyspnoea. Education of high-risk patients, such as those with a history of previous infarction, could reduce the tendency to delay seeking help. Responses and coping strategies, adaptive or maladaptive, are influenced by personality, family and medical factors. Persons who habitually deny or minimize the threatening significance of events tend to do so after a MI [29].

Minor Depression

The diagnosis of depression in medically ill patients is complex [45], and cardiac patients are no exception. Many investigators question if what we call depression in coronary patients is essentially the same disorder as depression in non medical population [46] to the extent that some researchers prefer "depressive symptomatology" over "depression" that could be better delineated as a spectrum of depressive symptoms, and even negative cognitive states, that may be associated with the development of coronary artery disease and thus worthy of clinical attention and management [47]. Other researchers are of the opinion that the mental state of coronary patients may be better thought of as a general negative affect, because of the substantial and consistent correlation of measures of depression, hostility, anxiety and fatigue [48]. Cardiac patients' reports of depressive symptoms are usually less direct and less typical than those in psychiatric setting [49]. They are likely to complain primarily of unusual tiredness or lack of energy and unexplained somatic symptoms, including atypical chest pain, dyspnoea and palpitations. Cardiac patients tend to normalize depression and attribute somatic symptoms of depression to their heart disease, making them less likely to consider emotional causes for their complaints. Also, the typical symptoms of depression in psychiatric patients, like sadness, low self-esteem, guilt, and wishes for death, are often replaced by less typical symptoms, like anxiety (chronic worries, hypervigilance, multiple somatic complaints) and irritability (sudden bursts of anger and hostility, frequent negative and unpleasant comment to others, hypersensitivity to noise [50]. Numerous studies suggest that not only major depressive disorder, but also minor depression, in addition to their effects on quality of life [50], are cardiac risk factors. The diagnosis of minor depression is based on criteria in the appendix to DSM-IV-TR and is performed when an "essential feature" of major depression (dysphoria or anhedonia) is present over a period of 2 weeks with at least 1 but not more than 3 additional symptoms of depression. The cardiac risk is referred not only for the development of CHD events in healthy patients [52], but also for recurrent events in patients with established CHD [53-55], and for adverse cardiovascular outcomes after artery by-pass grafting (CABG) surgery [56,57]. In the study by Rafanelli et al [57], clinical and sub-clinical distress was evaluated in a consecutive series of 47 patients with recent CABG surgery, referred to the Cardiac Rehabilitation Program of the hospital, both at a one month assessment as well as at a 6-8 year follow-up visit. One month after CABG, at the first psychological assessment, 6 patients (12.8%) received a diagnosis of minor depression, 5 (10.6%) of major depression. Among the variables examined as potential risk factors for coronary events (angina pectoris, myocardial infarction, cardiac death) only observer-rated minor depression attained statistical significance ($p < 0.01$). The available data suggest that depression in general, assessed by self-rated methods, could be a risk factor for cardiac events in this population. In the study by Connerney and collegues [58], only major depression was evaluated in CABG patients by clinical interview and was found to be related to cardiac events at the one year follow-up. The data of the study by Rafanelli et al [57] suggest the relevance of minor depression as potential cardiac risk factor in CABG patients at the 6-8 year follow-up. Clinical approach to these patients should then include not only an accurate investigation of severe depression, as outlined in the literature on cardiovascular patients, but also of minor depression. Blumenthal and collegues [59] showed that not only patients with moderate to severe depression before CABG but also patients with mild or moderate to severe depression that persisted 6 months after CABG, had higher rates of death than did those without depression. It is likely that depression is thought of as an understandable and inevitable reaction to the severe circumstances accompanying CABG surgery, and as a result, it is not always treated [58]. It is conceivable that minor depression could be underestimated and undertreated even more frequently compared to major depression and could thus represent a persistent factor incrementing psychological and physical vulnerability. Although the basis of the relationship between depression and cardiac morbidity and mortality remains speculative, there are various potential social, behavioral and biological mechanisms by which depression may confer this increased risk [59].

Future studies should investigate the degree of certain symptoms in association or not with other psychological or physical factors responsible for clinical outcomes. Even though the only randomised behavioral intervention trial attempting to reduce morbidity and mortality in depressed patients with existing coronary disease [60] showed that changes in depression did not translate into improved survival, there remains the need to further investigate if treating even minor depression can reduce the risk of morbidity and mortality in patients who underwent CABG.

Table 5. DCPR Illness denial

Illness Denial
A 1 Have you ever neglected to bring to your physician's attention serious symptoms or ignored your physician's diagnosis and recommendations? Yes   No 2 If the physician tells you that you have a disorder and prescribes you drugs, a suitable diet or an appropriate physical activity, do you follow the medical advice? Yes   No B Did the physician tell you that you have a medical disorder and provide a clear explanation of the medical situation and management to be followed? Yes   No
Diagnosis: If A (1 = yes and/or 2 = no; or 1 = yes and/or 2 =yes; or 1 = no and/or 2 = no) and B = yes

(From the Interview for the Diagnostic Criteria for Psychosomatic Research (DCPR) by L. Mangelli, C. Rafanelli, P. Porcelli, G.A. Fava, Department of Psychology, University of Bologna, Bologna, Italy, in : Rafanelli C, Roncuzzi R, Finos L, Tossani E, Tomba E, Mangelli L, Urbinati S, Pinelli G, Fava GA: Psychological assessment in cardiac rehabilitation. Psychother Psychosom 2003; 72: 343-349)

HEART FAILURE

Congestive Heart Failure (CHF) is the end stage of many diseases of the heart (ischemic heart disease, hypertensive heart disease, valvular heart disease and cardiomyopathy) and a major cause of morbidity and mortality. It is only in recent years that the psychological impact of heart failure has been explored, which is reflected by the absence of standardized psychological assessment for patients with CHF [61] and concerns about how to measure psychosocial factors in clinical practice [62]. In fact, despite extensive work, researchers have not even agreed among themselves on the best instrument to measure any of the major psychological or social constructs of interest. An example that illustrates the problem is that of quality of life [63]. Problems with lack of universally accepted definitions and standard instruments for assessing anxiety, depression, and social support are also common and limit the inclusion of these variables in clinical practice [62].

Regardless of the severity of the disease, a high level of psychological distress is a significant predictor of hospital readmission [64], poor quality of life [65] and high mortality [66] in cardiac patients. Psychosocial issues are then important variables that need to be addressed in patients with CHF. Unfortunely, these issues are often overlooked. Both depression and anxiety have been linked independently to recurrent cardiac events and increased mortality in post-MI patients, but few investigators have studied the impact of these emotions in patients with heart failure [62]. The study by Moser et al [67] outlines that patients newly discharged from hospitalization for CHF exhibit both behavioral and psychosocial risk factors for rehospitalization, although they have been judged clinically stable. Many findings in patients with CHD are relevant to patients with CHF because more than one half of patients with CHF have underlying CHD [68], and the two conditions often have shared characteristics. Nonetheless, CHF patients have to bear a chronic and life-threatening disease trajectory that is characterized by severe fatigue and dyspnoea, deteriorating functional status, episodic adverse cardiac events and repeated hospital readmission [69]. Thus, it is not only physically debilitating, but also psychologically distressing. Moreover, in CHF even more than in the case of ischemic heart disease, the situation is complicated by difficulties in deciding whether to ascribe symptoms like dyspnoea, fatigue, insomnia, anorexia, or even palpitation to disease of the heart or of the nervous system [70]. For example depression, when severe enough, can result in malnutrition. Acute mental stress, such as mental arithmetic or a stress interview, can induce transient changes in left ventricular systolic and diastolic function [71] and, in susceptible individuals, the hypertensive and tachycardic reactions are impressive.

Subclinical Psychological Aspects

DCPR Syndromes

In the study by Grandi et al [72], 129 patients were seen 1 month after the cardiac transplantation. DCPR diagnoses [6] were formulated independently of the DSM-IV diagnostic findings. Only 41 patients out of 129 (31%) received no DCPR diagnosis. In the remaining patients, there were 141 diagnoses. Demoralization, type A behavior, alexythimia and irritable mood were the most frequent diagnostic findings and accounted for roughly 75% of the diagnoses. Also common were health anxiety and illness denial diagnoses.

Feelings of demoralization (Table 1) in heart transplant population seem to be related to the loss of a working position, the reduction of social links and the dependence on other people's support, which creates in the patients a feeling of impotence and loneliness. Patients who were given a DSM diagnosis also presented a DCPR diagnosis. Demoralization was frequently associated with mood disorders and anxiety disorders.

As already shown in the literature in the previous chapters, subjects affected by cardiovascular disease seem to present a behavioral pattern characterized by hostility and a sense of being under the pressure of time. The results of the cited study confirm a high prevalence of type A behaviour (Table 4) in this sample.

Alexithymia, a concept introduced by Sifneos [73] to describe impoverished fantasy life with a resulting utilitarian way of thinking and a characteristic inability to use appropriate words to describe emotions, accounted for nearly 12% of DCPR diagnoses [6] (Table 6). This concept has stimulated two decades of psychosomatic research. It has been found that alexithymia is more common in patients with long-lasting psychosomatic conditions than in other subjects. The inhibition of emotional expression and particularly a life-long tendency to suppress anger, have been found to involve increased risk for a variety of health problems both using the alexithymia [74] or similar [75,76] psychological constructs. Alexithymia is generally considered as a stable personality trait [74,77,78]. Alexithymia was found to be present also in heart-transplant patients. The relationship between alexithymia and depression is still controversial [79,80]. Poor ability to be aware of and to cope with emotions may make an alexithymic individual vulnerable to continuous stress.

Table 6. DCPR Alexithymia

Alexithymia
The interviewer should assess the overall content of the interview and nonverbal behavior, in addition to the following questions:
A 1 When you experience something good or bad, are you able to describe your emotions (delight, joy, worry, sadness, anger)? <div align="center">Yes   No</div>
2 When you experience either good or bad events, do you talk about what has happened and what you feel inside of you? <div align="center">Yes   No</div>
3 Do you often day-dream and let your imagination run away? <div align="center">Yes   No</div>
4 Do your thoughts concern more often your internal emotions and feelings? <div align="center">Yes   No</div>
5 When you experience a strong emotion, do you also feel physical reactions (e.g. sick to stomach etc.)? <div align="center">Yes   No</div>
6 Have you ever had occasional but violent outbursts of anger, crying, or joy, that are inappropriate either in relationship with what was happening or your usual behavior? <div align="center">Yes   No</div>
Diagnosis: at least 3 characteristics: A1 = no; A2 = no; A3 = no; A4 = no; A5 = no; A6 = yes.

(From the Interview for the Diagnostic Criteria for Psychosomatic Research (DCPR) by L. Mangelli, C. Rafanelli, P. Porcelli, G.A. Fava, Department of Psychology, University of Bologna, Bologna, Italy, in : Rafanelli C, Roncuzzi R, Finos L, Tossani E, Tomba E, Mangelli L, Urbinati S, Pinelli G, Fava GA: Psychological assessment in cardiac rehabilitation. Psychother Psychosom 2003; 72: 343-349)

Irritable mood (Table 2) appears to be a long-standing syndrome in this population: patients admit to often feeling irritated by someone else's behavior and they declare to make a big effort to contain their anger, which sometimes explodes anyway. It is, however, important to keep in mind that the very stressful circumstances that they have to cope with could exacerbate and amplify an already existent attitude.

Health anxiety (Table 3), indicating preoccupations about health in the absence of a pathology or excessive concern in case pathology is present, seemed to be quite common among these patients. The main aspect of health anxiety seems to be the presence of dysfunctional beliefs about health and illnesses which could derive from past experiences of illness in oneself or others [81,82]. These worries are part of a vicious circle characterized by selective perception and misinterpretation of bodily symptoms which all together may increase health anxiety.

Illness denial (Table 5) is reported relatively often in this sample. In the literature it has been highlighted how this type of psychological defence is quite common among subjects who have to deal with a chronic illness. If denial does not reach excessive levels, it could be considered as an adaptive mechanism which could be helpful in the decrease of anxiety. An excessively strong denial, however, could interfere with a good compliance. A specific type of denial is characterized by too optimistic expectations towards the future and an underestimation of problems and complications [20,83].

Mood disorders appear to be related to irritable mood and alexithymia. The overlaps were smaller compared to the previous associations. Anxiety disorders were mostly associated with demoralization, type A behavior and irritable mood. Thirty-seven (28%) of the patients received neither a DCPR diagnosis nor a DSM diagnosis. There were fewer patients (31%) with no DCPR diagnosis than with no DSM-IV diagnosis (82%). Fifty-six patients (43%) who received a DCPR diagnosis were not identified by any DSM-IV diagnosis. Only 4 patients (3%) who received a DSM-IV diagnosis did not receive any DCPR diagnosis. The most frequent associations were between demoralization, type A behavior and irritable mood. The findings of the study by Grandi et al. [72] indicate that diagnostic criteria which may be viewed as encompassing psychosomatic and sub-clinical variable symptomatology (DCPR) fit better with a medical population than DSM criteria. The number of DCPR diagnoses has been, in fact, almost triple the number of DSM diagnoses. Only a small percentage of patients were not identified by DCPR criteria and this percentage was less than that entailed by DSM criteria. While patients who were given a DSM diagnosis frequently had additional DCPR diagnoses, many patients with DCPR syndromes did not fulfil any DSM criteria. These findings seem to suggest that the DCPR detect psychological dimensions which are not identified by DSM criteria. Finally, the joint use of DSM and DCPR criteria was found to improve the identification of psychological factors in a population of heart-transplanted patients. Even though it is possible to identify depressive and anxiety symptoms, in the majority of the cases, they are not severe enough in order to satisfy all the necessary criteria to make a diagnosis. Using DCPR criteria the authors outlined a more specific profile which seems to be characteristic of heart-transplant patients.

Minor Depression

As outlined in the previous chapters, in psychosomatic research there is an increasing attention on quantitative and qualitative aspects of depression. In recent studies, sub-clinical self-rated depressive symptoms resulted as clinically significant [84], highly prevalent [85] and with prognostic factor in CHF patients [86,87].

The aims of a study by Rafanelli et al. [88] were to assess clinical and subclinical depression in 68 CHF outpatients visited at Bellaria Hospital in Bologna, Italy, at the initial assessment and at 2 months follow-up routine visit. At the first evaluation, 22 patients (32.4%) reported major depression, 7 (10.3%) minor depression and 14 (20.6%) demoralization. Among the variables examined as potential risk factors for cardiovascular outcome events, based on rehospitalization and cardiac death, only minor depression attained statistical significance. Previous studies have reported that depression symptoms have an adverse effect on the physical outcomes of people with CHF [89-91]. In the cited study, results from survival analysis show that observer rated minor depression is a potential risk factor for cardiac outcome events 2 months after a first psychologic evaluation during routine outpatient visits. These data, resembling those of a previous study in CABG patients [56] suggest the relevance of the assessment of minor depression in CHF outpatients. The fact that minor depression, but not major depression, influenced survival, could be explained by means of qualitative differences between the two syndromes. It could be supposed that just a few symptoms diagnosed in patients with minor depression could be more important in terms of prognosis than the others, numerically superior, diagnosed in patients with major depression. On the other hand, we know that the symptomatic course of depression is dynamic and changeable, and major depression, minor depression and even depressive symptom levels commonly alternate over time in the same patients as a symptomatic continuum of illness activity of a single clinical disease [92]. The roll-back phenomenon by Detre and Jarecki [93] could explain the course of depression on the basis of prodromal and residual symptoms: as the illness remits, it progressively recapitulates, even though in reverse order, many of the stages and symptoms that were seen during the time it developed. For example, if an illness begins with slight symptoms of sadness, that are superseded some weeks later by depressive symptoms which then become progressively more severe until after several months the patient develops total insomnia and confusion, the symptoms tend, as the condition improves, to remit in reverse order, the confusion and insomnia diminishing first, and the depressed mood next. After the depression lifts, the patient may again experience residual depressive symptoms for several weeks, until finally these symptoms, too, disappear.

It is conceivable that minor depression could be underestimated and undertreated even more frequently compared to major depression and could thus represent a persistent factor incrementing psychological and physical vulnerability.

INTERVENTIONS FOR PSYCHOLOGICAL CONDITIONS

Research on the efficacy of interventions for psychological conditions in cardiac patients is quite limited, and much of the literature has been anecdotal, relying heavily on clinical experience and intuition to guide the selection of treatment strategies [94]. The issue of studying and integrating psychosocial interventions into clinical practice would benefit from important measures. The first step in managing cardiac patients should be routine screening to identify those who are distressed. Recent data, as strengthened in this article, outlines the need to evaluate not only clinical syndromes but also sub-clinical ones (such as irritable mood, demoralization, illness denial, Type A behavior). DCPR criteria could be thus added in routine screening to better identify specific needs of the patients in cardiac settings. More physicians need thus to be made aware of the recent developments that establish key psychosocial variables as risk factors for the development of CHD and as contributing factors to the expression of disease activity [95]. Secondly, the effectiveness of behavioral interventions for cardiac patients needs to be evaluated and implemented in clinical settings. Since very few studies have examined the efficacy of these interventions for cardiac patients. Patients with mild levels of anxiety or depression are likely to benefit from Cardiac Rehabilitation (CR) programs that combine psychosocial interventions with exercise training [96,97]. Psychosocial interventions offered by CR programs can vary widely [98], but interventions such as relaxation training, stress management, psychological support and cognitive restructuring are likely to be beneficial because they have been shown to reduce anxiety and depression in psychiatry patients [99]. In particular, the so-called cardiac stress management program is a method, based on principles of behavioral modification, aimed at two objectives: stress management training and change of habitual behavior. Stress management training involves teaching the person how to relax, identify situations inducing stress responses in him or her competitiveness, time pressure, achievement motivation, hostility, and other components of the type A behavior pattern. That pattern, however, is so strongly embedded in Western culture and occupational careers and is so often rewarded that it is liable to prove resistant to lasting change [28]. Other techniques used to treat sub-clinical anxious and depressive conditions could be incorporated easily into CR programs. For example, scheduling pleasant activities is an important component of some evidence-based interventions for depression [100,101]. Therefore, in addition to encouraging increased physical exercise, CR clinicians could encourage patients to become more engaged in pleasurable activities such as reading, visiting friends or gardening. Because the problem of lifestyle factors (e.g. smoking, alcohol use) and psychosocial stress frequently cluster together, treatment of patients who are noncompliant with lifestyle changes may benefit from consideration of concomitant psychosocial stresses. As outlined by Rozansky [95], the efficacy of psychosocial interventions may be improved by development of "patient-specific" treatment plans, based on the "profiling" of the major psychosocial risk factors in individual patients. Further studies will confirm if the pshychological management of sub-clinical syndromes as well could improve quality of life, through adverse health behaviors, lack of adherence, physical symptom perception, functional impairment and medical utilization. Moreover there remains the need to further investigate if the management of DCPR syndromes had prognostic implication preventing cardiac morbidity and mortality in these patients. Moreover, the pathophysiological mechanisms by which behavior therapies addressed to psychological risk factors reduce cardiac events need to be identified [95].

CONCLUSIONS

The findings of the present article indicate that DCPR diagnostic criteria which may be viewed as encompassing subclinical symptomatology do fit with a cardiac population and their use might expand the range of a psychological assessment in the setting of cardiovascular disease. There remains the need to further investigate if treating subsyndromal psychological conditions can improve quality of life and reduce the risk of morbidity and mortality in these patients. It is clear that further research on the interactions between mental and cardiac health is needed at the clinical, pathophysiological, biochemical and molecular levels if we are to understand the interactions of these two illnesses [102].

REFERENCES

[1]   *American Psychiatric Association. Diagnostic and Statistical Manual of Mental Disorders*. 4th Ed. Text revised. Washington, DC, American Psychiatric Press, 2000

[2]   Roy-Byrne P, Katon W, Broadhead WE, Lepine JP, Richards J, Brantley PJ, Russo J, Zinbarg R, Barlow D, Liebowitz M: Subsyndromal (mixed) anxiety-depression in primary care. *J Intern Med* 1994;9:507–512

[3]   Ketterer MW, Mahr G, Goldberg AD: Psychological factors affecting medical condition: ischemic coronary heart disease. *J Psychosom Res*. 2000; 48:357-67

[4]   Fava GA, Ruini C, Rafanelli C: Psychometric theory is an obstacle to the progress of clinical research. *Psychotherapy and Psychosomatics* 2004; 73: 145-148

[5]   Fava GA, Freyberger HJ, Bech P, Christodoulou G, Sensky T, Theorell T, Wise TN: Diagnostic criteria for use in psychosomatic research. *Psychother Psychosom* 1995; 63: 1-8

[6]   Rafanelli C, Roncuzzi R, Finos L, Tossani E, Tomba E, Mangelli L, Urbinati S, Pinelli G, Fava GA: Psychological assessment in cardiac rehabilitation. *Psychother Psychosom* 2003; 72: 343-349

[7]   Porcelli P, Sonino N (eds): *Psychological factors affecting medical conditions. A new classification for DSM-V*. Adv Psychosom Med. Basel, Karger, 2007, vol 28

[8]   Yusuf S, Hawken S, Ounpuu S, Dans T, Avezum A, Lanas F, McQueen M, Budaj A, Pais P, Varigos J, Lisheng L; INTERHEART Study Investigators study. Effect of potentially modifiable risk factors associated with myocardial infarction in 52 countries (the INTERHEART study): case-control study. *Lancet* 2004; 364:937-52

[9]   Rosengren A, Hawken S, Ôunpuu S, Sliwa K, Zubaid M, Almahmeed WA, Blackett KN, Sitthi-amorn C, Sato H, Yusuf S: Association of psychosocial risk factors with risk of acute myocardial infarction in 11119 cases and 13648 controls from 52 countries (the INTERHEART study): case-control study. *Lancet* 2004; 364:953-62

[10]   Rugulies R. Depression as a predictor for coronary heart disease: a review and meta-analysis. *Am J Prev Med* 2002; 23: 51–61

[11]   Everson SA, Goldberg DE, Kaplan GA, Cohen RD, Pukkala E, Tuomilehto J, Salonen JT: Hopelessness and risk of mortality and incidence of myocardial infarction and cancer. *Psychosom Med* 1996; 58: 113-121

[12]   Everson SA, Kaplan GA, Goldberg DE, Salonen JT: Hopelessness and 4-year progression of carothid atherosclerosis: the Kupio ischemic heart disease risk factor study. *Arteriosler Thromb Vasc Biol* 1997; 17: 1490-1495

[13]   Appels A, Mulder P: Excess fatigue as a precursor of myocardial infarction. *Eur Heart J* 1988; 9: 758-764

[14]   Schmale AH, Engel GL: The giving up-given-up complex illustrated on fil. *Arch Gen Psychiatry* 1967; 17: 135-145

[15]   Bech P. Measurement of psychological distress and well-being. *Psychother Psychosom* 1990; 54: 77-89

[16]   Rafanelli C, Roncuzzi R, Milaneschi Y, Tomba E, Colistro MC, Pancaldi LG, Di Pasquale G: Stressful life events, depression and demoralization as risk factors for acute coronary heart disease. *Psychother Psychosom* 2005; 74: 179-184

[17]   Ottolini F, Modena MG, Rigatelli M: Prodromal Symptoms in Myocardial Infarction. *Psychother Psychosom* 2005; 74:323-327

[18]   De Figuereido JM: Depression and demoralization: Phenomenological differences and research perspectives. *Comp Psychiatry* 1993; 34: 308–311

[19]   Fava GA: Screening and diagnosis of depression. *Dis Manage Health Outcomes* 1997; 2:1-7

[20]   Frank JD, Frank JB: *Persuasion and Healing*. Baltimore, Johns Hopkins University Press, 1991

[21]   Fava GA: Irritable mood and physical illness. *Stress Medicine* 1987; 3: 293-299

[22]   Mangelli L, Fava GA, Grassi L, Ottolini F, Paolini S, Porcelli P, Rafanelli C, Rigatelli M, Sonino N: Irritable mood in Italian patients with medical disease. *J Nerv Ment Dis* 2006; 194:1-3

[23]   Slater E, Roth M: Irritabilità. In Mayer-Gross, Slater and Roth *Clinical Psychiatry*. London, Bailliere, Tindall and Cassell, pp.137

[24]   Snaith RP, Taylor CM: Irritability. *Br J Psychiatry* 1985; 147: 127-136

[25]   Fava GA, Grandi S: Differential diagnosis of hypochondriacal fears and beliefs. *Psychother Psychosom* 1991; 55:114-119

[26]   Johnston DW: The current status of the coronary prone behaviour pattern. *Journal of the Royal Society of Medicine* 1993; 86: 406-409

[27]   Friedman M, Rosenman RH. Association of a specific overt behaviour pattern with increases in blood cholesterol: blood clotting time: incidence of arcus senilis and clinical coronary artery disease. *JAMA* 1959; 169:1286-96

[28]   Rosenman RH, Friedman M, Strauss R, Wurm M, Kositchek R, Hahn W, et aL A predictive study of coronary heart disease. *JAMA* 1964;189:15-22

[29]   Lipowski ZJ: Cardiovascular Disorders. In *Comprehensive Textbook of Psychiatry/III.* Kaplan HI, Freedman AM, Sadock BJ (eds), Baltimore/London, Williams & Wilkins, 1980

[30]   Friedman M, Powell LH. The diagnosis and quantitative assessment of Type A behaviour. *Integrative Psychiatry* 1984; 2: 123-129

[31]   Littman AB. Review of psychosomatic aspects of cardiovascular disease. *Psychother Psychosom.* 1993; 60: 148-167

[32]   Hemingway H, Marmot M: Evidence based cardiology: Psychosocial factors in the aetiology and prognosis of coronary heart disease: systematic review of prospective cohort studies. *BMJ* 1999; 318: 1460-1467

[33]   Nunes EV, Frank KA, Kornfield DS. Psychologic treatment for the type A behaviour pattern for coronary heart disease: a meta-analysis of the literature. *Psychosom Med* 1987; 48:159-73

[34]   Haynes SG, Feinleib M, Kannel WB. The relationship of psychosocial factors to
        coronary heart disease in the Framingham study: 3. Eight year incidence of coronary
        heart disease. *Am J Epidemiol* 1980; 111:37-58

[35]   Rosenman RH, Brand RJ, Sholtz RI, Friedman M: Multivariate prediction of coronary
        heart disease during 8.5 year follow-up in Western Collaborative Group Study. *Am J
        Cardiol* 1976; 37:903-9

[36]   Shekelle RB, Hulley SB, Neaton JD, Billings J, Borhani NO, Gerace TA, Jacobs DR,
        Lasser NL, Mittlemark MB, Stamler J: The MRFIT behavior pattern study. II. Type A
        behavior and incidence of coronary heart disease. *Am J Epidemiol* 1985;122:559-70

[37]   Johnston DW, Cook DG, Shaper AG: Type A behaviour and ischaemic heart disease
        in middle-aged British men. *BMJ* 1987; 295:86-9

[38]   Hearn M, Murray DM, Luepker RB: Hostility, coronary heart disease and total
        mortality: a 33 year follow up study of university students. *J Behav Med*
        1989;12:105-21

[39]   Pilowsky I: Abnormal illness behavior. *Psychother Psychosom* 1986; 46: 76-84

[40]   Wielgosz A., Nolan R, Earp J, Biro E, Wielgosz M: Reasons for patients' delay in
        response to symptoms of acute myocardial infarction. *Can Med Assoc J* 1988; 139:
        853-857

[41]   Levine J, Warrenburg S, Kerns R, Schwartz G, Delaney R, Fontana A, Gradman A,
        Smith S, Allen S, Cascione R: The role of denial in recovery from coronary heart
        disease. *Psychosomatic Medicine* 1987; 49: 109-117

[42]   Julkunen J, Saarinen T: Psychosocial predictors of recovery after a myocardial
        infarction: Development of a comprehensive assessment method. *The Irish Journal of
        Psychology* 1994; 15, 67-83.

[43]   Sirous F: Le deni dans la maladie coronarienne (Denial in coronary artery disease).
        Can Med Assoc J 1992; 147, 315-321

[44]   Jamner L, Schwartz G: Self-deception predicts self-report and endurance of pain.
        Psychosomatic Medicine 1986; 48: 211-223

[45]   Fava GA, Sonino N: Depression associated with medical illness. *CNS Drugs* 1996;
        5:175-189

[46]   Appels A: Depression and coronary artery disease: observations and question. *J
        Psychosom Res* 1997; 43:443-452

[47]   Sheps D, Rozansky A: From feeling blue to clinical depression: Exploring the
        pathogenicity of depressive symptoms and their management in cardiac practice.
        Psychosom Med 2005; 67:S2-S5

[48]   Denollet J, Brutsaert DL. Enhancing emotional well-being by comprehensive
        rehabilitation in patients with coronary heart disease. *Eur Heart J.* 1995; 16: 1070–
        1078

[49]   Freedland KE, Lustman PJ, Carney RM, Hong BA: underdiagnosis of depression in
        patients with coronary artery disease: the role of non-specific symptoms. *Int J
        Psychiatry Med* 1992; 22:221-229

[50]   Fava M, Abraham M, Pava J, Shuster J, Rosenbaum J: Cardiovascular risk factors in
        depression: the role of anxiety and anger. *Psychosomatics* 1996; 37:31-37

[51]   Lane D, Carroll D, Ring C et al: Mortality and quality of life 12 months after myocardial infarction: effects of depression and anxiety. *Psychosom Med* 2001; 63:221-230

[52]   Lett HS, Blumenthal JA, Babyak MA, Sherwood A, Strauman T, Robins C, Newman MF: Depression as a risk factor for coronary artery disease: evidence, mechanism and treatment. *Psychosom Med* 2004; 66:305-315

[53]   Barth J, Schumacher M, Herrmann-Lingen C: Depression as a risk factor for mortality in patients with coronary heart disease: a meta-analysis. *Psychosom Med.* 2004;66:802-13

[54]   Van Melle JP, de Jonge P, Spijkerman TA, Tijssen JGP, Ormel J, van Veldhuisen DJ, van den Brink RHS, van den Berg MP: Prognostic association of depression following myocardial infarction with mortality and cardiovascular events: a meta-analysis. *Psychosom Med* 2004; 66: 814–22

[55]   Evans DL, Charney DS, Lewis L, Golden RN, Gorman JM, Krishnan KR, et al. Mood disorders in the medically ill: scientific review and recommendations. *Biol Psychiatry.* 2005;58:175-89

[56]   Borowicz L, Royall R, Grega M, Selnes O, Lyketsos K, McKhann G: Depression and cardiac morbidity 5 years after coronary artery bypass surgery. *Psychosomatics* 2002; 43:464-71

[57]   Rafanelli C, Roncuzzi R, Milaneschi Y: Minor depression as a cardiac risk factor after Coronary Artery Bypass Surgery. *Psychosomatics* 2006; 47:289-295

[58]   Connerney I, Shapiro PA, McLaughlin JS, Bagiella E, Sloan RP: Relation between depression after coronary artery bypass surgery and 12-month outcome: a prospective study. *Lancet* 2001; 358: 1766-1771

[59]   Blumenthal JA, Lett HS, Babyak MA, White W, Smith PK, Mark DB, Jones R, Mathew JP, Newman MF and NORG Investigators. Depression as a risk factor for mortality after coronary artery bypass surgery. *Lancet* 2003; 362: 604-609

[60]   Writing Commettee for the ENRICHD Investigators. Effects of treating depression and low perceived social support on clinical events after myocardial infarction: the Enhancing Recovery in Coronary Heart Disease Patients (ENRICHD) randomized trial. *JAMA* 2003; 289: 3106-3116

[61]   MacMahon KM, Lip GY: Psychological factors in heart failure: a review of the literature. *Arch Int Med* 2002, 162: 509-516

[62]   Moser DK: Psychosocial factors and their association with clinical outcomes in patients with heart failure: why clinicians do not seem to care. *Eur J Card Nursing* 2002; 1:183-188

[63]   Kinney MR, Burfitt SN, Stullenbarger E, Rees B, DeBolt MR: Quality of life in cardiac patient research: a meta-analysis. *Nurs Res* 1996; 45:173-180

[64]   Levine JB, Covaino NA, Slack VW et al: psychological predictors of subsequent medical care among patients hospitalized with cardiac disease. *J Cardiopulm Rehab* 1996; 16:109-116

[65]   Lane D, Carroll D, Ring C, Beevers DG, Lip GYH: Mortality and quality of life 12 months after myocardial infarction. *Psychosom Med* 2001; 63:221-230

[66]   Vaccarino V, Kasl SV, Abramson J, Krumholz HM: Depressive symptoms and risk of functional decline and death in patients with heart failure. *J Am Coll Cardiol* 2001; 38:199-205

[67]   Moser DK, Doering LV, Ching ML: Vulnerabilities of patients recovering from an exacerbation of chronic heart failure. *Am Heart J* 2005; 150:7-13

[68]   Kannel WB, Ho K, Thom T: Changing epidemiological features of cardiac failure. *Br Heart J* 1994; 72:S3-S9

[69]   Yu DS, Lee DT, Woo J, Thompson DR: Correlates of psychological distress in elderly patients with congestive heart failure. *J Psychosom Res* 2004; 57: 573-581

[70]   Skotzko CE, Krichten C, Zietowski G, Alves L, Freudenberger R, Robinson S, Fisher M, Gottlieb SS: Depression is common and precludes accurate assessment of functional status in elderly patients with congestive heart failure. *J Card Fail* 2000; 6:300-305

[71]   Giannuzzi P, Shabetai R, Imparato A, Temporelli PL, Bhargava V, Cremo R, Tavazzi L: Effects of mental exercise in patients with dilated cardiomyopathy and congestive heart failure: an echocardiographic Doppler Study. *Circulation* 1991; 83: 155-165

[72]   Grandi S, Fabbri S, Tossani E, Mangelli L, Branzi A, Magelli C: Psychological evaluation after cardiac transplantation: the integration of different criteria. *Psychother Psychosom* 70: 176-183, 2001

[73]   Sifneos PE. The prevalence of "alexithymic" characteristics in psychosomatic patients. *Psychother Psychosom* 1973; 22: 255-262

[74]   Taylor GJ, Bagby RM, Parker JDA: *Disorders of affect regulation: alexithymia in medical and psychiatric illness.* Cambridge, UK, Cambridge University Press, 1997

[75]   Greer J. Cancer and the mind. *Br J Psychiatry* 1983; 143: 535-543

[76]   Berry DS, Pennebaker JW. Nonverbal and verbal emotional expression and health. *Psychother Psychosom* 1993; 59: 11-19

[77]   Kauhanen J, Julkunen J, Salonen JT: Validity and reliability of the Toronto Alexithymia Scale (TAS) in a population study. *J Psychosom Res* 1992; 36:687-69480. 253.

[78]   Salminen JK, Saarijarvi S, Toikka T, Kauhanen J. Prevalence of alexithymia and its association with sociodemographic variables in the general population of Finland. *J Psychosom Res* 1999; 46:75-82

[79]   Honkalampi A, Saarinen P, Hintikka J, Virtanen V, Vinamaki H: Factors associated with alexithymia in patients suffering from depression. *Psychother Psychosom* 1999;68:270–275

[80]   Honkalampi A, Hintikka J, Saarinen P, Sehtonen J, Vinamaki H: Is alexithymia a permanent feature in depressed patients? *Psychother Psychosom* 2000;69:305–308

[81]   Lucock MP, Morley S: The Health Anxiety Questionnaire. *Br J Health Psychol* 1996;1: 137–150

[82]   Wells A, Hackmann A: Imagery and core beliefs in health anxiety: Content and origins. *Behav Cogn Psychother* 1993;21:265–273

[83]   Fraizer OH, Cooley DA: Cardiac transplantation. *Surg Clin North Am* 1986; 66:477–489

[84]   Turvey CL, Klein DM, Pies CJ, Arndt S: Attitudes about impairment and depression in elders suffering from chronic heart failure. *Int J Psychiatry Med* 2003; 33: 117-32.

[85]   Koenig HG, Vandermeer J, Chambers A, Burr-Crutchfield L, Johnson JL: Comparison of major and minor depression in older medical inpatients with chronic heart and pulmonary disease. *Psychosomatics* 2006; 47: 296-303.

[86]   Frasure-Smith N, Lesperance F, Talajic M: Depression and 18-month prognosis after myocardial infarction. *Circulation* 1995; 91: 999-1005.

[87]   Penninx BW, Beekman AT, Honig A, Deeg DJ, Schoevers RA, van Eijk JT, van TilburgW: Depression and cardiac mortality: results from a community-based longitudinalstudy. *Arch Gen Psychiatry* 2001; 58: 221-7.

[88]   Rafanelli C, Milaneschi Y, Roncuzzi R: Minor depression as short term risk factor in congestive heart failure outpatients. *Psychosomatics*, in press.

[89]   Rumsfeld JS, Havranek E, Masoudi FA, Peterson ED, Jones P, Tooley JF, Krumholz HM, Spertus JA: Depressive symptoms are the strongest predictors of short-term declines in health status in patients with heart failure. *JACC* 2003; 42:1811–1817.

[90]   de Denus S, Spinler SA, Jessup M, Kao A. History of depression as a predictor of adverse outcomes in patients hospitalized for decompensated heart failure. *Pharmacotherapy.* 2004;24:1306-1310.

[91]   Sullivan M, Levy WC, Russo JE, Spertus JA: Depression and health status in patients with advanced heart failure: a prospective study on tertiary care. *J Card Fail* 2004; 10: 390-396.

[92]   Judd LL, Akiskal HS, Maser JD, Zeller PJ, Endicott J, Coryell W: A prospective 12-year study of subsyndromal and syndromal depressive symptoms in unipolar major depressive disorders. *Arch of General Psychiatry* 1998, 55: 694-700.

[93]   Detre TP, Jarecki H: *Modern Psychiatric Treatment.* Philadelphia, Lippincott, 1971.

[94]   Doerfler LA, Paraskos JA: Anxiety, posttraumatic stress disorder, and depression in patients with coronary heart disease: A practical review for cardiac rehabilitation professionals. *J Cardiopulm Rehab* 2004; 24: 414-421

[95]   Rozanski A, Blumenthal JA, Kaplan J: Impact of psychological factors on the pathogenesis of cardiovascular disease and implications for therapy. *Circulation* 1999; 99: 2192-2217

[96]   Linden W, Stossel C, Maurice J: Psychosocial interventions for patients with coronary artery disease. *Arch Intern Med* 1996; 156:745-752

[97]   World Health Organization: Needs and action priorities in cardiac rehabilitation and secondary prevention in patients with coronary heart disease. Geneva, WHO regional Office for Europe, 1993

[98]   Barlow DH: *Anxiety and its disorders.* 2nd ed. New York: Guilford; 2002

[99]   Nathan PE, Gorman JM, eds: *A guide to treatments that work.* 2nd ed. New York: Oxford, 2002

[100]   Beck AT, Rush AJ, Shaw BF, Emery G. *Cognitive Therapy of depression.* New York, Guiford, 1979

[101]   Levinsohn PM, Gotlib IH: Behavioral theory and treatment of depression. In: Beckam EE, Leber WR, eds. *Handbook of depression.* 2nd ed. New York, Guilford, 1995, pp.352-375

[102]   Shabetai R: Depression and heart failure. *Psychosomatic Medicine* 2002; 64: 13-14.

In: Psychological Factors and Cardiovascular Disorders   ISBN: 978-1-60456-871-4
Editor: Leo Sher   © 2008 Nova Science Publishers, Inc.

Chapter XIV

PERIPHERAL ARTERIAL DISEASE AND COGNITIVE FUNCTION IN OLDER PEOPLE

Snorri Bjorn Rafnsson

Department of Public Health Sciences, University of Edinburgh Medical School,
Edinburgh, United Kingdom.

ABSTRACT

With the ongoing demographic aging of most Western societies, cognitive impairment is predicted to become a major cause of the burden of ill health in older people. The search for preventable risk factors has revealed the importance of various cardiovascular risk factors and atherosclerotic disease for the onset and progression of cognitive decline. As a marker of generalised atherosclerosis, peripheral arterial disease (PAD) constitutes a major risk factor for both secondary cardiovascular events and vascular mortality. In addition, there is growing evidence that PAD increases the risk of both cognitive impairment and progressive cognitive decline in older people independently of other vascular comorbidity and concomitant cardiovascular risk factors.

INTRODUCTION

Cognitive function constitutes a critical dimension of the health and well-being of older people [1,2]. Whereas subtle age-related cognitive decline may prevent a person from performing at the highest possible level of ability, cognitive impairment, manifested as mild to severe pathological changes in different cognitive functions, is a major determinant of long-term institutionalisation and dependency in old age [2,3]. With the demographic ageing of populations, cognitive impairment is predicted to become a major cause of the burden of ill health in many societies [4]. Any strategies designed to prevent or delay the onset of cognitive impairment need to acknowledge the potential role of preventable cardiovascular risk factors and atherosclerotic vascular disease in both the initiation and progression of cognitive decline [4,5,6,7].

As a result, this chapter aims to review findings from published studies on the association between PAD and cognitive function in older people. A second objective is to describe the possible mechanisms and neuropathological changes underlying cognitive decline in individuals with PAD. The scope for strategies aimed at maintaining cognitive function in persons with PAD is then briefly discussed. The chapter concludes by highlighting the current needs for further research in this area within the field of cognitive epidemiology.

PERIPHERAL ARTERIAL DISEASE

Peripheral arterial disease, which is synonymous with the term 'peripheral vascular disease', mainly refers to atherosclerotic disease in the arteries supplying the upper and the lower extremities, and is much more rarely used to denote atherosclerotic disease in the carotid arteries of the neck [8]. However, since disease in the upper extremities is proportionately rare, PAD is generally used to indicate atherosclerosis of the arteries supplying the lower limbs. In more precise terms, PAD refers to atherosclerotic disease of the distal aorta and the lower extremity arteries that induces lumen narrowing and disruption of blood flow in the legs [9].

The gradual progression of atherosclerotic disease from an early age in the distal aorta, the iliac, femoral, and popliteal arteries may eventually lead to arterial narrowing in the lower extremities [10,11]. Only when the atherosclerotic disease is relatively advanced, symptoms of ischemia may appear. The most common clinical presentation of transient ischemia in the lower limbs is intermittent claudication (sometimes referred to as angina of the legs), which is manifested as pain or tightness in the calf, or the thigh, on physical exertion and is relieved by rest [9,10]. Whereas most claudicants either improve with the disappearance of symptoms or stay about the same, still as many as 16% experience worsening of symptoms, 5-10% have critical limb ischemia and 5% undergo major amputation within 5 years of diagnosis [12].

The clinical diagnosis of PAD is usually made on the basis of presenting symptoms [9]. Similarly, self-reporting of symptoms has been employed in epidemiological research for detecting atherosclerotic disease in the lower extremities [10]. For example, the WHO Intermittent Claudication Questionnaire has been widely used for the identification of symptomatic PAD in the general population [13]. More recently, the Edinburgh Claudication Questionnaire was constructed with the aim of improving the validity of the WHO questionnaire [14]. Other methods may be more objective in diagnosing PAD and several non-invasive tests may be used for confirming the clinical history. Thus, the measurement of the ratio of systolic blood pressure in the ankle to the upper arm (the ankle-brachial index or ABI), has commonly been used for the non-invasive assessment of PAD [15]. A resting ABI equal or less than 0.9 is diagnostic of PAD and has 98% sensitivity and 99% specificity in identifying angiogram positive disease [16]. Other techniques include palpitation of peripheral pulses, the use of stress tests, and Doppler ultrasonography [15]. Arteriography, where specific arterial segments can be directly visualized in living subjects, is still the best objective method of quantifying atherosclerotic disease and is used as reference against which non-invasive techniques of existing disease are validated [17]. Apart from the ABI, however, important limitations with regard to validity, costs, and patient tolerance have precluded many of these methods from being widely used in population-based studies.

Epidemiological studies have collected data on the prevalence of symptomatic PAD in different populations [18]. Frequently, the WHO questionnaire has been administered for the purpose of determining prevalence rates of intermittent claudication. Prevalence estimates have been found to differ widely across studies, which in addition to reflecting true differences in levels of disease, might be due to variation in age distributions and other population characteristics [19]. Overall, the prevalence of intermittent claudication has been found to increase with age in both sexes. For example, the Rotterdam Study [20] described a prevalence ranging from 1.0% in men aged 55-59 years to 6.0% in those 85 years and older. Similarly, the prevalence increased from 0.7% to 2.5% in the corresponding age categories for women. Furthermore, the use of non-invasive measures of PAD has resulted in prevalence rates several times higher than that observed using a symptom-based questionnaire, highlighting the fact that most individuals with PAD tend to be symptom-free [8,19]. In the Rotterdam study, the prevalence of PAD diagnosed on the presence of an ABI less than 0.9 increased from 6.6% in men aged 55-59 years to 52.0% in those 85 years and older [20]. For women, the prevalence increased from 9.5% to 59.6% across these same age bands. Also, in the Edinburgh Artery Study, approximately 17.0% of men and women had an ABI less than 0.9 compared to about 4.5% having intermittent claudication [21]. When a reactive hyperemia stress test was added, the prevalence rate for PAD rose to 24.6% for both sexes.

The main risk factors for atherosclerosis tend to be similar regardless of its anatomical location, although predilection of certain risk factors to the development and progression of atherosclerosis in different vascular sites has been observed [22]. Thus, smoking is a major modifiable risk factor for both the development and progression of PAD [23]. Cigarette smoking is prevalent in up to 90% of arteriographically-diagnosed patients and the amount of risk is related to the number of cigarettes smoked while smoking cessation reduces the probability of clinical disease [8,19]. Similarly, diabetes is associated with an increased risk of PAD and impaired glucose tolerance possibly so as well [19,23]. Systolic blood pressure levels also seem to correlate positively with the occurrence of PAD; a 2.5 and 3.9-fold increased risk of developing PAD have been reported for hypertensive men and women, respectively [23]. Additional factors, including physical inactivity, abnormal blood lipids, and elevated levels of various atherothrombotic biomarkers have been linked to an increased risk of PAD in several investigations [19].

Peripheral arterial disease has implications that pertain not only to the affected lower extremity but also to overall cardiovascular health [17]. The occurrence of PAD is associated with an increased risk of both non-fatal and fatal vascular events, independently of coexisting ischemic heart disease [19,24]. Even in initially asymptomatic patients, the risk of subsequent vascular events is higher than in normal subjects, and has been shown to increase steeply with the severity of PAD. More importantly, PAD may be a particularly strong predictor of comorbid atherosclerotic disease in the cerebrovascular circulation but a finely tuned relationship exists between the brain and the circulatory system which, if upset by vascular pathology, may disrupt normal neurological and cognitive function [25].

Table 1. Published studies of peripheral arterial disease and cognitive function

Author and publication date	Sample origin	Sample size	Age	Study type	Patient group/Risk factor	Cognitive measures*	Results
Pinzur et al. 1986 (ref 27)	Clinic	60†	60.3§	Cross-sectional	Leg amputees	TMFE, AVLT, RCF	Comparison with controls not available
Shaw et al. 1987 (ref 28)	Clinic	50‡	57.4§	Cross-sectional	PAD surgery candidates	Trail Making Test B, WMS, WAIS	No difference on any cognitive measure between CABG patients and PAD surgery candidates
Phillips et al. 1993 (ref 30)	Clinic	14‡	67.4§	Cross-sectional	PAD amputees	WMS, WAIS, RCF, RMTFW, GNT, COWAT, MCST	Amputees performed significantly worse on measures of psychomotor speed, problem solving, and abstract reasoning than healthy controls
Breteler et al. 1994 (ref 38)	Community	4791†	55-94	Cross-sectional	ABI<0.9	MMSE	Low ABI associated with lower average mental status scores and shift in score distribution
Phillips and Mate-Kole 1997 (ref 31)	Clinic	29‡	64.8§	Cross-sectional	ABI<0.8/PAD amputees	WCST, COWAT, WFT, WAIS, CVLT, Digit Span, RCF, Trail Making Test A/B, GNT, PEG, TPD	PAD patients performed significantly worse on measures of attention, psychomotor speed, executive functioning, visuospatial ability, and visual memory than healthy controls
Haan et al. 1999 (ref 39)	Community	~5000†	≥65	Prospective (7-year follow-up)	ABI<0.9	MMSE, WAIS	Low ABI associated with a greater decline in psychomotor speed
Rao et al. 1999 (ref 29)	Community	25‡	≥65	Cross-sectional	PAD surgery candidates	CAMCOG, Trail Making Test A/B, BDCS, COWAT	20% of PAD patients fell within the bottom 5% of orthopaedic surgery controls on measures of attention, memory and frontal lobe function
Elwood et al. 2002 (ref 36)	Community	31-38‡	55-69	Cross-sectional	Intermittent claudication	MMSE, CAMCOG, AH4, CRT	No difference between claudicants and non-vascular controls

Table 1. (Continued)

Author and publication date	Sample origin	Sample size	Age	Study type	Patient group/Risk factor	Cognitive measures*	Results
Waldstein et al. 2003 (ref 34)	Community	38‡	69.8§	Cross-sectional	Intermittent claudication/low ABI	WAIS, WMS, Trail Making Test A/B, Stroop, PEG, JOLT	PAD patients performed significantly worse on measures of non-verbal memory, concentration, perceptual-motor speed, manual dexterity and executive functioning than normotensive controls
Piguet et al. 2003 (ref 33)	Community	63‡	80.4§	Prospective (6-year follow-up)	Intermittent claudication	MMSE	No difference between claudicants and non-claudicants
Singh-Manoux et al. 2003 (ref 35)	Community	5822†	46-68	Cross-sectional	Intermittent claudication	Short-term memory test, AH4, Mill Hill Test, VFT	Claudicants performed significantly worse on measures of verbal memory, verbal and non-verbal reasoning, knowledge, comprehension, lexical and semantic verbal fluency than non-vascular controls
Tilvis et al. 2004 (ref 32)	Community	159‡	75,80,85¶	Prospective (1, 5, and 10-year follow-up)	Intermittent claudication	MMSE	Claudication associated with decline in mental status over 1-year of follow-up only.
Price et al. 2006 (ref 40)	Community	717†	55-74	Cross-sectional	ABI	WMS, RPM, VFT, WAIS, NART	ABI predictive of decline in information processing speed
Rafnsson et al. 2007 (ref 37)	Community	57‡	73.1§	Prospective (4-year follow-up)	Intermittent claudication	WMS, RPM, VFT, WAIS	Significantly greater 4-year decline in verbal memory among claudicants

*AH4=Alice Heim Reasoning Test; AVLT=Auditory Verbal Learning Task; BDCS=Behavioural Dyscontrol Scale; CVLT=California Verbal Learning Test; CAMCOG=Cambridge Examination for Mental Disorders of the Elderly; CRT=Choice Reaction Test; COWAT=Controlled Oral Word Association Test; GNT=Graded Naming Test; JOLT=Judgment of Line Orientation Test; MMSE=Mini-Mental State Examination; MCST=Modified Card Sorting Test; PEG=Pegboard Test; PMA=Primary Mental Abilities; RPM=Raven's Progressive Matrices; RMTFW=Recognition Memory Test for Faces and Words; RCF=Rey's Complex Figure; TMFE=Test of Mental Functions for the Elderly; TPD=Two-point Discrimination; VFT=Verbal Fluency Test; WAIS=Wechsler Adult Intelligence Scale; WMS=Wechsler Memory Scale; WCST=Wisconsin Card Sorting Test; WFT=Word Fluency Test. †Total study sample; ‡ Number of PAD patients. §Mean age of the total number of subjects. ¶Age cohorts.

Further to the biological plausibility of an association with cognitive function, the relatively recent interest taken in the potential role of atherosclerotic vascular disease in cognitive decline is also reflects the importance of vascular disease as a cause of ill health in the adult population, the possibility for prevention and modification of both cardiovascular diseases and risk factors, and the availability of valid methods for their diagnosis and detection in the research setting. The next section reviews results from published clinical and community-based studies of PAD and cognitive function. An overview of these studies is given in table 1.

PERIPHERAL ARTERIAL DISEASE AND COGNITIVE FUNCTION

Cognitive Function in Vascular Surgical Patients and Amputees

Although a rare event, PAD may progress to critical limb ischemia and gangrene which is a major cause of lower extremity amputation, representing a "terminal" event for the patient involved. At this stage of the disease, advanced atherosclerosis is likely to be present in other parts of the arterial system as well. Indeed, vascular amputees are at a significantly higher risk of further cardiovascular events and have very poor survival rates [26]. Among older vascular amputees going on to receive rehabilitation, the successful use and maintenance of a prosthetic limb may in part be influenced by cognitive status.

Only a few studies have examined cognitive function in PAD vascular surgical candidates and amputees. A further limitation is reflected in the fact that some early studies were not designed specifically to address this problem. For example, Pinzur et al [27] noted that 10% of 60 leg amputees undergoing evaluation for prosthetic limb fitting and rehabilitation had cognitive deficits of enough severity to limit the patients' capacity to learn how to use a prosthetic limb successfully. The study, however, was methodologically limited in several important ways. In particular, the sample was restricted to male patients only (some as young as 34 years of age) and no control group was used. More seriously, the patient sample included patients who differed with regard to the underlying cause for amputation. Although the majority of amputees had peripheral vascular insufficiency, subjects undergoing amputation as a result of trauma or from other causes were also included. Furthermore, not all patients received the same set of cognitive function tests since those below 60 years of age were administered different tests from older subjects. Since no data on actual cognitive test outcomes were reported, no firm conclusions can be drawn about the level of cognitive performance in this sample of predominantly vascular amputees.

In a second investigation [28] 50 PAD surgical candidates were included as controls in a study where the aim was to examine cognitive function following major surgery in 312 coronary artery bypass graft (CABG) electives. When compared, the two groups did not differ significantly in mean levels of pre-surgery cognitive test scores. Whereas the PAD group was older and included relatively more women, as expected, the CABG patients had more pre-operative coronary heart disease. Also, the proportion of cases and controls with history of hypertension, diabetes, previous transient ischemic episode (TIA), or clinical stroke proved to be similar, but the PAD group had evidence of more carotid arterial disease.

Although not confirming the intactness of cognitive function in PAD patients, the results rather suggest that the level of cognitive impairment in these patients may be at a par with that in patients with advanced coronary artery disease. In a subsequent investigation, Rao et al [29] noted that PAD surgery candidates showed similar patterns of cognitive impairment as those with a previous history of TIA. Specifically, in comparison to non-diseased controls, 25% of PAD patients had scores on tests assessing attention, arithmetic, and frontal lobe function lying within the bottom 5% of the control group.

The addition of two more studies was partly to serve a twofold purpose: firstly to add to the almost non-existing literature on the present topic, and secondly to improve the methodological quality of available data. In the former report [30] investigators administered a comprehensive cognitive test battery to 14 stroke-free PAD amputees and 14 healthy community-drawn controls. Whereas differing only minimally in age (mean age 69.9 versus 67.4 years), the amputees reported higher smoking rates, more diabetes, hypertension and obesity. On cognitive testing, the amputees performed significantly worse on tests of psychomotor speed, problem solving and abstract reasoning compared to the controls. Moreover, there were non-significant trends pointing to lower scores on tests assessing verbal fluency, concentration, and visuoperceptual skills.

In the second investigation [31] the performance on cognitive tests was compared in three groups: patients comprising both PAD amputees (n=13) and non-amputees (n=16), 29 controls with stroke, and 30 healthy community controls. All groups were age and education matched. By using two control groups, the authors aimed at determining whether PAD patients performed worse than healthy controls on cognitive tests, and moreover, whether the pattern of cognitive deficits observed matched that of stroke patients. The findings revealed that the patients with PAD performed significantly worse on tests of attention and psychomotor speed, executive function, visuospatial ability, and visual memory. In contrast, no differences were found on tests of language ability or verbal memory. Furthermore, the PAD patients showed deficits in similar cognitive functions as those with stroke, only of less severity. Specifically, the performance of the two patient groups was comparable on six out of the eight cognitive tests administered.

Following further analyses of the data, the severity of PAD and history of ischemic heart disease were the only significant predictors of cognitive impairment in patients with PAD. In contrast, none of the conventional cardiovascular risk factors independently predicted cognitive test performance once disease severity was accounted for in multivariate analyses. In sum, these findings provide further cross-sectional data of widespread cognitive deficits in patients with greatly advanced PAD. Moreover, the results suggest that, in such patients, any direct cognitive effects of cardiovascular risk factors themselves may be minimal once progressive, generalised atherosclerotic disease has established itself.

Intermittent Claudication and Cognitive Function

A major advantage of population-based studies over investigations of selected samples of vascular amputees and surgical candidates stems in part from the insight they provide into cognitive function in patients with less severe manifestations of the disease. In such investigations, intermittent claudication has been used as a marker of underlying PAD [8]. For example, the Helsinki Aging Study [32] reported that older claudicants performed significantly worse on a general mental status test at baseline compared to those without PAD. Similarly, the claudicants had more than a twofold greater risk of either increasing in Clinical Dementia Rating class or declining at least four points on the mental status test during the first year of follow-up. In contrast, claudication at baseline was not associated with an elevated risk of cognitive decline over five years of follow-up.

Similarly, the Sydney Older Persons Study [33] failed to find significant differences between subjects with and without intermittent claudication at baseline with regard to the rate of change in overall cognitive function over a six-year follow-up. Whereas the null-findings were based on those scoring at least 25 or more on a mental status test at baseline, and therefore unlikely to be cognitively impaired at the time, identical results occurred when the analysis was restricted to subjects having a baseline score of less than 25.

In other research settings, tests assessing particular cognitive domains have been administered in order to examine cross-sectionally the extent to which particular cognitive abilities may be affected in individuals with PAD. As an example, Waldstein et al [34] compared the cognitive performance of 38 community-resident stroke-free subjects with PAD to that of stroke patients and normotensive individuals. The study found that relative to the stroke patients, those with PAD performed better on all tests. In comparison to the normotensive controls, however, those with PAD scored significantly worse on seven tests of nonverbal memory, concentration, executive function, perceptuo-motor speed, and manual dexterity. Similarly, Singh-Manoux and colleagues [35] demonstrated that both stroke-free male and female (aged 46-68 years) claudicants performed significantly worse when administered an inventory of cognitive tests for the first time 11 years since baseline. Specifically, the male claudicants scored low on tests assessing short-term memory, verbal and mathematical reasoning, word recognition and knowledge, and executive function. Whereas relative to the males no effects on either short-term memory or semantic fluency were observed for the females, weaker effects were seen on lexical fluency but stronger on measures of knowledge and word recognition. In contrast, the Caerphilly study [36] failed to observe a significant relationship between intermittent claudication and cognitive test performance in older stroke-free males. However, the claudicants did obtain lower scores on tests of mental speed, general cognitive function, and non-verbal and verbal reasoning, suggesting the lack of statistical significance might have been a consequence of low statistical power associated with a relatively small sample of subjects with PAD (n=31 to 38 depending on the cognitive test).

Few studies have determined the extent to which persons with PAD may be vulnerable to change in different cognitive functions over time, although data from the Edinburgh Artery Study revealed that claudicants may be at an increased risk of cognitive decline as recently reported by Rafnsson and colleagues [37]. Specifically, in this population study of 452 older males and females who attended cognitive testing on two separate occasions four years apart, intermittent claudication was found to be associated with a significantly greater decline in verbal memory performance in particular. Importantly, the relationship with cognitive decline was neither accounted for by previous stroke nor concomitant major cardiovascular risk factors emphasising to some extent its dependence on the underlying atherosclerotic process.

The Ankle-Brachial Index and Cognitive Function

The measurement of the ABI provides one of the most effective, accurate and practical means to objectively documenting both the presence and severity of PAD [8,23]. Yet, only a few population-based studies examining cognitive function in relation to PAD have reported on the ABI. In the earliest of such investigations, the Rotterdam Study [38] demonstrated that an ABI of less than 0.9 was associated with moderately lower mental status scores and a shift in the overall distribution of test scores among 4971 individuals aged between 55 and 94 years. Moreover, the association proved to be independent of differences in both age and education. Furthermore, in a subsequent study of 5888 persons aged 65 years and older, a baseline ABI of less than 0.9 was associated with a significantly steeper decline in mental status performance over a seven-year follow-up [39]. Multivariate analyses confirmed that the relationship was independent of both demographic confounding factors as well as incident stroke during follow-up.

More recently, Price and colleagues [40] analysed data from 717 older men and women participating in the Edinburgh Artery Study. In age and sex-adjusted analyses, significant, positive, linear associations emerged between ABI measured at baseline and performance on tests of non-verbal intelligence, executive function, and information processing speed, administered 10 years later. In multivariate analyses, the association between ABI and information processing speed remained significant, suggesting the ABI may be an early predictor of cognitive decline and of potential value in identifying older people at increased risk of cognitive impairment.

PATHOPHYSIOLOGY OF COGNITIVE DECLINE IN PERIPHERAL ARTERIAL DISEASE

There is widespread agreement that atherosclerosis in the lower extremities represents just one manifestation of similar pathology in other arterial systems [41,42]. In fact, the presence of PAD should prompt an inquiry into ischemic manifestations in other vascular territories, particularly those involving the brain and the heart [43].

In patients with evidence of PAD, the prevalence of atherosclerosis in the carotid arteries is increased several fold compared to the general population [44,45]. Whereas angiographically-determined coronary artery atherosclerosis may be demonstrated in as many as 90% of patients, cerebrovascular disease may be present in up to a half [19]. Severe narrowing of the carotid or major cerebral arteries may possibly interfere with blood flow to the brain, thus leading to cerebral hypoperfusion. In addition, atherosclerosis in the carotid arteries is also associated with a significantly elevated risk of thromboembolic events. For example, for each 10% increase in the degree of arterial stenosis, the risk of acute cerebrovascular episode is increased by as much as 26% [45].

Depending in part on its size and the artery in which it will ultimately lodge, the impact of circulating embolic material on neurological function is likely to vary widely. Even in the absence of clinical stroke, ongoing discharge of cerebral microemboli (detected using transcranial Doppler ultrasound) from ulcerous atheromatous lesions may be observed over time in most, if not all, patients with significant carotid stenosis [46]. Whereas asymptomatic circulating emboli strongly predict both TIAs as well as clinical strokes [47], it has been suggested they may also have a role to play in progressive cognitive decline [48].

NEUROPATHOLOGY OF COGNITIVE DECLINE IN PERIPHERAL ARTERIAL DISEASE

Cortical Damage

The absence of structural neuroimaging data in currently published studies prevents the identification of the neuropathological substrates of cognitive decline in individuals with PAD. In the absence of overt stroke, however, isolated ischemic damage to the cerebral cortex is an unlikely (although possible) neuropathological feature of cognitive decline in such individuals. In the general population, approximately one third of symptomatic strokes occur in the cerebral cortex [49]. While a similar frequency has been described for infarcts in subcortical grey matter areas (the basal ganglia and thalamus), the same data show that only a small proportion of cortical infarcts are in fact asymptomatic as compared to approximately 80% of subcortical lesions.

Even focal cortical lesions, however, as opposed to extensive cortical infarcts or those traversing both cortical and subcortical structures, may result in neurological dysfunction in both adjacent and distant cortical regions [50,51]. Experimentally, small cortical infarcts in the territory of the middle cerebral artery (localised within the parietal lobe) can induce an immediate depression of metabolic activity in both the frontal and parietal cortex adjacent to the infarct [52]. Although such stroke-induced cortical hypometabolism tends to improve over time, full recovery to pre-stroke levels may not occur, particularly in cortical areas adjacent to the lesion.

Further to inducing a long-lasting depression in cortical metabolism, spreading neuronal dysfunction may activate multiple molecular cascades in remote areas, characterised by increased microglial cellular activity and up-regulation of proinflammatory proteins. Despite the limited and sometimes contradictory findings with regard to the independent influence of cortical hypometabolism on neurological and cognitive outcomes resulting from ischemic damage [51,53], such a process, possibly mediated through a neuroinflammatory response, should not be rule out as a potential underlying reason for the diffuse cognitive deficits that may occur following isolated cortical infarcts.

Subcortical Grey Matter Lesions

Symptomatic infarcts may involve subcortical areas, either in combination with superficial cortical structures or in isolation. Regarding the latter, substantial evidence exists to show that a direct ischemic injury to subcortical grey matter structures occurs significantly more often without any apparent neurological symptoms i.e. clinically silent infarcts [49,54]. Neuroimaging shows that subcortical infarcts are manifested as areas of focal hyperintensity of less than 15 mm in diameter in the deep territory of small, non-branching end arteries, arising directly from larger cerebral arteries. It has been suggested that atherosclerosis may contribute directly to subcortical grey matter infarcts. For example, microatheromatous vessel pathology may induce lumen stenosis or occlusion of small penetrating arterioles, leading to ischemia and necrosis. Similarly, an atherothrombotic lesion at the origin of the penetrating arteriole, or at the wall of a large, proximal cerebral artery, might lead to an obstruction of its opening. In other circumstances, artery-to-artery embolism or cardiogenic embolic material may be suspected as the underlying etiology.

Signs of asymptomatic infarcts are commonly observed in stroke-free patients with manifested atherosclerotic vascular disease, including in the lower extremities. Recent data from the Second Manifestations of Arterial Disease (SMART) Study demonstrated positively, albeit non-significantly, that the frequency of clinically silent brain infarcts was related to having an ABI equal or less than 0.9 [55]. In contrast, the mean level of carotid artery intima-media thickness, possibly being the more sensitive marker of generalised atherosclerosis in younger individuals, proved to be significantly greater in those having evidence of silent brain lesions.

In modestly-sized samples of healthy older people, there is a suggestion of an association between the presence of subcortical brain infarcts and worse performance on specific cognitive tests, including measures of perceptual speed, episodic, working, and semantic memory, and visuospatial abilities, but not with reduced overall cognitive function as based on summarising the scores of all tests [56]. In other cross-sectional studies, silent infarcts in the basal ganglia were associated with slower verbal memory retrieval speed and worse executive function [57]. Similarly, thalamic lesions were related to worse focused attention in addition to both slower verbal memory retrieval speed and executive functioning. Specifically, in the Rotterdam Scan Study, silent thalamic infarcts present at baseline predicted four-year decline in verbal memory performance, whereas non-thalamic infarcts (mostly restricted to the basal ganglia) were associated with decline in psychomotor speed [54]. Relative to a single lesion, multiple silent infarcts were more strongly associated with cognitive decline. Importantly, in this study, the effects were confined to patients who suffered silent infarcts during the follow-up, irrespective of whether they presented with silent lesions at baseline, suggesting progressive deterioration in cognitive function following incident lesions.

Subcortical White Matter Changes

Alterations to the subcortical white matter, visualised as bright, hyperintensive periventricular or deep white matter regions on neuroimaging, are frequently observed in studies of people with atherosclerotic vascular disease. For example, as many as 20% of older patients with myocardial infarction have evidence of white matter changes, either in periventricular or deep white matter regions [58]. In the same data, about 30% of patients with intermittent claudication had evidence of white matter changes. Specifically, in the

Rotterdam Study, an ABI of less than 0.9 and a diagnosis of either possible or definite myocardial infarction were associated with two to threefold increased probability of visible structural alterations to the cerebral white matter [59].

The significance of the integrity of the cerebral white matter for intact cognitive function is well established [60]. Importantly, changes to the white matter are associated with lower overall cognitive function, reduced processing speed, delayed memory, and worse executive function [61]. More specifically, the presence of hyperintensities in both periventricular and deep regions has been related to specific deficits in implicit learning of sequences [62]. Other studies have associated white matter lesions with a greater decline in particular aspects of cognitive function, including mental processing speed [63]. White matter lesions also contribute significantly to lifetime decline in overall cognitive ability rather than individual cognitive functions [64]. In addition, the decline in performance on tests of memory, conceptualisation and visuopractical skills may be directly related to the progression of the burden of white matter lesions [65]. In studies using highly sensitive diffusion tensor magnetic resonance imaging, whereby the detection of markers sensitive to the ultrastructural integrity of the cerebral white matter is made possible, strong and consistent, inverse relationships between white matter structural parameters and performance on tests of executive function have been observed [66]. Interestingly, these associations proved not to be limited to any of the anatomical regions studied, including the frontal brain area, suggesting that the cognitive impact of white matter changes might in particular implicate those cognitive functions that are largely dependent on either the speed of information processing or the integrity of sub-cortical neural structures [60,61].

PRESERVATION OF COGNITIVE FUNCTION IN INDIVIDUALS WITH PERIPHERAL ARTERIAL DISEASE

Cognitive decline is often progressive and a high proportion of individuals showing signs of mild cognitive symptoms continues to progress to overt cognitive impairment [67]. Already there is evidence to suggest that both cardiovascular risk factors and atherosclerotic vascular diseases may be important to the occurrence and progression of cognitive decline in older people, thereby opening up the possibility for strategies aimed at either preventing or delaying its onset. In individuals with PAD, in particular, secondary preventive measures directed at decreasing the long-term systemic complications are of outmost importance and also likely to be key to the preservation of cognitive function [8,68].

Specifically, medical treatment regimens involving antiplatelet therapy, antihypertensive medication, and lipid-lowering drugs are important in reducing the risk of secondary events and mortality in coronary heart disease and stroke patients, and may possibly benefit patients with PAD as well [8,17]. Moreover, direct positive influence of such therapies on cognitive function has also been documented [4]. Beyond the benefits of lowering blood lipid levels per se, however, the pleiotropic effects of statins may favourably influence the progression of atherosclerosis which may be particularly relevant to patients with PAD as its extent or severity may be associated with level of cognitive deficits [43,69,70]. In addition influencing atherogenesis, such medical therapies may further lead to reduction in inflammation and blood thrombogenicity, both of which may be responsible for thrombotic complications of atherosclerotic plaques [71]. Complementing pharmacologic interventions, complete and permanent cessation of smoking is one of the most important determinants of prognosis in individuals with PAD [23]. Importantly, smoking is also an independent modifiable risk factor for cognitive decline in adults [72].

In comparison to coronary heart disease patients, however, individuals with PAD tend to be undertreated with regard to atherosclerotic risk factor modification [73,74]. This lack of strict risk factor management may partly be due because most interventions to lower atherosclerotic risk factors to date have not been tested in clinical trials involving these patients but also to an extent by the seemingly overwhelming emphasis on symptom relief than essential risk factor reduction in these individuals [74]. Obviously, a major goal regarding reducing the risk for secondary vascular events and for guarding against cognitive decline in individuals with PAD should be the prompt diagnosis and management of PAD in line with existing national treatment guidelines.

Further to the above, the use of antioxidant vitamins [75,76], reducing stress levels [77], engaging socially [78], adopting a healthy diet [79,80], and exercising regularly [81,82] are other low-risk approaches to maintaining vascular and cognitive health that possibly might benefit patients with PAD. For example, physical exercise is favourably associated with pain-free walking distance in these patients [83], and may also directly or indirectly protect against cognitive decline.

CONCLUSION

Peripheral arterial disease is a common disease entity with the potential to affect considerably the quality of life of millions of older people. In addition, PAD directly affects functional capacity by restricting ambulation, sometimes through lower extremity amputation. Perhaps more importantly, PAD is a marker of generalised atherosclerosis and a powerful predictor of coronary heart disease and cerebrovascular events and mortality from vascular causes. Furthermore, there is growing evidence that PAD may also increase the risk of cognitive impairment and cognitive decline. Current priorities in the management of individuals with PAD relate to increasing the numbers of patients receiving adequate treatment the objective of which is the reduction of the long-term risk of systemic vascular complications. These strategies are also likely to be important in guarding against continuing cognitive decline in this high-risk population. Adequate support and follow-up of individuals with PAD should be provided in order to ensure treatment compliance.

Future studies should aim at determining the cumulative effects of atherosclerotic risk factors on cognitive function in PAD patients and whether strict risk factor control relates to positive cognitive outcomes. While in selected samples of patients with advanced PAD the severity of disease may be the most important predictor of cognitive function, it is important that similar work is carried out in large, representative population samples involving individuals with less advanced vascular disease. Also, in the light of the increased risk of cognitive decline in persons with PAD, it is necessary to determine the neuropathological substrate underlying such cognitive changes in future studies. In particular, the careful assessment of both the location and extent of brain lesions as well as the detailed examination of cognitive functions must be the minimum in such investigations. Moreover, there is need for more community-based studies determining whether subtle cognitive alterations are related to everyday functioning of individuals with PAD. The potential effects of subtle cognitive decrements on everyday activities, including adherence to medical regimens would need particular attention. Lastly, more prospective studies are required to determine the predictive value of mild cognitive changes for progressive cognitive decline in individuals with systemic atherosclerotic vascular disease. Specifically, more information is needed on changes in which cognitive domains may be predictive of future cognitive impairment as well as other adverse events, including the likelihood of premature mortality or institutionalisation in such high-risk individuals.

REFERENCES

[1]   Fried LP. Epidemiology of aging. *Epidemiol Rev* 2000; 22: 95-106.

[2]   Waldstein SR, Elias MF. Introduction to the special section on health and cognitive function. *Health Psychol* 2003; 22: 555-558.

[3]   Melzer D, Ely M, Brayne C. Cognitive impairment in elderly people: population based estimate of the future in England, Scotland, and Wales. *Brit Med J* 1997; 315: 462.

[4]   Alagiakrishnan K, McCracken P, Feldman H. Treating vascular risk factors and maintaining vascular health: Is this the way towards successful cognitive ageing and preventing cognitive decline? *Postgrad Med J* 2006; 82: 101-105.

[5]   Haan MN, Wallace R. Can dementia be prevented? Brain aging in a population-based context. *Annu Rev Pub Health* 2004; 25: 1-24.

[6]   Newman SD, Just MA. The neural bases of intelligence: a perspective based on functional neuroimaging. In Sternberg RJ, Pretz J (Eds.). *Cognition and intelligence: identifying the mechanisms of the mind.* New York: Cambridge University Press, 2005. pp. 88-103.

[7]   Rockwood K. Vascular cognitive impairment and vascular dementia. *J Neurol Sci* 2002; 203-204: 23-27.

[8]   Ouriel K. Peripheral Arterial Disease. *Lancet* 2001; 358: 1257-1264.

[9]   Fowkes FGR. Peripheral vascular disease, 2004. http://hcna.radcliffe-oxford.com/pvd.htm.

[10]   Dawber T. *The Framingham Heart Study. The epidemiology of atherosclerotic disease.* Cambridge MA: Harvard University Press, 1980.

[11]   Rauch U, Osende JI, Fuster V, Badimon JJ, Fayad Z, Chesebro JH. Thrombus formation on atherosclerotic plaques: pathogenesis and clinical consequences. *Ann Intern Med* 2001; 134: 224-238.

[12]   Meru AV, Mittra S, Thyagarajan B, Chugh A. Intermittent claudication: An overview. *Atherosclerosis* 2006; 187: 221-237.

[13]   Rose GA. The diagnosis of ischaemic heart pain and intermittent claudication in field surveys. *B World Health Organ* 1962; 27: 645-58.

[14] Leng GC, Fowkes FG. The Edinburgh Claudication Questionnaire: an improved version of the WHO/Rose Questionnaire for use in epidemiological surveys. *J Clin Epidemiol* 1992; 45: 1101-1109.

[15] Fowkes FGR. Review of simple measurement techniques. In: Fowkes FGR (Ed). *Epidemiology of peripheral vascular disease*. London: Springer-Verlag, 1991. pp. 3-15.

[16] Watson K, Watson BD, Pater KS. Peripheral arterial disease: A review of disease awareness and management. *Am J Geriatr Pharmacother* 2006; 4: 365-379.

[17] Federman DG, Kravetz JD. Peripheral arterial disease: diagnosis, treatment, and systemic implications. *Clin Dermatolog* 2007; 25: 93-100.

[18] Diehm C, Kareem S, Lawall H. Epidemiology of peripheral arterial disease. *J Vasc Dis* 2004; 33: 183-189.

[19] Vogt MT, Wolfson SK, Kuller LH. Lower extremity arterial disease and the aging process: a review. *J Clin Epidemiol* 1992; 45: 529-542.

[20] Meijer WT, Hoes AW, Rutgers D, Bots ML, Hofman A, Grobbee DE. Peripheral arterial disease in the elderly. The Rotterdam Study. *Arterioscler Thromb Vasc Biol* 1998; 18: 185-192.

[21] Fowkes FGR, Housley E, Cawood EHH, Macintyre CCA, Ruckley CV, Prescott RJ. Edinburgh Artery Study: prevalence of asymptomatic and symptomatic peripheral arterial disease in the general population. *Int J Epidemiol* 1991; 20: 384-392.

[22] Kannel WB. Risk factors for atherosclerotic cardiovascular outcomes in different arterial territories. *J Cardiovasc Risk* 1994; 1: 333-339.

[23] Baumgartner I, Schainfeld R, Graziani L. Management of peripheral vascular disease. *Annu Rev Med* 56: 249-272.

[24] Pasternak RC, Criqui MH, Benjamin EJ, Fowkes FGR, Isselbacher EM, McCullough PA, Wolf PA, Zheng Z-J. Atherosclerotic Vascular Disease Conference: writing group I: epidemiology. *Circulation* 2004; 109: 2605-2612.

[25] Tarter RE, Edwards KL, van Thiel DH. Perspective and rationale for neuropsychological assessment of medical disease. In Tarter RE, Edwards KL, van Thiel DH (Eds.). *Medical neuropsychology. The impact of disease on behaviour*. New York: Plenum Press, 1988. pp.1-10.

[26] Kulkarni J, Pande S, Morris J. Survival rates in dysvascular lower limb amputees. *Int J Surg* 2006; 4: 217-221.

[27] Pinzur MS, Graham G, Osterman H. Psychologic testing in amputation rehabilitation. *Clin Orthoped* 1986; 229: 236-240.

[28] Shaw PJ, Bates D, Cartlidge NEF, French JM, Heaviside D, Julian DG, Shaw DA. Neurologic and neuropsychological morbidity following major surgery: comparison of coronary artery bypass and peripheral vascular surgery. *Stroke* 1987; 18: 700-707.

[29] Rao R, Jackson S, Howard R. Neuropsychological impairment in stroke, carotid stenosis, and peripheral vascular disease. A comparison with healthy community residents. *Stroke* 1999; 30: 2167-2173.

[30] Phillips NA, Mate-Kole CC, Kirby RL. Neuropsychological function in peripheral vascular disease amputee patients. *Arch Phys Med Rehab* 1993; 74: 1309-1314.

[31]   Phillips NA, Mate-Kole CC. Cognitive deficits in peripheral vascular disease. A comparison of mild stroke patients and normal control subjects. *Stroke* 1997; 28: 777-784.

[32]   Tilvis RS, Kähönen-Väre MH, Jolkkonen J, Valvanne J, Pitkala KH, Strandberg TE. Predictors of cognitive decline and mortality of aged people over a 10-year period. *J Gerontol* 2004; 59: 268-74

[33]   Piguet O, Grayson DA, Creasey H, Bennett HP, Brooks WS, Waite LM, Broe GA. Vascular risk factors, cognition and dementia incidence over 6 years in the Sydney Older Persons Study. *Neuroepidemiology* 2003; 22: 165-71.

[34]   Waldstein SR, Tankard CF, Maier KJ, Pelletier JR, Snow J, Gardner AW, Macko R, Katzel LI. Peripheral arterial disease and cognitive function. *Psychosom Med* 2003; 65: 757-763.

[35]   Singh-Manoux A, Britton AR, Marmot M. Vascular disease and cognitive function: evidence from the Whitehall II study. *J Am Geriatr Soc* 2003; 51: 1445-50.

[36]   Elwood PC, Pickering J, Bayer A, Gallacher JE. Vascular disease and cognitive function in older men in the Caerphilly cohort. *Age Ageing* 2002; 31: 43-8.

[37]   Rafnsson SB, Deary IJ, Smith FB, Whiteman MC, Fowkes FGR. Cardiovascular diseases and decline in cognitive function in an elderly community population: The Edinburgh Artery Study. *Psychosom Med* 2007; 69: 425-34.

[38]   Breteler MMB, Claus JJ, Grobbee DE, Hofman A. Cardiovascular disease and distribution of cognitive function in elderly people: the Rotterdam study. *Brit Med J* 1994; 308: 1604-1608.

[39]   Haan MN, Shemanski L, Jagust WJ, Manolio TA, Kuller L. The role of APOE ε4 in modulating effects of other risk factors for cognitive decline in elderly persons. *J Amer Med Assoc* 1999; 282: 40-46.

[40]   Price JF, McDowell S, Whiteman MC, Deary IJ, Stewart MC, Fowkes FGR. Ankle brachial index as a predictor of cognitive impairment in the general population: ten-year follow-up of the Edinburgh Artery Study. *J Am Geriatr Soc* 2006; 54: 763-769.

[41]   Drouet L. Atherothrombosis as a systemic disease. *Cerebrovasc Dis* 2002; 13: 1-6.

[42]   Golomb BA, Dang TT, Criqui MH. Peripheral arterial disease. Morbidity and mortality implications. *Circulation* 2006; 114: 688-699.

[43]   Phillips NA. Thinking on your feet: a neuropsychological review of peripheral vascular disease. In: Waldstein SR, Elias MF (Eds). *Neuropsychology of cardiovascular disease*. New Jersey: Lawrence Erlbaum Associates, 2001. pp. 121-142.

[44]   Cheng SWK, Wu LLH, Lau H, Ting ACW, Wong J. Prevalence of significant carotid stenosis in Chinese patients with peripheral and coronary artery disease. *Austral New Zeal J Surg* 1999; 69: 44.

[45]   Mathiesen EB, Joakimsen O, Bønaa KH. Prevalence of and risk factors associated with carotid artery stenosis: the Tromsø Study. *Cerebrovasc Dis* 2001; 12: 44-51.

[46]   Hutchinson S, Riding G, Coull S, McCollum CN. Are spontaneous cerebral microemboli consistent in carotid disease? *Stroke* 2002; 33: 685-688.

[47]   Molloy J, Markus HS. Asymptomatic embolization predicts stroke and TIA in patients with carotid artery stenosis. *Stroke* 1999; 30: 1440-1443.

[48]   Russell D. Cerebral microemboli and cognitive impairment. *J Neurol Sci* 2002; 203-204: 211-214.

[49]   Vermeer SE, Koudstaal PJ, Oudkerk M, Hofman A, Breteler MMB. Prevalence and risk factors of silent brain infarcts in the population-based Rotterdam Scan Study. *Stroke* 2002; 33: 21-25.

[50]   Brown GG, Eyler Zorilla LT. Neuropsychological aspects of stroke. In: Waldstein SR and Elias MF (Eds). *Neuropsychology of cardiovascular disease*. New Jersey: Lawrence Erlbaum Associates, Publishers, 2001. pp. 301-324.

[51]   Witte OW, Bidmon HJ, Schiene K, Redecker C, Hagemann G. Functional differentiation of multiple perilesional zones after focal cerebral ischemia. *J Cereb Blood Flow Metabol* 2000; 20: 1149-1165.

[52]   Carmichael ST, Tatsukawa K, Katsman D, Tsuyuguchi N, Kornblum HI. Evolution of diaschisis in a focal stroke model. *Stroke* 2004; 35: 758-763.

[53]   Bowler JV, Wade JP, Jones BE, Nijran K, Jewkes RF, Cuming R, Steiner TJ. Contribution of diaschisis to the clinical deficit in human cerebral infarction. *Stroke* 1995; 26: 1000-1006.

[54]   Vermeer SE, Prins ND, den Heijer T, Hofman A, Koudstaal PJ, Breteler MMB. Silent brain infarcts and the risk of dementia and cognitive decline. *New Engl J Med* 2003; 348: 1215-1222.

[55]   Giele JLP, Witkamp TD, Mali WPTM, van der Graaf Y, for the SMART study group. Silent brain infarcts in patients with manifest vascular disease. *Stroke* 2004; 35: 742-746.

[56]   Schneider JA, Wilson RS, Cochran EJ, Bienias JL, Arnold SE, Evans DA, Bennett DA. Relation of cerebral infarctions to dementia and cognitive function in older persons. *Neurology* 2003; 60: 1082-1088.

[57]   O'Brien JT, Wiseman R, Burton EJ, Barber B, Wesnes K, Saxby B, Ford GA. Cognitive associations of subcortical white matter lesions in older people. *Ann NY Acad Sci* 2002; 977: 436-444.

[58]   Gerdes VE, Kwa VI, Ten Cate H, Brandjes DP, Buller HR, Stam J; Amsterdam Vascular Medicine Group. Cerebral white matter lesions predict both ischemic strokes and myocardial infarctions in patients with established atherosclerotic disease. *Atherosclerosis* 2006; 186: 166-172.

[59]   Bots ML, van Swieten JC, Breteler MM, de Jong PT, van Gijn J, Hofman A, Grobbee DE. Cerebral white matter lesions and atherosclerosis in the Rotterdam Study. *Lancet* 1993; 341: 1232-1237.

[60]   Malloy P, Correia S, Stebbins G, Laidlaw DH. Neuroimaging of white matter in aging and dementia. *Clin Neuropsychol* 2007; 21: 73-109.

[61]   Gunning-Dixon FM, Raz N. The cognitive correlates of white matter abnormalities in normal aging: a quantitative review. *Neuropsychology* 2000; 14: 224-232.

[62]   Aizenstein HJ, Nebes RD, Meltzer CC, Fukui MB, Williams RL, Saxton J, Houck PR, Carter CS, Reynolds CF, DeKosky ST. The relation of White Matter Hyperintensities to implicit learning in healthy older adults. *Int J Geriatr Psych* 2002; 17: 664-669.

[63]   van den Heuvel DM, ten Dam VH, de Craen AJ, Admiraal-Behloul F, Olofsen H, Bollen EL, Jolles J, Murray HM, Blauw GJ, Westendorp RG, van Buchem MA.

Increase in periventricular white matter hyperintensities parallels decline in mental processing speed in a non-demented elderly population. *J Neurol Neurosur Ps* 2006; 77: 149-153.

[64]   Deary IJ, Leaper SA, Murria AD, Staff RT, Whalley LJ. Cerebral white matter abnormalities and lifetime cognitive change: a 67-year follow-up of the Scottish Mental Survey of 1932. *Psychol Aging* 2003; 18: 140-148.

[65]   Schmidt R, Ropele S, Enzinger C, Petrovic K, Smith S, Schmidt H, Matthews PM, Fazekas F. White matter lesion progression, brain atrophy, and cognitive decline: the Λustrian Stroke Prevention Study. *Ann Neurol* 2005; 58: 610-616.

[66]   Shenkin SD, Bastin ME, MacGillivray TJ, Deary IJ, Starr JM, Rivers CS, Wardlaw JM. Cognitive correlates of cerebral white matter lesions and water diffusion tensor parameters in community-dwelling older people. *Cerebrovasc Dis* 2005; 20: 310-318.

[67]   Rockwood K, Moorhouse PK, Song X, MacKnight C, Gauthier S, Kertesz A, Montgomery P, Black S, Hogan DB, Guzman A, Bouchard R, Feldman H. Disease progression in vascular cognitive impairment: Cognitive, functional and behavioural outcomes in the Consortium to Investigate Vascular Impairment in Cognition (CIVIC) cohort study. *J Neurol Sci* 2007; 252: 106-112.

[68]   O'Brien JT, Erkinjuntti T, Reisberg B, Roman G, Sawada T, Pantoni L, Bowler JV, Ballard C, DeCarli C, Gorelick PB, Rockwood K, Burns A, Gauthier S, DeKosky ST. Vascular cognitive impairment. *Lancet* 2003; 2: 89-98.

[69]   Aung PP, Maxwell HG, Jepson RG, Price JF, Leng GC. Lipid-lowering for peripheral arterial disease of the lower limb. *Cochrane Database Syst Rev* 2007; 4: CD000123.

[70]   Kang S, Wu Y, Li X. Effects of statin therapy on the progression of carotid atherosclerosis: a systematic review and meta-analysis. *Atherosclerosis* 2004; 177: 433-442.

[71]   Tunon J, Blanco-Colio LM, Martín-Ventura JL, Egido J. Intensive treatment with statins and the progression of cardiovascular diseases: the beginning of a new era? *Nephrol Dial Transpl* 2004; 19: 2696-2699.

[72]   Richards M, Jarvis MJ, Thompson N, Wadsworth MEJ. Cigarette smoking and cognitive decline in midlife: Evidence from a prospective birth cohort study. *Am J Pub Health* 2003; 93: 994-998.

[73]   McDermott MM, Mehta S, Ahn H, Greenland P. Atherosclerotic risk factors are less intensively treated in patients with peripheral arterial disease than in patients with coronary artery disease. *J Gen Int Med* 1997; 12: 209-215.

[74]   Rehring TF, Sandhoff BG, Stolcpart RS, Merenich JA, Hollis HW. Atherosclerotic risk factor control in patients with peripheral arterial disease. *J Vasc Surg* 2005; 41: 816-822.

[75]   Riviere S, Birlouenz-Aragon I, Nourhasheni F, et al. Low plasma vitamin C in Alzheimer's patients despite an adequate diet. Int J Geriatr Psychiatry 1998;13:749–54.

[76]   Morris MC, Evans DA, Bienias JL, et al. Vitamin E and cognitive decline in older persons. *Arch Neurol* 2002; 59: 1125–1132.

[77]   Berr, C : Balansard, B : Arnaud, J : Roussel, A M : Alperovitch, A. Cognitive decline is associated with systemic oxidative stress: the EVA study. Etude du Vieillissement Arteriel. *J Am Geriatr Soc* 2000; 48: 1285-1291.

[78]   Barnes LL, Mendes de Leon CF, Wilson RS, Bienias JL, Evans DA. Social resources and cognitive decline in a population of older African Americans and whites. *Neurology* 2004; 63: 2322-2326.

[79]   Panza F, Solfrizzi V, Colacicco AM, D'Introno A, Capurso C, Torres F, Del Parigi A, Capurso S, Capurso A. Mediterranean diet and cognitive decline. *Pub Health Nutrit* 2004; 7: 959–963.

[80]   Solfrizzi V, Panza F, Capurso A. The role of diet in cognitive decline. *J Neural Transm* 2003; 110: 95–110.

[81]   van Gelder BM, Tijhuis MA, Kalmijn S, Giampaoli S, Nissinen A, Kromhout D. Physical activity in relation to cognitive decline in elderly men: the FINE Study. *Neurology* 2004; 63: 2316–2321.

[82]   Yaffe K, Barnes D, Nevitt M, Lui LY, Covinsky K. A prospective study of physical activity and cognitive decline in elderly women: women who walk. *Arch Int Med* 2001; 161: 1703-1708.

[83]   Mika P, Spodaryk K, Cencora A, Unnithan VB, Mika A. Experimental model of pain-free treadmill training in patients with claudication. *Am J Phys Med Rehabil* 2005; 84: 756-762.

In: Psychological Factors and Cardiovascular Disorders   ISBN: 978-1-60456-871-4
Editor: Leo Sher   © 2008 Nova Science Publishers, Inc.

Chapter XV

THE EPIDEMIOLOGY OF TYPE D PERSONALITY: A NEW CARDIOVASCULAR RISK FACTOR – FACT OR FICTION?

Susanne S. Pedersen and Helle Spindler

CoRPS – Center of Research on Psychology in Somatic diseases,
Tilburg University, Tilburg, The Netherlands;
Department of Psychology, University of Aarhus, Aarhus, Denmark.

ABSTRACT

Personality factors tend to have been neglected in the context of cardiovascular disease, since inconsistent findings published in relation to the Type A Behavior Pattern. With the emergence of the Type D personality construct, personality factors may again find their way into cardiovascular disease, as Type D has been associated with adverse health outcomes in cardiac patients independent of mood states, disease severity and other clinical risk factors. The question remains whether the time is ripe for labeling Type D as a risk factor on par with traditional biomedical risk factors, or whether further research is warranted before risk factor status can be acquired.

INTRODUCTION

Type D personality is a relatively new personality taxonomy that has been associated with adverse health outcomes, including mortality and morbidity, in patients with cardiovascular disease (CVD). This chapter focuses on the underpinnings of the construct, its overlap with and distinctiveness from other constructs and CVD risk factors, assessment issues, prevalence, and its associations with clinical and patient-centered outcomes, culminating in a discussion that seeks to answer the question: *Is Type D personality a new cardiovascular risk factor – fact or fiction?*

UNDERPINNINGS OF THE TYPE D CONSTRUCT: *OLD WINE IN NEW BOTTLES?*

The Type D (distressed) personality construct was developed in cardiac patients in the beginning of the 1990's by Denollet and derived from a combination of theory, empirical evidence (including factor and cluster analyses), and clinical observations of patients attending cardiac rehabilitation [1-3]. The construct is comprised of two normal and stable personality traits, that is *negative affectivity* (tendency to experience increased negative emotions) and *social inhibition* (tendency to nonexpression of emotions in social interaction due to fear of rejection) [4]. Type D personality typifies individuals who tend to experience more feelings of dysphoria and tension (i.e. worry, feel down in the dumps and are irritable), have a negative view of self, report more distress and somatic symptoms, and tend to scan the world for impending trouble, while at the same time feeling insecure, closed, and inhibited when together with others, fearing rejection and disapproval [4,5].

The Type D construct has been met with some skepticism, and was in 1997 labeled as *old wine in new bottles* [6] and is almost a decade later still criticized for being a *reinvention of an old construct under a new label* [7]. In this context, it is important to note, however, that Denollet never argued that Type D would be *the* psychosocial risk factor in CVD nor that Type D would cover all facets of personality [5]. In addition, empirical evidence and the theoretical underpinnings of the construct indicate that Type D personality is different from other personality factors (e.g. traits) and mood states (e.g. anxiety and depression), but also from coping styles, including repression, defensiveness, denial, and alexithymia.

Given that the Type D personality construct is based on the two normal and stable traits *negative affectivity* and *social inhibition,* it is not surprising that there is some overlap with neuroticism and extraversion of the Five-Factor Model of Personality [4,8]. However, the shared variance between DS14 *negative affectivity* and neuroticism of 32-46%, and DS14 *social inhibition* and extraversion of 27-35%, indicates that 54-73% of the variance in Type D cannot be explained by the Five-Factor Personality characteristics [4,8]. Ultimately, in order to deal with the criticism of being a *reinvention of an old construct under a new label* [7], studies are warranted that investigate whether the interaction of the Five-Factor traits neuroticism and extraversion is also predictive of adverse health outcomes in patients with CVD. If the interaction of neuroticism and extraversion also predicts mortality (as does Type D), then the criticism must be heeded. For now, evidence from a Danish study of patients with a first myocardial infarction (MI) and healthy controls shows that Type D personality is associated with posttraumatic stress disorder independent of the traits neuroticism and extraversion [8]. Results of a recent study, although not in patients with established CVD but in older patients seen in primary care, confirm that personality types in general and Type D in particular has added value compared to traits, as measured by the Five-Factor Model of Personality, when predicting health outcomes [9]. The authors state that: "This raises the possibility that perhaps this type (*referring to Type D*) embodies unique intraindividual information relevant to health that is not captured by multiple trait ratings. Such information probably arises not just from the particular constellation of traits, but from their levels in relation to one another."

Type D personality has also been shown to predict mortality and other adverse health outcomes in patients with CVD, despite statistical adjustment for measures of anxiety and depression [10-12]. Studies using patient-centered outcome measures, such as anxiety and fatigue, provide additional evidence that Type D is different from mood states, with Type D personality remaining independently associated with these outcomes adjusting for the patient-centered measure at baseline [13,14]. For example, in patients treated with percutaneous coronary intervention (PCI) with the paclitaxel-eluting stent as the default strategy, Type D was shown to add significantly to the prediction of anxiety at 12 months follow-up compared to a model comprising demographic and clinical characteristics, and anxiety and depressive symptoms at the time of the index PCI [14]. Moreover, Type D is considered a chronic risk factor, with the duration being ≥2 years compared to mood states, such as depression, reflecting more episodic factors with a duration of <2 years [15,16]. Taken together, these studies indicate that Type D personality has unique prognostic and predictive value over and above measures of emotional distress. In turn, this confirms the validity of the Type D construct and that it is more than a measure of negative affect, as it also stipulates how individuals deal with this negative affect, due to the inclusion of the *social inhibition* component [4].

The Type D construct also distinguishes itself from coping styles, with repression and defensiveness referring to *low distress* and the *unconscious* suppression of negative emotions [17], whereas Type D patients experience high levels of distress while simultaneously keeping these emotions in check at a conscious level [4]. In patients with CVD, *social inhibition* correlates -0.06 with the Marlowe-Crowne measure of defensiveness, confirming that these constructs are unrelated [17]. A recent study of 731 patients with coronary artery disease confirms that repression and Type D comprise different constructs, with both Type D and repressive coping being independent predictors of adverse clinical events at 6-10 years follow-up [18]. Similarly, individuals high in *social inhibition*, such as Type D's, are not prone to underreport their levels of emotional distress [19,20], which is characteristic of denial [21]. Conceptually the Type D construct is also different from alexithymia, with difficulty identifying feelings being the primary feature of alexithymia [22], whereas Type D's, due to their high score on *negative affectivity,* seem to be able to label their feelings even though they choose not to express them.

Finally, it seems appropriate to contrast Type D personality with the Type A Behavior Pattern (TABP), since TABP was the first psychosocial factor to gain status as a risk factor in CVD [23] and is often misconceived of as a personality type, even though it was designed to avoid any associations with global personality traits [24]. TABP is defined as the tendency to be competitive, impatient, time-urgent, restless, and hostile, with insecurity likely forming the nucleus of TABP [25]. As such, TABP reflects a 'heterogeneous hodgepodge' of behavioral symptoms [25], whereas Type D is a more homogenous construct that is based on existing personality theory [1,2].

WHY STUDY PERSONALITY FACTORS IN THE CONTEXT OF CVD?

Improvement in treatment options and clinical care of patients with CVD has led to a significant reduction in mortality [26], paving the way for the adoption of other outcome measures, such as quality of life. A recent report from the National Heart, Lung and Blood Institute in the US emphasizes the study of patient-centered outcomes, such as quality of life, and its determinants as a means by which to bridge the gap between research and clinical practice [27].

There is increasing evidence that Type D personality is an important determinant of a wide range of adverse health outcomes, including mortality, morbidity, and poor quality of life, indicating that patients with this personality disposition comprise high-risk patients [15]. In other words, personality factors, such as Type D, may be important explanatory factors of individual differences in emotional distress and health outcomes [5,15]. The adoption of a personality approach in the context of somatic disease in general and CVD in particular may also be advantageous over a mood stage approach, as personality factors are stable and hence less prone to be influenced by disease severity and acute events, such as myocardial infarction [28-30]. In addition, given the stable effects of personality on outcome across time and situations, using personality measures as screening tools in clinical practice in order to identify high-risk patients may also be advantageous in comparison to the use of mood state measures. Recently, the Third Joint Task Force of European and other Societies on Cardiovascular Disease Prevention updated the European guidelines on CVD prevention in clinical practice, emphasizing the importance of assessing psychosocial risk factors, due to their influence on adherence, life style changes, and prognosis [31]. In connection with the publication of these updated guidelines, an international expert committee provided recommendations for the assessment of psychosocial risk factor, and recommended the use of the Type D Scale as one of the measures to use in clinical cardiology practice to identify high-risk patients [32].

ASSESSMENT AND NATURE OF TYPE D

Type D personality can be assessed with the standardized and validated Type D Scale (DS14), which consists of 14-items rated on a 5-point Likert scale ranging from 0 (false) to 4 (true) [4]. The 14 items are divided into two 7-item sub scales, reflecting *negative affectivity* and *social inhibition*. The psychometric properties of the DS14 are good, with Cronbach's α =.88/.86 and 3-month test-retest reliability r = .72/.82 for the *negative affectivity* and the *social inhibition* sub scales, respectively [4]. Type D caseness is determined by a high score (cut-off $\geq$10) on both sub scales [4], with item-response theory showing this cut-off to be the most optimal for both sub scales [33]. A recent study of patients in the Rapamycin-Eluting Stent Evaluated At Rotterdam Cardiology Hospital (RESEARCH) registry, treated with percutaneous coronary intervention (PCI) with either bare metal stents or sirolimus-eluting stents, confirmed the theoretical underpinnings of the Type D construct, showing that the cardio-toxicity of Type D is incurred by the combination of a high score on both *negative affectivity* and *social inhibition* rather than the single traits [12]. In the latter study, *social inhibition* moderated the effects of *negative affectivity* on clinical prognosis, emphasizing that Type D is more than negative affect but also the added value of the *social inhibition* component, that is how patients deal with their negative emotions.

There is also evidence to suggest that Type D personality is not confounded by disease severity. Martens and colleagues administered the DS14 to 475 patients post myocardial infarction (MI) at 3 time points (i.e. during hospitalization, 12 months, and 18 months) and found that Type D was stable over an 18-month period and not confounded by demographic and clinical characteristics, including indicators of disease severity [34]. Similarly, a recent study based on MI patients from the Myocardial Infarction and Depression-Intervention Trial (MIND-IT) showed that depressive symptoms, as measured by the Beck Depression Inventory, but not Type D was confounded by left ventricular dysfunction [35].

PREVALENCE OF TYPE D ACROSS CARDIOVASCULAR DISEASES

The prevalence of Type D personality varies from 18-36% in patients with ischemic heart disease [4,34,36-40], 24-45% in chronic heart failure [41-43], 34-35% in patients with peripheral arterial disease [44,45], 23-25% in patients receiving implantable cardioverter defibrillator (ICD) therapy [46,47], 18-29% in heart transplantation recipients [48,49] to 53% in hypertensives [4]. Overall, these studies indicate that 25-33% of cardiac patients have a Type D personality disposition. The prevalence of Type D in patients with CVD compares to that found in the general population [4,8,44].

TYPE D AND ADVERSE CLINICAL OUTCOME

There is increasing evidence that Type D personality is an independent predictor of adverse clinical outcome, including mortality and morbidity, in patients with established CVD (Table 1). Although the majority of these studies have been conducted in patients with ischemic heart disease (IHD) [3,10-12,18,37,50-53], there is preliminary evidence showing that the cardio-toxicity of Type D may also extend to heart transplantation recipients [48] and patients experiencing a sudden cardiac arrest [54] and that Type D personality may also be associated with incident cancer [50].

The risk associated with Type D in patients with IHD is consistent across studies, with the average risk being 4-fold and the range from 2- to 9-fold [3,10-12,18,37,50-53]. These risks are adjusted for disease severity and demographic and clinical risk factors, indicating that the cardio-toxicity related to Type D personality cannot be attributed to patients with this personality disposition being more severely ill. It should also be noted that Type D is associated with adverse clinical outcome despite state-of-the art medical treatment, such as PCI with the use of drug-eluting stents [12,37,52]. The latter studies are sub studies of the

RESEARCH registry, which was conducted in the 'real world', with no patients being excluded on the basis of anatomical and clinical criteria [55]. A post-hoc analysis of the RESEARCH registry population indicated that 68% of the patients would not have qualified for inclusion in clinical trials due to a more complex clinical profile, confirming that the patient sample represented those seen in daily clinical practice [56].

Table 1. The impact of Type D personality on adverse clinical outcome in patients with cardiovascular disease

Authors	Reference	Patients	Study design	Follow-up	Endpoint	Adjusted risk
Appels et al (2000)	54	99 SCA 119 IHD	Case-control	-	Sudden cardiac arrest	OR: 9.4
Denollet et al (1995)	53	105 MI	Prospective	2-5 years (mean 3.8)	All-cause death, cardiac death	Type D added significantly to the level of prediction of clinical outcome compared to baseline characteristics
Denollet et al (1996)	3	303 IHD	Prospective	6-10 years (mean: 7.9)	All-cause death	OR: 4.1
Denollet et al (1998)	10	87 MI	Prospective	6-10 years (mean: 7.9)	Cardiac death/MI	RR: 4.7
Denollet (1998)	50	246 IHD	Prospective	6-10 years (mean: 7.8)	Incident cancer	OR: 7.2
Denollet et al (2000)	11	319 IHD	Prospective	5 years	Cardiac death/MI, MACE	ORs: 4.5 - 8.9
Denollet et al (2006)	12	875 PCI/SES	Prospective	9 months	MACE	HR: 1.9
Denollet et al (2006)	51	337 CAD	Prospective	5 years	All-cause death/MI, MACE	ORs: 2.9 - 4.8
Denollet et al (2007)	48	51 HTX	Prospective	1-10 years (mean 5.4)	Combined all-cause death, grade ≥3A rejection, number of rejection free days	OR: 6.8
Denollet et al (In Press)	18	731 CAD	Prospective	5-10 years (mean 6.6)	All-cause death/MI, cardiac death/MI	ORs: 3.8 - 4.0
Pedersen et al (2004)	37	875 PCI/SES	Prospective	9 months	All-cause death/MI	OR: 5.3
Pedersen et al (2007)	52	358 PCI/SES	Prospective	2 years	All-cause death/MI	HR: 2.6

CAD = coronary artery disease; IHD = ischemic heart disease; HR = hazard ratio; HTX = heart transplantation; MACE = major adverse cardiac event; MI = myocardial infarction; OR = odds ratio; PCI = percutaneous coronary intervention; SCA = sudden cardiac arrest; SES = sirolimus-eluting stent

Table 2. The impact of Type D personality on patient-centered outcomes in patients with cardiovascular disease

Authors	Reference	Patients	Study design	Follow-up	Endpoint	Adjusted risk
Chronic Heart Failure						
Schiffer et al (2005)	41	84 CHF	Cross-sectional	-	QoL, NA, depression, PA	ORs: 3.3 - 7.1 for all NA measures; OR: 0.3 for PA
Schiffer et al (2007)	42	178 CHF	Prospective	2 months	Cardiac symptoms	OR: 6.4
Schiffer et al (2008)	57	149 CHF	Prospective	1 year	Anxiety	OR: 5.7
Smith et al (2007)	58	136 CHF	Prospective	1 year	Fatigue	$\beta = .17; p = .03$
Heart Transplantation						
Pedersen et al (2006)	49	186 HTX	Cross-sectional	-	QoL	ORs: 3.5 - 6.1; BP and GH: ns
Implantable Cardioverter Defibrillator						
Pedersen et al (2004)	46	182 ICD 144 partners	Cross-sectional	-	Anxiety Depression	ORs: 4.4 - 8.8
Pedersen et al (2007)	47	154 ICD	Prospective	3 months	QoL	Independent predictor ($p < .001$)
Ischemic Heart Disease						
Al-Ruzzeh et al (2005)	40	437 CABG	Cross-sectional	-	QoL	ORs: 2.3 - 5.5
Martens et al (2007)	59	287 MI patients	Prospective	1 year	Course of depression	Log ORs: 1.7 - 4.2
Pedersen et al (2001)	36	171 IHD	Prospective	6 weeks	Vital exhaustion	ORs: 4.7 - 6.4
Pedersen et al (2004)	8	112 first MI 114 healthy controls	Case-control	-	PTSD	OR: 4.5
Pedersen et al (2006)	60	542 PCI/SES	Prospective	6 months	New onset depression	OR: 3.0
Pedersen et al (2007)	61	692 PCI/SES	Prospective	6 months	QoL	ORs: 1.60 - 3.99; PF: ns
Pedersen et al (2007)	13	419 PCI/PES	Prospective	1 year	Vital exhaustion	OR: 3.5
Spindler et al (2007)	62	167 PCI/SES	Prospective	6 months	Chronic anxiety	OR: 3.3
Van Gestel et al (2007)	14	416 PCI/SES	Prospective	1 year	Anxiety	OR: 2.9
Whitehead et al (2006)	39	135 ACS	Prospective	3 months	PTSD symptoms	ns
Peripheral Arterial Disease						
Aquarius et al (2005)	44	150 PAD 150 healthy controls	Case-control	-	Perceived stress, QoL	ORs: 6.5 - 7.4
Aquarius et al (2007)	63	150 PAD	Prospective	6 months	QoL, depression	ORs: 3.9 - 8.6
Aquarius et al (2007)	45	203 PAD	Prospective	1 year	QoL	ORs: 3.7 - 6.0

ACS = acute coronary syndrome; BP = bodily pain (SF-36); CABG = coronary artery bypass graft surgery; CHF = chronic heart failure; GH = general health (SF-36); HTX = heart transplantation; ICD = implantable cardioverter defibrillator; IHD = ischemic heart disease; MI = myocardial infarction; NA = negative affect; NS = not significant; OR = odds ratio; PA = positive affect; PAD = peripheral arterial disease; PCI = percutaneous coronary intervention; PES = paclitaxel-eluting stent; PF = physical functioning (SF-36); PTSD = posttraumatic stress disorder; QoL = quality of life; SES = sirolimus-eluting stent.

TYPE D AND PATIENT-CENTERED OUTCOMES

Compared to studies on clinical endpoints, research examining the impact of Type D personality on patient-centered outcomes has been more plentiful and covers a broader range of CVD groups, extending from ischemic heart disease, chronic heart failure, heart transplantation, and peripheral arterial disease to patients implanted with an ICD (Table 2). Across studies, quality of life is the most frequently studied endpoint, followed by symptoms of depression, anxiety, and fatigue (including vital exhaustion, which is a broader concept than fatigue).

The risks associated with Type D personality and these outcomes range from 3- to 8-fold, with results being consistent across studies and CVD groups with little exception [39,49,61]. The results of two studies focusing on quality of life in heart transplant recipients [49] and PCI patients [61], respectively, showed that Type D was independently associated with impaired quality of life for the majority of the quality of life facets, as measured by the Short-Form Health Survey (SF-36), but not with bodily pain nor general health in heart transplant recipients [49], nor with physical functioning in PCI patients [61]. Whitehead and colleagues could not confirm that Type D personality was an independent predictor of posttraumatic stress disorder (PTSD) at 3 months, even though Type D patients were at a substantially greater risk of PTSD than non-Type D patients (61.1% versus 30.9%; $p = .013$) [39]. This is contrary to a cross-sectional study of first MI patients and healthy controls, showing that individuals with a Type D personality were more likely to have PTSD adjusting both for personality traits (i.e. neuroticism and extraversion) and disease status (i.e. MI) [8].

TYPE D – A NEW RISK FACTOR – FACT OR FICTION?

In a recent review, Pedersen and Denollet delineated a list of 7 external criteria for evaluating Type D as a potential risk factor in the context of CVD [15]. This list was partly derived from criteria developed to help clinicians evaluate the importance of new risk markers in cardiology practice [64] and partly from the general psychosomatic literature. An additional criterion could be added to this list when evaluating the role of psychological factors in the pathogenesis of CVD, namely that the psychological factor in question should not be confounded by disease severity, leading to a list comprised of 8 criteria as shown in Table 3.

In essence, Type D fulfils 6 of the 8 criteria, as follows: Criterion 1: Type D provides independent information about risk, as it is associated with clinical and patient-centered outcomes independent of demographic and clinical risk factors, including disease severity. Criterion 2: The prevalence of Type D is relatively frequent, ranging from 25-33%, and the risk of a clinically relevant magnitude, with Type D being associated with a 4-fold risk of clinical outcome and a 3- to 8-fold risk of patient-centered outcomes. Criterion 3: The measure (i.e. the DS14) is reproducible, remains fairly stable over time, and consistent in multiple groups of patients, as shown by the 3-month test-retest reliability $r = .72/.82$ for the *negative affectivity* and the *social inhibition* sub scales [4], the stable prevalence rates over 18 months [34], and the consistent findings across CVD groups [15]. Criterion 5: There is a standardized test available with which to assess Type D, namely the DS14 [4], with emerging evidence that the Type D personality construct is also cross-culturally valid, as shown in validation studies in Danish [8], German [38], and Italian patients with CVD [65]. Criterion 6: Type D seems not to be confounded by indicators of somatic disease, including left ventricular dysfunction, as indicated by two studies of MI patients [34,35] and studies that have adjusted for disease severity in multivariable analysis [15]. Criterion 7: There are plausible mechanisms that may explain the cardio-toxicity of Type D personality in relation to mortality and morbidity. The first studies are available showing that these mechanisms likely consist of an amalgam of behavioral and physiological pathways, including self-care management [42], inflammatory markers [66,67], and genetics [68].

Table 3. External criteria for evaluating Type D as a potential risk factor in cardiovascular disease

	Criterion	Fulfilled
1	Independent information about risk	√
2	Frequency of risk factor and the associated risk – a given magnitude	√
3	Measure should be reproducible, remain fairly stable within a patient over time, be consistent in multiple groups of patients in a variety of clinical settings	√
4	Measure should be sensitive, specific, have high predictive value for diagnostic purposes	?
5	A standardized test available to assess the risk factor	√
6	Unconfounded by disease severity	√
7	Plausible mechanisms linking risk factors to adverse prognosis	√
8	The risk factor should be modifiable	?

As yet, Type D personality does not comply with criteria 4 and 8. Criterion 4 is not fulfilled due to the simple reason that there is no diagnostic interview with which to assess Type D, but only a self-report measure. It could be argued, however, that the development of an interview would be nonsensical, given that *social inhibition* is one of the key features of Type D personality. In other words, even if a diagnostic interview would be developed, its validity would probably be questionable, as patients with this personality disposition would feel threatened and insecure in a face-to-face interview and more likely to provide what they deem as socially desirable answers. Criterion 8 is not complied with, since no intervention trial to date has targeted Type D personality as a risk factor. Such an intervention trial would be a logical and pertinent next step in Type D research, given the increasing wealth of observational data that appear consistent across studies and CVD groups. It does, however, comprise a major challenge, in particular in the aftermath of the mixed results of large-scale intervention trials, including the Sertraline Antidepressant Heart Attack Randomized Trial (SADHART) [69], the Enhancing Recovery in Coronary Heart Disease (ENRICHD) trial [70], Exhaustion Intervention Trial (EXIT) [71], MIND-IT [72], and the Canadian Cardiac Randomized Evaluation of Antidepressant and Psychotherapy Efficacy (CREATE) trial [73], showing that it may be possible to reduce levels of distress, but that this does not translate into a concomitant beneficial impact on survival.

CONCLUSION

Current evidence indicates that Type D personality is associated with a multitude of adverse health outcomes, ranging from increased emotional distress, poor quality of life, to adverse prognosis, including an increased risk of mortality, across CVD patient groups. Weighing this evidence against a set of 8 external criteria that may be used to evaluate new risk factors shows that Type D personality complies with 6 of these criteria. Nevertheless, despite increasing and consistent evidence that Type D personality may be associated with the pathogenesis of CVD, it may be too premature to provide an answer to or even pose the question: *Is Type D personality a new cardiovascular risk factor – fact or fiction?* Neither an affirmative *Yes* (or *No* for that matter) would seem appropriate, simply due to as yet unexplored issues. First of all, it is not known whether Type D can be modified and thereby its adverse effects on clinical and patient-centered outcomes. Furthermore, this personality disposition may exert differential cardio-toxic effects within the Type D subgroup of patients, with the likelihood that Type D's comprise a heterogeneous group. A recent study showed that Type D patients with a partner had fewer symptoms of anxiety and depression compared to Type D patients without a partner, indicating that having a partner may serve as a buffer [74]. There may be many more as yet unexplored factors that may moderate the effects of Type D on clinical and patient-centered outcomes, including hostility, attachment, self-esteem, etc. Perhaps most importantly, the possibility exists that Type D is not a risk factor but a risk marker that lies on the causal pathway between another variable and adverse clinical outcome. Hence, given that Type D shows promise as a potential risk factor in CVD, it may be wise to proceed with caution and first try to fill these gaps in Type D research. In turn, this may help prevent that Type D personality suffers the same fate as TABP, providing yet again a set back to personality factors in the context of somatic disease. This scenario would be worth pre-empting, given that personality factors in general and Type D personality in particular may have a lot to offer both to psychosomatic research but also to clinical cardiology practice [25].

REFERENCES

[1]   Denollet J. Negative affectivity and repressive coping: Pervasive influence on self-reported mood, health, and coronary-prone behavior. *Psychosom Med* 1991;53:538-556.

[2]   Denollet J, De Potter B. Coping subtypes for men with coronary heart disease: Relationship to well-being, stress, and Type A behavior. *Psychol Med* 1992;22:667-684.

[3]   Denollet J, Sys SU, Stroobant N, Rombouts H, Gillebert TC, Brutsaert DL. Personality as independent predictor of long-term mortality in patients with coronary heart disease. *Lancet* 1996;347:417-421.

[4]   Denollet J. DS14: Standard assessment of negative affectivity, social inhibition, and Type D personality. *Psychosom Med* 2005;67:89-97.

[5]   Denollet J. Type D personality: A potential risk factor refined. *J Psychosom Res* 2000;49:255-266.

[6]   Lespérance F, Frasure-Smith N. Negative emotions and coronary heart disease: getting to the heart of the matter. *Lancet* 1996;347:414-415.

[7]   Smith TW, MacKenzie J. Personality and risk of physical illness. *Annu Rev Clin Psychol* 2006;2:435-467.

[8]   Pedersen SS, Denollet J. Validity of the Type D personality construct in Danish post-MI patients and healthy controls. *J Psychosom Res* 2004;57:265-272.

[9]   Chapman BP, Duberstein PR, Lyness JM. The distressed personality type: replicability and general health associations. *Eur J Pers* 2007;21:911-929.

[10]   Denollet J, Brutsaert DL. Personality, disease severity, and the risk of long-term cardiac events in patients with decreased ejection fraction after myocardial infarction. *Circulation* 1998;97:167-173.

[11]   Denollet J, Vaes J, Brutsaert DL. Inadequate response to treatment in coronary heart disease. Adverse effects of Type D personality and younger age on 5-year prognosis and quality of life. *Circulation* 2000;102:630-635.

[12]   Denollet J, Pedersen SS, Ong ATL, Erdman RAM, Serruys PW, van Domburg RT. Social inhibition modulates the effect of negative emotions on cardiac prognosis following percutaneous coronary intervention in the drug-eluting stent era. *Eur Heart J* 2006;27:171-177.

[13]   Pedersen SS, Daemen J, van de Sande M, Sonnenschein K, Serruys PW, Erdman RA, van Domburg RT. Type-D personality exerts a stable, adverse effect on vital exhaustion in PCI patients treated with paclitaxel-eluting stents. *J Psychosom Res* 2007;62:447-453.

[14]   van Gestel YR, Pedersen SS, van de Sande M, de Jaegere PP, Serruys PW, Erdman RA, van Domburg RT. Type-D personality and depressive symptoms predict anxiety 12 months post-percutaneous coronary intervention. *J Affect Disord* 2007;103:197-203.

[15]   Pedersen SS, Denollet J. Is Type D personality here to stay? Emerging evidence across cardiovascular disease patient groups. *Curr Cardiol Rev* 2006;2:205-213.

[16]   Kop WJ. Chronic and acute psychological risk factors for clinical manifestations of coronary artery disease. *Psychosom Med* 1999;61:476-487.

[17]   Denollet J. Personality and coronary heart disease: the type D Scale-16 (DS16). *Ann Behav Med* 1998;20:209-215.

[18] Denollet J, Martens EJ, Nyklicek I, Conraads VM, de Gelder G. Clinical events in coronary patients who report low distress: Adverse effect of repressive coping. *Health Psychol*, In Press.

[19] Eisenberg N, Fabes RA, Murphy BC. Relations of shyness and low sociability to regulation and emotionality. *J Pers Soc Psychol* 1995;68:505-517.

[20] Gest SD. Behavioral inhibition: stability and associations with adaptation from childhood to early adulthood. *J Pers Soc Psychol* 1997;72:467-475.

[21] Ketterer MW, Huffman J, Lumley MA, Wassef S, Gray L, Kenyoon L, Kraft P, Brymer J, Rhoads K, Lovallo WR, Goldberg AD. Five-year follow-up for adverse outcomes in males with a at least minimally positive angiograms: importance of "denial" in assessing psychosocial risk factors. *J Psychosom Res* 1998;44:241-250.

[22] Garssen B. Repressing: Finding our way in the maze of concepts. *J Behav Med* 2007;30:471-481.

[23] Cooper T, Detre T, Weiss SM. Coronary-prone behaviour and coronary heart disease: a critical review. *Circulation* 1981;63:1199-1215.

[24] Dimsdale JA. A perspective on Type A Behaviour and coronary disease. *N Engl J Med* 1988;318:310-312.

[25] Pedersen SS, Denollet J. Type-D personality, cardiac events, and impaired quality of life: A review. *Eur J Cardiovasc Prev Rehabil* 2003;10:241-248.

[26] Levi F, Lucchini F, Negri E, La Vecchia C. Trends in mortality from cardiovascular and cerebrovascular diseases in Europe and other areas of the world. *Heart* 2002;88:119-124.

[27] Krumholz HM, Peterson ED, Ayanian JZ, Chin MH, DeBusk RF, Goldman L, Kiefe CI, Powe NR, Rumsfeld JS, Spertus JA, Weintraub WS. Report of the National Heart, Lung, and Blood Institute Working Group on Outcomes Research in Cardiovascular Disease. Circulation 2005;111:3158-3166.

[28] de Jonge P, Ormel J, van den Brink RH, van Melle JP, Spijkerman TA, Kuijper A, van Veldhuisen DJ, van den Berg MP, Honig A, Crijns HJ, Schene AH. Symptom dimensions of depression following myocardial infarction and their relationship with somatic health status and cardiovascular prognosis. *Am J Psychiatry* 2006;163:138-144.

[29] van Melle JP, de Jonge P, Ormel J, Crijns HJ, van Veldhuisen DJ, Honig A, Schene AH, van den Berg MP; MIND-IT investigators. Relationship between left ventricular dysfunction and depression following myocardial infarction: data from the MIND-IT. *Eur Heart J* 2005;26:2650-2656.

[30] Nicholson A, Kuper H, Hemingway H. Depression as an aetiologic and prognostic factor in coronary heart disease: a meta-analysis of 6362 events among 146 538 participants in 54 observational studies. *Eur Heart J* 2006;27:2763-2774.

[31] De Backer G, Ambrosioni E, Borch-Johnsen K, Brotons C, Cifkova R, Dallongeville J, Ebrahim S, Faergeman O, Graham I, Mancia G, Cats VM, Orth-Gomer K, Perk J, Pyorala K, Rodicio JL, Sans S, Sansoy V, Sechtem U, Silber S, Thomsen T, Wood D; European Society of Cardiology Committee for Practice Guidelines. European guidelines on cardiovascular disease prevention in clinical practice: third joint task force of European and other societies on cardiovascular disease prevention in clinical

practice (constituted by representatives of eight societies and by invited experts). *Eur J Cardiovasc Prev Rehabil* 2003;10:S1-S10.

[32] Albus C, Jordan J, Herrmann-Lingen C. Screening for psychosocial risk factors in patients with coronary heart disease – recommendations for clinical practice. *Eur J Cardiovasc Prev Rehabil* 2004;11:75-79.

[33] Emons WHM, Meijer RR, Denollet J. Negative affectivity and social inhibition in cardiovascular disease: evaluating Type D personality and its assessment using item response theory. *J Psychosom Res* 2007;63:27-39.

[34] Martens EJ, Kupper N, Pedersen SS, Aquarius AE, Denollet J. Type-D personality is a stable taxonomy in post-MI patients over an 18-month period. *J Psychosom Res* 2007;63:545-550.

[35] De Jonge P, Denollet J, van Melle JP, Kuyper A, Honig A, Schene AH, Ormel J. Associations of type-D personality and depression with somatic health in myocardial infarction patients. *J Psychosom Res* 2007;63:477-482.

[36] Pedersen SS, Middel B. Increased vital exhaustion among Type D patients with ischemic heart disease. *J Psychosom Res* 2001;51:443-449.

[37] Pedersen SS Lemos PA, van Vooren PR, Liu T, Daemen J, Erdman RAM, Serruys PW, van Domburg RT. Type D personality predicts death or myocardial infarction after bare metal stent or sirolimus-eluting stent implantation: A Rapamycin-Eluting Stent Evaluated At Rotterdam Cardiology Hospital (RESEARCH) registry sub-study. *J Am Coll Cardiol* 2004:44:997-1001.

[38] Grande G, Jordan J, Kummel M, Struwe C, Schubmann R, Schulze F, Unterberg C, von Kanel R, Kudielka BM, Fischer J, Herrmann-Lingen C. Evaluation of the German Type D Scale (DS14) and prevalence of the Type D personality pattern in cardiological and psychosomatic patients and healthy subjects. *Psychother Psych Med* 2004;54:413-422.

[39] Whitehead DL, Perkins-Porras L, Strike PC, Magid K, Steptoe A. Post-traumatic stress disorder in patients with cardiac disease: predicting vulnerability from emotional responses during admission for acute coronary syndromes. Heart 2006;92:1225-1229.

[40] Al-Ruzzeh S, Athanasiou T, Mangoush O, Wray J, Modine T, George S, Amrani M. Predictors of poor mid-term health related quality of life after primary isolated coronary artery bypass grafting surgery. Heart 2005;91:1557-1562.

[41] Schiffer AA, Pedersen SS, Widdershoven JW, Hendriks EH, Winter JB, Denollet J. Type D personality is independently associated with impaired health status and increased depressive symptoms in chronic heart failure. *Eur J Cardiovasc Prev Rehabil* 2005;12:341-346.

[42] Schiffer AA, Denollet J, Widdershoven JW, Hendriks EH, Smith OR. Failure to consult for symptoms of heart failure in patients with a type-D personality. *Heart* 2007;93:814-818.

[43] Scherer M, Stanske B, Wetzel D, Koschack J, Kochen MM, Herrmann-Lingen C. Psychische kosymptomatik von hausärztlichen patienten mit herzinsuffizienz. *Herz* 2006;31:347-354.

[44]   Aquarius AE, Denollet J, Hamming JF, De Vries J. Role of disease status and Type D personality in outcomes in patients with peripheral arterial disease. *Am J Cardiol* 2005;96;996-1001.

[45]   Aquarius AE, Denollet J, de Vries J, Hamming JF. Poor health-related quality of life in patients with peripheral arterial disease: type D personality and severity of peripheral arterial disease as independent predictors. *J Vasc Surg* 2007;46:507-512.

[46]   Pedersen SS, van Domburg RT, Theuns DAMJ, Jordaens L, Erdman RAM. Type D personality: A determinant of anxiety and depressive symptoms in patients with an implantable cardioverter defibrillator and their partners. *Psychosom Med* 2004;66:714-719.

[47]   Pedersen SS, Theuns DAMJ, Muskens-Heemskerk A, Erdman RAM, Jordaens L. Type-D personality but not ICD indication is associated with impaired health-related quality of life 3 months post implantation. *Europace* 2007;9:675-680.

[48]   Denollet J, Holmes RV, Vrints CJ, Conraads VM. Unfavorable outcome of heart transplantation in recipients with type D personality. *J Heart Lung Transplant* 2007;26:152-158.

[49]   Pedersen SS, Holkamp PG, Caliskan K, van Domburg RT, Erdman RA, Balk AH. Type D personality is associated with impaired health-related quality of life 7 years following heart transplantation. *J Psychosom Res* 2006;61:791-795.

[50]   Denollet J. Personality and risk of cancer in men with coronary heart disease. *Psychol Med* 1998;28:991-995.

[51]   Denollet J, Pedersen SS, Vrints CJ, Conraads VM. Usefulness of type D personality in predicting five-year cardiac events above and beyond concurrent symptoms of stress in patients with coronary heart disease. *Am J Cardiol* 2006;97:970-973.

[52]   Pedersen SS, Denollet J, Ong AT, Sonnenschein K, Erdman RA, Serruys PW, van Domburg RT. Adverse clinical events in patients treated with sirolimus-eluting stents: the impact of Type D personality. *Eur J Cardiovasc Prev Rehabil* 2007;14:135-140.

[53]   Denollet J, Sys SU, Brutsaert DL. Personality and mortality after myocardial infarction. *Psychosom Med* 1995;57:582-591.

[54]   Appels A, Golombeck B, Gorgels A, de Vreede J, van Breukelen G. Behavioral risk factors of sudden cardiac arrest. *J Psychosom Res* 2000;48:463-469.

[55]   Lemos PA, Serruys PW, van Domburg RT, Saia F, Arampatzis CA, Hoye A, Degertekin M, Tanabe K, Daemen J, Liu TK, McFadden E, Sianos G, Hofma SH, Smits PC, van der Giessen WJ, de Feyter PJ. Unrestricted utilization of sirolimus-eluting stents compared with conventional bare stent implantation in the "real world": the Rapamycin-Eluting Stent Evaluated At Rotterdam Cardiology Hospital (RESEARCH) registry. *Circulation* 2004;109:190-195.

[56]   Lemos PA, Serruys PW, van Domburg RT. In: Serruys PW, Lemos PA Eds. Sirolimus-eluting stents: From RESEARCH to clinical practice. London, Taylor & Francis 2005; 17.

[57]   Schiffer A, Pedersen SS, Broers H, Widdershoven JW, Denollet J. Type-D personality but not depression predicts severity of anxiety in heart failure patients at 1-year follow-up. *J Affect Disord* 2008;106:73-81.

[58] Smith OR, Michielsen HJ, Pelle AJ, Schiffer AA, Winter JB, Denollet J. Symptoms of fatigue in chronic heart failure patients: clinical and psychological predictors. *Eur J Heart Fail* 2007;9:922-927.

[59] Martens EJ, Smith OR, Winter J, Denollet J, Pedersen SS. Cardiac history, prior depression and personality predict course of depressive symptoms after myocardial infarction. *Psychol Med* 2007;17:1-8.

[60] Pedersen SS, Ong ATL, Serruys PW, Erdman RAM, van Domburg RT. Type D personality and diabetes predict the onset of depressive symptoms in patients following percutaneous coronary intervention. *Am Heart J* 2006;151:367e1-6.

[61] Pedersen SS, Denollet J, Ong AT, Serruys PW, Erdman RA, van Domburg RT. Impaired health status in Type D patients following PCI in the drug-eluting stent era. *Int J Cardiol* 2007;114:358-365.

[62] Spindler H, Pedersen SS, Serruys PW, Erdman RA, van Domburg RT. Type-D personality predicts chronic anxiety following percutaneous coronary intervention in the drug-eluting stent era. *J Affect Disord* 2007;99:173-179.

[63] Aquarius AE, Denollet J, Hamming JF, Van Berge Henegouwen DP, De Vries J. Type-D personality and ankle brachial index as predictors of impaired quality of life and depressive symptoms in peripheral arterial disease. *Arch Surg* 2007;142:662-667.

[64] Manolio T. Novel risk markers and clinical practice. *New Engl J Med* 2003;349:1587-1589.

[65] Gremigni P, Sommaruga M. Pesonalità di Tipo D, un costrutto rilevante in cardiologia. Studio preliminare di validazione del questionario italiano. *Psicoterapia Cognitiva e Comportamentale* 2005;11:7-18.

[66] Denollet J, Conraads VM, Brutsaert DL, De Clerck LS, Stevens WJ, Vrints CJ. Cytokines and immune activation in systolic heart failure: the role of Type D personality. *Brain Behav Immun* 2003;17:304-309.

[67] Conraads VM, Denollet J, De Clerck LS, Stevens WJ, Bridts C, Vrints CJ. Type D personality is associated with increased levels of tumour necrosis factor (TNF)-alpha and TNF-alpha receptors in chronic heart failure. *Int J Cardiol* 2006;26;113:34-38.

[68] Kupper N, Denollet J, de Geus EJ, Boomsma DI, Willemsen G. Heritability of type-D personality. *Psychosom Med* 2007;69:675-681.

[69] Glassman AH, O'Connor CM, Califf RM, Swedberg K, Schwartz P, Bigger JT Jr, Krishnan KR, van Zyl LT, Swenson JR, Finkel MS, Landau C, Shapiro PA, Pepine CJ, Mardekian J, Harrison WM, Barton D, Mclvor M; Sertraline Antidepressant Heart Attack Randomized Trial (SADHART) Group. Sertraline treatment of major depression in patients with acute MI or unstable angina. *JAMA* 2002;288:701-709.

[70] Berkman LF, Blumenthal J, Burg M, Carney RM, Catellier D, Cowan MJ, Czajkowski SM, DeBusk R, Hosking J, Jaffe A, Kaufmann PG, Mitchell P, Norman J, Powell LH, Raczynski JM, Schneiderman N; Enhancing Recovery in Coronary Heart Disease Patients Investigators (ENRICHD). Effects of treating depression and low perceived social support on clinical events after myocardial infarction: The Enhancing Recovery in Coronary Heart Disease Patients Investigators (ENRICHD) Randomized Trial. *JAMA* 2003;289:3106-3116.

[71] Appels A, Bär F, van der Pol G, Erdman R, Assman M, Trijsburg W, van Diest R, van
      Dixhoorn J, Mendes de Leon C. Effects of treating exhaustion in angioplasty patients
      on new coronary events: results of the randomized Exhaustion Intervention Trial
      (EXIT). *Psychosom Med* 2005;67:217-223.

[72] Honig A, Kuyper AM, Schene AH, van Melle JP, de Jonge P, Tulner DM, Schins A,
      Crijns HJ, Kuijpers PM, Vossen H, Lousberg R, Ormel J; MIND-IT investigators.
      Treatment of post-myocardial infarction depressive disorder: a randomized, placebo-
      controlled trial with mirtazapine. *Psychosom Med* 2007;69:606-613.

[73] Lespérance F, Frasure-Smith N, Koszycki D, Laliberté MA, van Zyl LT, Baker B,
      Swenson JR, Ghatavi K, Abramson BL, Dorian P, Guertin MC; CREATE
      Investigators. Effects of citalopram and interpersonal psychotherapy on depression in
      patients with coronary artery disease: the Canadian Cardiac Randomized Evaluation of
      Antidepressant and Psychotherapy Efficacy (CREATE) trial. *JAMA* 2007;297:367-379.

[74] van den Broek KC, Martens EJ, Nyklícek I, van der Voort PH, Pedersen SS. Increased
      emotional distress in type-D cardiac patients without a partner. *J Psychosom Res*
      2007;63:41-49.

In: Psychological Factors and Cardiovascular Disorders   ISBN: 978-1-60456-871-4
Editor: Leo Sher   © 2008 Nova Science Publishers, Inc.

Chapter XVI

POTENTIAL MECHANISMS THAT MAY EXPLAIN ADVERSE HEALTH OUTCOMES IN PATIENTS WITH A TYPE D PERSONALITY

Johan Denollet and Nina Kupper

CoRPS – Center of Research on Psychology in Somatic diseases,
Tilburg University, Tilburg, The Netherlands.

ABSTRACT

Cardiac patients with a Type D personality (high negative affectivity and social inhibition) have a poor prognosis, and recent evidence points to biological and behavioral pathways that may explain this relationship. Physiological hyperreactivity, as indicated by increased heart rate, blood pressure and cardiac output, may be one link between Type D personality and cardiovascular health. Type D personality is also related to greater cortisol reactivity in healthy adults and in cardiac patients. Immune activation and increased activity of the pro-inflammatory cytokine tumor necrosis factor-α is another pathway that has been observed in heart failure patients with a Type D personality. Possible behavioral mechanisms include an unhealthy lifestyle, low adherence to treatment, impaired communication with health care providers, and reluctance to consult clinical staff. These findings suggest that assessment of Type D personality in clinical research may significantly improve our understanding of pathways that mediate individual differences in stress-related heart disease.

INTRODUCTION

Emotional stress may increase the risk of coronary artery disease (CAD) and hypertension [1,2], but people differ substantially in their level of vulnerability to emotional stress-related disease [3]. Initially, research on individual differences in stress-related cardiovascular disease focused on Type A behavior [4]. This behavior pattern, characterized by time-urgency and anger-proneness, was found to predict the incidence of CAD, but later research showed that only parts of Type A behavior had toxic effect and that Type A behavior did not predict prognosis in patients with CAD [5]. This controversy surrounding Type A made it unfashionable to study personality types, and subsequent research focused on specific negative emotional states such as depression [6], anger [7], and anxiety [8]. In 1995 and 1996, the 'distressed' [9] or Type D [10] personality construct was introduced to fill this gap in research on broad personality traits that may increase vulnerability to stress-related progression of cardiovascular disease. Hence, the Type D construct was specifically designed to extend our knowledge of personality as a chronic psychological risk factor in cardiovascular disease.

TYPE D PERSONALITY

"Despite myriad studies during the past five decades, the precise role of personality types in producing coronary artery disease awaits clarification. Meanwhile, current evidence suggests that Type D has displaced Type A as the dominant personality risk factor" (Fred & Hariharan, Texas Heart Institute Journal, 2002) [11].

Type D personality refers to the individuals who are high in both negative affectivity and social inhibition. Negative affectivity denotes the stable tendency to experience negative emotions [12], and has also been conceptualized as neuroticism. Because both traits are centrally defined by the tendency to experience negative affect [13], the label "negative affectivity" was used to designate this disposition in patients with CAD [14]. Social inhibition denotes the stable tendency to inhibit the expression of emotions and behaviors in social interaction [15], and is related, but not identical, to the interpersonal dimension of introversion. As such, Type D personality is a global personality cluster that manifests itself across time and situations. Cognitively, individuals with a Type D personality are inclined to be worrying a lot and to take a pessimistic view of things. Affectively, they are more likely to feel unhappy and to be tensed and easily irritated. However, given their inhibited behavior, these intrapsychic phenomena may not be acknowledged by others. Type D persons may perceive the social world as 'threatening' in the sense that they are more likely to anticipate negative reactions from others. To avoid these reactions, they adopt self-enhancing strategies such as inhibition of self-expression. Hence, on an *interpersonal* level, Type D persons frequently experience negative emotions but may be unable to express their true thoughts and feelings towards others. This combination of experiencing and inhibiting emotional distress renders them liable to a chronic form of psychological stress.

By definition, global and stable personality constructs, such as Type D personality, may have much explanatory and predictive power [16]. In fact, several studies have shown that Type D personality predicts adverse cardiac events and poor quality of life in patients with coronary artery disease [10,17,18], heart failure [19], and peripheral arterial disease [20]. Evidence also suggests that Type D personality predicts poor outcomes after invasive cardiac interventions such as coronary stent implantation [21,22], coronary bypass surgery [23], implantation of an cardioverter defibrillator [24], and heart transplantation [25]. Importantly,

Type D personality has been shown to predict cardiac prognosis [26] and anxiety [27], after adjustement of co-occurring symptoms of depression. An overview of the epidemiological evidence on Type D personality can be found in the chapter by Pedersen and Spindler in this book [28], or in a number of recent review articles on Type D personality [29,30].

In contrast to this growing epidemiological evidence on the role of Type D personality in the context of heart disease, relatively little is known about biological, behavioral, or other mechanisms that may account for this personality-disease relationship. It is unlikely that only one mechanism can explain the link between Type D personality and cardiac prognosis, because adverse cardiac events are known to be perpetuated by multiple factors [31]. Moreover, research on potential pathways linking psychological factors to cardiovascular disease still is in its infancy, and Type D personality is no exception. Nevertheless, there is some recent evidence suggesting a number of pathways that may help to explain the observed association between Type D personality and poor prognosis in heart disease.

The way individuals with a Type D personality experience the ongoing situations in their lifes may have *direct physiological effects* that impact on the cardiovascular system. Type D patients tend to experience a wide range of interpersonal and social situations as being potentially stressful. It has been suggested that social situations may elicit negative emotional reactions such as feelings of insecurity or tension in Type D individuals [32]. This may result in physiological hyperreactivity every time a potentially "threatening" situation is encountered [33]. In fact, laboratory research shows that Type D personality may affect cardiovascular health through higher subjective feelings of stress following an acute stressor [34]. Psychological stress may induce cardiovascular effects such as high blood pressure [35] or decreased heart rate variability [36,37]. Disruption of the hypothalamic-pituitary-adrenal (HPA) axis has been suggested as one of the main mechanisms linking increased feelings of stress to physiological hyperreactivity [38,39]. Other physiological mediators of the relation between psychological stress and heart disease include dysfunctions in the *immune system* [40]. Apart from these direct physiological effects, psychological stress may also promote heart disease indirectly through *health-related behaviors* [41]. These mechanisms may help to explain the adverse health outcomes in Type D patients, and are discussed more in detail in the following paragraphs.

PHYSIOLOGICAL REACTIVITY

"Findings are consistent with the noted relationship between Type D and cardiovascular disease, and suggest a possible pathway to disease via an association with physiological hyperreactivity" (Habra, Linden, Anderson & Weinberg, 2003) [33].

Chronic stress may exert its deleterious effect on cardiovascular health through a wide variety of physiological reactions such as, for example, high blood pressure [35], altered hemostasis [42] and increased platelet reactivity [43]. Markers of autonomic activity such as heart rate and heart rate variability have also been studied in the relationship between emotional distress and cardiovascular disease. Increased heart rate as well as decreased heart rate variability have been associated with a significantly greater risk of cardiovascular morbidity and mortality [37,44]. Evidence suggests that depression following myocardial infarction is related to decreased heart rate variability [36]. From a conceptual point of view, these markers of autonomic activity are potential pathways that may also help to explain the relationship between Type D personality and poor outcome in patients with CAD. Studies have shown that behaviorally or emotionally inhibited individuals display increased sympathetic nervous system activity, as indicated by increased stress reactivity [45], prolonged recovery time following stress [46], and decreased heart rate variability [47,48]. For example, emotional inhibition has been associated with impaired autonomic functioning in a cross-sectional study of healthy women, and was evident through reduced heart rate variability in inhibited women [47].

As noted by researchers from the University of British Columbia when discussing their study on laboratory stress in healthy undergraduate students [33], it is possible that Type D personality is also associated with altered physiological reactions that promote the onset and course of CAD. These researchers showed that negative affectivity, one of the two subcomponents of the Type D construct, was related to a *dampened change in heart rate* in reaction to mental stress in young adult men, but not in women [33]. They also found that social inhibition, the other subcomponent of the Type D construct, was associated with *heightened blood pressure reactivity*. Recently, Williams and colleagues [34] also investigated the relationship between Type D personality and cardiovascular reactivity. They used a taxing mental arithmetic task to experimentally induce stress in a sample of 84 healthy, young adults. These researchers found that men with a Type D personality exhibited *higher cardiac output* during the stressor phase compared to non-Type D men [34]. Type D personality was not related to cardiac output in women. Unlike the findings of Habra and colleagues [33], they did not find associations with heart rate or blood pressure.

Although evidence from these experimental studies suggests that there may be a link between Type D personality and cardiovascular health through physiological hyperreactivity, it is not clear whether this operates through increased heart rate and blood pressure [33] or increased cardiac output [34] following acute stress. Little is also know about Type D characteristics and *heart rate variability*. In their 8-year follow-up study of myocardial infarction patients, Carpeggiani and colleagues found that social inhibition and decreased heart rate variability were independent risk factors for poor prognosis [49]. Patients with both social inhibition and decreased heart rate variability had a markedly higher mortality rate of 62% as compared to only 6% in patients with no risk factors. Clearly, more research is needed to investigate the role of these cardiovascular effects as mediators of the relation between Type D personality and cardiovascular health, as well as any different autonomic effects of Type D personality in men as compared to women. Moreover, it still is unclear how findings from research on experimentally induced stress in young, healthy adults can be related to daily life stress in middle-aged adults with established heart disease.

Regarding HPA axis activity, there are two studies that have related Type D personality to greater *cortisol reactivity* in healthy adults [33] and in CAD patients [50], respectively. These findings corroborate the theoretical rationale for the role of cortisol as a mediating mechanism in the relationship between Type D personality, stress and heart disease [39]. Cortisol is a steroid hormone that plays an important role both in the regulation of normal physiology, and in the response of the human body to stress. At the time of stress, different physiological processes are being activated. During the first seconds of the stress response, catecholamines are being released by the sympathetic nervous system. During the ensuing minutes that follow this initial stress response, information is also sent from the brain to the HPA axis, which sets a chain reaction in motion [51]. The hypothalamus produces corticotrophin-releasing factor that acts on the pituitary to activate the release of adrenocorticotropin releasing hormone into the circulation. In response to this initial hormonal reaction, the adrenal glands enhance cortisol production as part of the acute stress reaction of the HPA axis [32]. Importantly, continued or frequently repeated stress challenges may result in chronically elevated levels of basal cortisol.

Cortisol is an effector hormone that influences many areas of the human body, including the cardiovascular system. As a consequence, continued or frequently repeated increases in cortisol levels may have potentially harmful effects on the heart, and has been associated with cardiovascular disease risk factors like high blood pressure, hypercholesterolemia, hypertriglyceridemia and elevated heart rate [38,52,53]. Individual differences such as personality factors and genetic factors have been shown to influence the HPA-mediated response to chronic stress [54]. Miller and colleagues examined the relationship between personality and basal neuroendocrine serum markers in 276 healthy adults, and found that higher levels of neuroticism, or negative affectivity, were associated with higher plasma cortisol levels [55]. Kagan and colleagues found that behavioral inhibition was associated with a larger cortisol awakening response and a larger cortisol response to stress [56]. Interestingly, both these subcomponents of Type D personality have also been associated with greater cortisol reactivity to experimentally induced stress in young, healthy adults [33].

To test this hypothesis that a dysfunctional HPA axis is a biological pathway that may explain the link between emotional distress and cardiac events, Whitehead and colleagues assessed Type D personality and depressive symptoms (as measured by the Beck Depression Inventory) while patients were hospitalized for an acute coronary syndrome [50]. They found that depressive symptoms were not related to cortisol, but that Type D personality was independently associated with the cortisol awakening response, adjusting for age, sex and body mass index. According to these investigators, disruption of the HPA axis function is a pathway that helps to explain the increased risk for adverse clinical events in coronary patients with a Type D personality [50]. Overall, these findings clearly indicate that more research is warranted to further investigate the role of increased cortisol reactivity as an intermediating mechanism that links Type D personality with adverse health outcomes in cardiac patients [32,39].

IMMUNE DYSFUNCTION

"After adjustment for age, Type D personality was independently associated with significant immune activation, and the increase in TNF-α activity observed among Type D patients paralleled the increase in TNF-α activity seen with ageing" (Denollet, Vrints & Conraads, 2008) [57].

During the past decade, the understanding of the etiology of CAD has shifted from exclusive emphasis on the role of major risk factors (e.g. lipids, smoking, hypertension) to the inclusion of *immune factors*. Accumulating evidence indicates that atherosclerosis and CAD also involve an ongoing, low-grade inflammatory process in the coronary arteries [58]. Accordingly, inflammatory status prior to percutaneous coronary intervention has been shown to be an important determinant of clinical outcome following this intervention [59]. Ongoing inflammatory processes have also been implicated in the pathogenesis of chronic heart failure. Chronic heart failure is the end-stage of many cardiac disease processes that carries a grim prognosis and severely impacts on quality of life [19]. However, chronic heart failure not only is a serious cardiac condition, but can also be considered to be a multi-facetted systemic disease that includes several maladaptive physiological processes [60,61].

Cytokines are key elements of immune activation and modulation because these proteins coordinate and stimulate the cellular interactions of the immune system and mediate the inflammatory response [62]. As such, pro-inflammatory cytokines are invaluable in terms of normal adaptive physiologic responses. However, pro-inflammatory cytokines are now also considered to be novel biomarkers of CAD [63]; these cytokines activate the immune system, causing inflammatory reactions in the coronary arteries that may incite acute coronary events [58,62]. There is now abundant evidence that pro-inflammatory cytokines are involved in the development and progression of chronic diseases, including atherosclerotic disease and chronic heart failure [58,64,65,66]. Increased plasma levels of pro-inflammatory cytokines have also been shown to be powerful predictors of mortality in elderly people [67].

One of most studied pro-inflammatory cytokines in chronic heart failure is Tumor Necrosis Factor-α (TNF-α) [68]. TNF-α plays a major role in the instability of an atherosclerotic plaque, the rupture of this plaque, and superimposed thrombosis as consecutive stages in the manifestation of acute coronary events [62]. Increased levels of TNF-α have been shown to predict recurrent cardiac events in patients who survived an acute myocardial infarction [69], as well as an increased mortality risk in patients with chronic heart failure [70]. The effects of TNF-α are mediated through its cell surface receptors; binding of these receptors with TNF-α results in shedding of the extracellular domain, referred to as soluble receptors 1 (sTNFR1) and 2 (sTNFR2). The reproducibility of sTNFR1 and sTNFR2 levels is higher than that of TNF-α because plasma levels of these TNF-α receptors vary less than those of TNF-α itself [68,71]. This may also explain why elevated circulating plasma levels of sTNFR1 and sTNFR2 have emerged among all cytokine parameters as the strongest and most accurate predictors of poor clinical outcome in patients with chronic heart failure [70,72].

There is evidence to suggest that psychological stress may promote immune dysregulation [73]. For example, psychological stress has been shown to reduce lymphocyte proliferation and natural killer cell activity, thereby increasing the individual's vulnerability to infections and disease [74]. It has been suggested that psychological stress may also promote low-grade inflammation in the coronary arteries [62]. But perhaps most convincingly, there is now growing evidence that emotional distress promotes immune dysregulation that is implicated in the pathophysiology of chronic heart failure [75,76,77]. Of note, Type D personality may also affect the chronic inflammatory condition in chronic heart failure patients. In a pilot study of 42 men with chronic heart failure, preliminary findings indicated that circulating levels of TNF-α and its receptors sTNFR1 and sTNFR2 were significantly higher in Type D patients as compared to non-Type D patients [75]. Moreover, Type D personality was an independent correlate of increased pro-inflammatory cytokine levels, adjusting for the etiology and severity of heart failure. This association between Type D personality and increased TNF-α acitivity was replicated in a subsequent study of 91 patients with chronic systolic heart failure [78].

With increasing age, there is a significant increase in levels of pro-inflammatory cytokines in the context of chronic heart failure. A large study of 1200 heart failure patients showed that TNF-α levels increased linearly with age in men, and that these levels abruptly increased in woman after the age of 50 [70]. Von Haehling and colleagues also showed that ageing is associated with an altered immune response in patients with advanced chronic heart failure [79]. Importantly, some have argued that chronic psychological stress may accelerate the rate of this age-related immune dysregulation [80]. In fact, a study of 130 outpatients with chronic heart failure showed that the mean circulating levels of sTNFR1 and sTNFR2 levels in younger Type D patients were equivalent to those in older non-Type D patients who were on average 18 years older [57]. In this study, younger non-Type D patients had the lowest sTNFR1/sTNFR2 levels, and older Type D patients the highest sTNFR1/sTNFR2 levels. Hence, these findings indicated that the disease-promoting effect of Type D personality did match the well-known effect of ageing, and that Type D personality and older age may have similar effects in terms of an increased pro-inflammatory TNF-α activity in chronic heart failure [57].

Overall, these findings suggest that Type D individuals may be more prone to chronic inflammatory dysregulation that is known to be cardiotoxic. Cortisol is often considered to be an anti-inflammatory agent, but it actually has both anti- and pro-inflammatory properties and may increase the expression of cytokine receptors [81]. Hence, the fact that Type D personality is associated with increased cortisol levels [50] may also contribute to the pro-inflammatory state of Type D patients. Of course, the findings from cross-sectional studies on Type D and cytokine activity discussed in this chapter need to be interpreted with some caution, and prospective follow-up research is needed to further investigate the notion that Type D personality has the capacity to accelerate the rate of immune dysfunction in patients with chronic heart failure.

BEHAVIORAL PATHWAYS

"Overall, this evidence provides further support for the utility of Type D personality as a risk factor for CVD by demonstrating that Type D is associated with a reduction in health-related behaviors and low perceived social support" (Williams et al., 2008) [82].

Apart from physiological mechanisms, there are also a number of behavioral mechanisms that might partially explain the link between Type D personality and adverse health outcomes in CAD and chronic heart failure. Psychological risk factors may promote progression of heart disease indirectly through their adverse effect on health-related behaviors [41]. Arguably, a failure to change unhealthy life styles [83] and poor treatment adherence [84] are related to a greater extent of coronary disease and increased mortality risk in CAD patients. Individuals with high levels of emotional distress may be at risk for cardiac events because they are more inclined to engage in disease-promoting health behaviors, such as smoking, sedentary life-style, or failure to adhere to dietary advice [85], and evidence suggests that depression is associated with poor compliance with treatment [41,86]. Hence, unhealthy life style factors, poor compliance with treatment, and a more passive stance to self-management constitute behavioral mechanisms that may mediate the relationship between Type D personality and poor cardiac prognosis.

Recent evidence supports the notion that *health-related behavior* may partly explain the link between Type D personality and cardiovascular disease. In a large cross-sectional study of 1012 healthy young adults from the British and Irish population, Williams and colleagues showed that individuals with a Type D personality reported performing significantly fewer health-related behaviors than other individuals [82]. More specifically, Type D individuals were less likely to eat sensibly, tended to spend less time outdoors, failed to avoid letting things get them down, and were less likely to get a regular medical checkup compared with non-Type D individuals. Interestingly, this relationship between Type D and health-related behavior remained significant after controlling for neuroticism. In addition, Type D individuals also reported lower levels of social support than non-Type D individuals [82].

Apart from an unhealthy lifestyle, evidence suggests that *low adherence to treatment* and *a more passive stance towards self-management* are other behavioral factors that may mediate the relationship between Type D personality and poor health outcomes. Adherence to treatment and active self-management are important patient characteristics that promote effective treatment of cardiac disease [83,84]. With reference to this issue, Broström and colleagues investigated the association of Type D personality with adherence to continuous positive airway pressure (CPAP) treatment in 247 patients with obstructive sleep apnoea syndrome [87]. In this study, Type D personality significantly increased the perceived frequency and severity of side effects of CPAP. Importantly, the objective assessment of adherence to CPAP was significantly lower for Type D patients than for other patients. On the basis of their findings, these investigators concluded that healthcare professionals should account for the adverse effect of Type D personality on adherence to CPAP treatment when treating patients with sleep apnoea [87].

In a Hungarian study on 358 patients who enrolled in cardiac rehabilitation after their first coronary artery bypass surgery, Simon and colleagues examined the influence of Type D personality on test results from the six minutes walking test [88]. This test is a frequently used method for estimating the physical exercise capacity of cardiac patients. However, as noted by these investigators, not only somatic but also psychological factors can influence the results of this exercise test because it requires active cooperation of the patient in order to yield a valid assessment of physical exercise capacity. In this study, CAD patients with a Type D personality covered significantly shorter distance than non-Type D patients, without any substantial differences in heart rate or rating of perceived exertion. These authors concluded that inadequate patient effort was responsible for the fact that Type D patients had a considerably shorter walking distance after coronary artery bypass surgery than other patients [88]. Stulemeijer and colleagues investigated cognitive performance in 110 patients with a mild traumatic brain injury, and found that Type D personality was associated with poor effort of the patient on a memory test [89]. These authors also concluded that Type D personality was strongly associated with inferior test performance because of inadequate effort. Not only do these findings suggest that Type D personality should be considered as a potential threat to the validity of effort-based assessments of physical and cognitive functioning [88,89], they also raise the question whether a more passive stance and insufficient mobilization of effort may impede adequate self-management of cardiovascular disease in Type D patients. With reference to this issue, personality variables have been shown to predict adherence to cardiac rehabilitation [90]. Hence, it is possible that cardiac patients with a Type D personality may be less likely to actively participate in an outpatient rehabilitation program. There is also evidence to suggest that an inhibited interpersonal style is associated with poor adherence to scheduled clinic visits [91].

Another line of research suggests that patients with a Type D personality may *refrain from discussing their emotional* [92] *and physical* [93] *problems* with their attending physician or nurse. By definition, Type D patients score high on social inhibition, and this inhibited interpersonal style of the Type D personality profile may impede effective communication between patient and physician. Roter and Ewart studied 203 patients with essential hypertension and found that these patients appear to have an inhibited pattern of self-presentation that could present an obstacle to effective communication with their physicians [92]. Hypertensive patients were less likely to exhibit signs of emotional distress during the visit to their attending physician as compared to patients with a normal blood pressure. As a consequence, physicians were less accurate in characterizing the emotional state of hypertensive patients, and paid little attention to psychosocial concerns but rather concentrated more on biomedical matters [92]. Hence, physicians' disinclination to probe for emotional difficulty in inhibited patients likely results in the undertreatment of psychological stress, which could be potentially damaging to health.

Impaired communication with health care providers can also promote disease progression through interference with adequate consultation for cardiac symptoms. In a study of 178 outpatients with chronic heart failure, Schiffer and colleagues found that patients with a Type D personality may delay medical consultation [93]. Type D patients experienced more cardiac symptoms such as chest pain or shortness of breath, and more often appraised these symptoms as worrisome compared with non-Type D patients. Paradoxically, however, they stated that they would be *less likely to report* these symptoms to their cardiologist or nurse than would other patients. In a cross-sectional study on voice complaints among female teachers and student teachers, Thomas and colleagues also showed that individuals with a Type D personality sought less voice care than non-Type D individuals, despite the fact that they were actually more bothered by their voice than other individuals [94]. This reluctance of Type D patients to consult clinical staff most likely is the consequence of increased levels of social inhibition [93], and may increase the likelihood of adverse clinical outcomes by jeopardizing appropriate adjustments in clinical care [95]. It also suggests that chronic heart failure patients with a Type D personality may require more detailed information about the consequences of ignoring cardiac symptoms, and guidance with adequate consultation behavior after the onset of these symptoms [95].

CONCLUDING REMARKS

"There has been vigorous debate among psychosocial researchers about the validity and usefulness of the Type D construct. One issue is whether it adds to the better-established evidence concerning depression" (Steptoe and Molloy, 2007) [95].

As indicated by this quote, it is often questioned whether Type D personality has incremental value above and beyond other psychological risk factors such as hostility or depression. Research on mechanisms that can explain the Type D – heart disease link are also important in this perspective. For example, Habra and colleagues pointed out that for a new personality risk factor to be useful, it should add to our ability to understand what contributes to physiological hyperresponsivity, rather than merely replicate was has been shown with already existing constructs [33]. Therefore, it is important to note that in their experimental study, Type D personality did emerge as a stronger predictor of stress reactivity as compared to hostility. Whitehead and colleagues provided more evidence for the notion that Type D may operate through distinctly different pathways as compared to more established psychological risk factors [50]. In their clinical study among patients with CAD, Type D was positively associated with the cortisol awakening response, whereas depression was not. This observation is in line with findings from other recent studies showing that Type D personality is distinctly different from depression in terms of prognostic power [26], susceptibility to anxiety [27], and somatic confounding [96].

The studies reviewed in this chapter may contribute to our understanding of the various mechanisms that may explain the possible pathogenic nature of Type D personality in cardiac patients. Nevertheless, the exact mediating mechanisms by which Type D personality affects cardiovascular health still await further clarification. Hence, it is important to keep on examining mechanisms that may explain the link between Type D and cardiac outcomes [95]. For example, it is also possible that Type D personality and the physiological alterations seen in cardiovascular disease reflect a similar underlying biological susceptibility that is conveyed by the same genetic factors [97].

Given their inhibited behavior, Type D patients are less likely to display overt evidence of stress. As a result, Type D patients may often go unrecognized by health care providers. Bridging this gap between the recognition of Type D and the provision of appropriate care is imperative for improving the health status of cardiac patients with a Type D personality. The systematic identification of personality traits related to treatment response may also improve the impact of innovations in treatments of cardiac disorder. The availability of the 14-item Type D Scale (DS14) as a brief assessment tool facilitates integration of the Type D construct in medical research and practice [98,99]. The DS14 has already been recommended in order to screen for Type D personality in the clinical care of patients with CAD [100]. The evidence presented in this chapter indicates that use of the DS14 scale in clinical research may also significantly improve our understanding of mechanisms that may explain the link between emotional distress and cardiac prognosis.

REFERENCES

[1]   Kop, W.J. (1999). Chronic and acute psychological risk factors for clinical manifestations of coronary artery disease. *Psychosomatic Medicine, 61*, 476-487.

[2]   al'Absi, M. & Wittmers, L.E. Jr. (2003). Enhanced adrenocortical responses to stress in hypertension-prone men and women. *Annals of Behavioral Medicine, 25*, 25-33.

[3]   Charney, D.S. (2004). Psychobiological mechanisms of resilience and vulnerability: Implications for successful adaptation to extreme stress. *American Journal of Psychiatry, 161*, 195-216.

[4]   Friedman, M., & Rosenman, R. H. (1974). *Type A Behavior and Your Heart*. New York: Fawcett Books.

[5]   Dimsdale, J.E. (1988). A perspective on Type A behavior and coronary disease. *New England Journal of Medicine, 318*, 110-112.

[6]   Frasure-Smith, N., Lesperance, F., & Talajic, M. (1995). Depression and 18-month prognosis after myocardial infarction. *Circulation, 91*, 999-1005.

[7]   Miller, T.Q., Smith, T.W., Turner, C.W., et al. (1996). A meta-analytic review of research on hostility and physical health. *Psychological Bulletin, 119*, 322-348.

[8]   Kawachi, I., Sparrow, D., Vokonas, P., et al. (1994). Symptoms of anxiety and risk of coronary heart disease: The Normative Aging Study. *Circulation, 90*, 2225-2229.

[9]   Denollet, J., Sys, S. U., & Brutsaert, D. L. (1995). Personality and mortality after myocardial infarction. *Psychosomatic Medicine, 57*, 582-591.

[10]   Denollet, J., Sys, S. U., Stroobant, N., Rombouts, H., Gillebert, T. C., & Brutsaert, D. L. (1996). Personality as independent predictor of long-term mortality in patients with coronary heart disease. *Lancet, 347,* 417-421.

[11]   Fred, H.L. & Hariharan, R. (2002). To be B or not to be B - Is that the question? (Editorial). *Texas Heart Institute Journal, 29*, 1-2.

[12]   Watson, D., & Clark, L. A. (1984). Negative affectivity: The disposition to experience aversive emotional states. *Psychological Bulletin, 96*, 465-490.

[13]   McCrae, R.R. & Costa, P.T. (1987). Validation of the five factor model of personality across instruments and observers. *Journal of Personality and Social Psychology, 52,* 81-90.

[14]   Denollet, J. (1991). Negative affectivity and repressive coping: pervasive influence on self-reported mood, health, and coronary-prone behavior. *Psychosomatic Medicine, 53*, 538-556.

[15]   Denollet, J., Pedersen, S. S., Ong, A. T., Erdman, R. A., Serruys, P. W., & van Domburg, R. T. (2006). Social inhibition modulates the effect of negative emotions on cardiac prognosis following percutaneous coronary intervention in the drug-eluting stent era. *European Heart Journal, 27*, 171-177.

[16]   Funder, D.C. (1991). Global traits: a neo-Allportian approach to personality. *Psychological Science, 2*, 31-39.

[17]   Denollet, J., Vaes, J., & Brutsaert, D. L. (2000). Inadequate response to treatment in coronary heart disease: Adverse effects of type D personality and younger age on 5-year prognosis and quality of life. *Circulation, 102*, 630-635.

[18] Denollet, J., Pedersen, S. S., Vrints, C. J., & Conraads, V. M. (2006). Usefulness of Type D personality in predicting five-year cardiac events above and beyond concurrent symptoms of stress in patients with coronary heart disease. *American Journal of Cardiology, 97*, 970-973.

[19] Schiffer, A. A., Pedersen, S. S., Widdershoven, J. W., Hendriks, E. H., Winter, J. B., & Denollet, J. (2005). The distressed (type D) personality is independently associated with impaired health status and increased depressive symptoms in chronic heart failure. *European Journal of Cardiovascular Prevention and Rehabilitation, 12*, 341-346.

[20] Aquarius, A. E., Denollet, J., Hamming, J. F., & De Vries, J. (2005). Role of disease status and type D personality in outcomes in patients with peripheral arterial disease. *American Journal of Cardiology, 96*, 996-1001.

[21] Pedersen, S. S., Lemos, P. A., van Vooren, P. R., Liu, T. K., Daemen, J., Erdman, R. A., et al. (2004). Type D personality predicts death or myocardial infarction after bare metal stent or sirolimus-eluting stent implantation: A rapamycin-eluting stent evaluated at Rotterdam cardiology hospital (RESEARCH) registry substudy. *Journal of the American College of Cardiology, 44*, 997-1001.

[22] Pedersen, S. S., Ong, K., Sonnenschein, P., Serruys, P. W., Erdman, R. A., & van Domburg, R. T. (2006). Type D personality and diabetes predict the onset of depressive symptoms in patients after percutaneous coronary intervention. *American Heart Journal, 151*, 367.e1-367.e6.

[23] Al-Ruzzeh, S., Athanasiou, T., Mangoush, O., Wray, J., Modine, T., George, S., et al. (2005). Predictors of poor mid-term health related quality of life after primary isolated coronary artery bypass grafting surgery. *Heart, 91*, 1557-1562.

[24] Pedersen, S. S., Van Domburg, R. T., Theuns, D. A., Jordaens, L., & Erdman, R. A. (2004). Type d personality is associated with increased anxiety and depressive symptoms in patients with an implantable cardioverter defibrillator and their partners. *Psychosomatic Medicine, 66*, 714-719.

[25] Denollet, J., Holmes, R.V., Vrints, C.J., Conraads, V.M. (2007). Unfavorable outcome of heart transplantation in recipients with Type D personality. *Journal of Heart and Lung Transplantation, 26*, 152-158.

[26] Denollet, J. & Pedersen, S. S. (2008). Prognostic value of Type D personality compared with depressive symptoms. *Archives of Internal Medicine, 168*, 431-432.

[27] Schiffer, A.A., Pedersen, S.S., Broers, H., Widdershoven, J.W., Denollet, J. (2008). Type D personality but not depression predicts severity of anxiety in heart failure patients at 1-year follow-up. *Journal of Affective Disorder, 106*, 73-81.

[28] Pedersen, S.S. & Spindler, H. (2008). The epidemiology of Type D personqlity: A new cardiovascular risk factor – fact or fiction? *This book*.

[29] Type D personality as a prognostic factor in heart disease: assessment and mediating mechanisms. *Journal of Personality Assessment, 89*, 265-276.

[30] Pedersen, S. S., & Denollet, J. (2006). Is Type D personality here to stay? Emerging evidence across cardiovascular disease patient groups. *Current Cardiology Reviews, 2*, 205-213.

[31]   Hellstrom, H.R., Rozanski, A., Blumenthal, J.A., Kaplan, J. (2000). Psychological factors and ischemic heart disease: Response. *Circulation, 101*, e177-e178.

[32]   Denollet, J. & Kupper, N. (2007). Type D personality, depression, and cardiac prognosis: cortisol dysregulation as a mediating mechanism. *Journal of Psychosomatic Research, 62*, 607-609.

[33]   Habra, M. E., Linden, W., Anderson, J. C., & Weinberg, J. (2003). Type D personality is related to cardiovascular and neuroendocrine reactivity to acute stress. *Journal of Psychosomatic Research, 55*, 235-245.

[34]   Williams, L., O'Carroll, R.E., O'Connor, R.C. (2008). Type D personality and cardiac output in response to stress. *Psychology and Health, 00*, 000-000, in press.

[35]   Verdecchia, P., Schillaci, G., Reboldi, G., Franklin, S. S., & Porcellati, C. (2001). Ambulatory monitoring for prediction of cardiac and cerebral events. *Blood Pressure Monitoring, 6*, 211-215.

[36]   Carney, R.M., Blumenthal, J.A., Stein, P.K., et al. (2001). Depression, heart rate variability, and acute myocardial infarction. *Circulation, 104*, 2024-2028.

[37]   Dekker, J. M., Crow, R. S., Folsom, A. R., Hannan, P. J., Liao, D., Swenne, C. A., et al. (2000). Low heart rate variability in a 2-minute rhythm strip predicts risk of coronary heart disease and mortality from several causes: The ARIC study. Atherosclerosis risk in communities. *Circulation, 102*, 1239-1244.

[38]   Rosmond, R., & Bjorntorp, P. (2000). The hypothalamic-pituitary-adrenal axis activity as a predictor of cardiovascular disease, type 2 diabetes and stroke. *Journal of Internal Medicine, 247*, 188-197.

[39]   Sher, L. (2005). Type D personality: The heart, stress, and cortisol. *Quarterly Journal of Medicine, 98*, 323-329.

[40]   Kop, W. J., & Gottdiener, J. S. (2005). The role of immune system parameters in the relationship between depression and coronary artery disease. *Psychosomatic Medicine, 67*(Suppl. 1), S37-S41.

[41]   Carney, R.M., Freedland, K.E., Eisen, S.A., et al. (1995). Major depression and medication adherence in elderly patients with coronary artery disease. *Health Psychology, 14*, 88-90.

[42]   Von Känel, R., Mills, P.J., Fainman, C., Dimsdale, J.E. (2001). Effects of psychological stress and psychiatric disorders on blood coagulation and fibrinolysis: A biobehavioral pathway to coronary artery disease? *Psychosomatic Medicine, 63*, 531-544.

[43]   Kuijpers, P.M., Hamulyak, K., Strik, J.J., et al. (2002). Beta-thromboglobulin and platelet factor 4 levels in post-myocardial infarction patients with major depression. *Psychiatry Research, 109*, 207-210.

[44]   Palatini, P., Casiglia, E., Julius, S., & Pessina, A. C. (1999). High heart rate: A risk factor for cardiovascular death in elderly men. *Archives of Internal Medicine, 159*, 585-592.

[45]   Gross, J. J., & Levenson, R. W. (1997). Hiding feelings: The acute effects of inhibiting negative and positive emotion. *Journal of Abnormal Psychology, 106*, 95-103.

[46]   Brosschot, J. F., & Thayer, J. F. (1998). Anger inhibition, cardiovascular recovery, and vagal function: A model of the link between hostility and cardiovascular disease. *Annals of Behavioral Medicine, 20*, 326-332.

[47]   Horsten, M., Ericson, M., Perski, A., Wamala, S. P., Schenck-Gustafsson, K., & Orth-Gomer, K. (1999). Psychosocial factors and heart rate variability in healthy women. *Psychosomatic Medicine, 61*, 49-57.

[48]   Marshall, P. J., & Stevenson-Hinde, J. (1998). Behavioral inhibition, heart period, and respiratory sinus arrhythmia in young children. *Developmental Psychobiology, 33*, 283-292.

[49]   Carpeggiani, C., Emdin, M., Bonaguidi, F., et al. (2005). Personality traits and heart rate variability predict long-term cardiac mortality after myocardial infarction. *European Heart Journal, 26*, 1612-7.

[50]   Whitehead, D.L., Perkins-Porras, L., Strike, P.C., Magid, K., Steptoe, A. (2007). Cortisol awakening response is elevated in acute coronary syndrome patients with Type D personality. *Journal of Psychosomatic Research, 62*, 419-425.

[51]   Chrousos, G.P. (1995). The hypothalamic-pituitary-adrenal axis and immune-mediated inflammation. *New England Journal of Medicine, 332*, 1351-1362.

[52]   Girod, J. P., & Brotman, D. J. (2004). Does altered glucocorticoid homeostasis increase cardiovascular risk? *Cardiovascular Research, 64*, 217-226.

[53]   Mantero, F. & Boscaro, M. (1992). Glucocorticoid-dependent hypertension. *Journal of Steroid Biochemical Molecular Biology, 43*, 409–413.

[54]   McEwen, B.S. (2000). Allostasis and allostatic load: Implications for neuropsychopharma-cology. *Neuropsychopharmacology, 22*, 108-124.

[55]   Miller, G. E., Cohen, S., Rabin, B. S., Skoner, D. P., & Doyle, W. J. (1999). Personality and tonic cardiovascular, neuroendocrine, and immune parameters. *Brain, Behavior, and Immunity, 13*(2), 109-123.

[56]   Kagan, J., Reznick, J. S., & Snidman, N. (1987). The physiology and psychology of behavioral inhibition in children. *Child Development, 58*, 1459-1473.

[57]   Denollet, J., Vrints, C.J., Conraads, V.M. (2008). Comparing Type D personality and older age as correlates of tumor necrosis factor-α dysregulation in chronic heart failure. *Brain, Behavior and Immunity, 22*, 736-743..

[58]   Libby, P., Ridker, P.M., Maseri, A. (2002). Inflammation and aherosclerosis. *Circulation, 105*, 1135-1143.

[59]   Toutouzas, K., Colombo, A., Stefanadis, C. (2004). Inflammation and restenosis after percutaneous coronary intervention. *European Heart Journal, 25*, 1679-1687.

[60]   Conraads, V.M., Bosmans, J.M., Vrints, C.J. (2002). Chronic heart failure: an example of a systemic chronic inflammatory disease resulting in cachexia. *International Journal of Cardiology, 85*, 33-49.

[61]   Torre-Amione, G. (2005). Immune activation in chronic heart failure. *The American Journal of Cardiology, 95*(11, Supplement 1), 3-8.

[62]   Gidron, Y., Gilutz, H., Berger, R., et al. (2002). Molecular and cellular interface between behavior and acute coronary syndromes. *Cardiovascular Research, 56*, 15-21.

[63]   Morrow, D.A. & Braunwald, E. (2003). Future of biomarkers in acute coronary syndromes: moving toward a multimarker strategy. *Circulation, 108*, 250-252.

[64]   Hansson, G.K. (2005). Inflammation, atherosclerosis, and coronary artery disease. *New England Journal of Medicine, 352*, 1685-1695.

[65]   Tedgui, A., Mallat, Z. (2006). Cytokines in atherosclerosis: pathogenic and regulatory pathways. *Physiological Review, 86*, 515-581.

[66]   Vasan, R.S., Sullivan, L.M., Roubenoff, R., Dinarello, C.A., Harris, T., Benjamin, E.J., Sawyer, D.B., Levy, D., Wilson, P.W., D'Agostino, R.B. (2003). Inflammatory markers and risk of heart failure in elderly subjects without prior myocardial infarction: the Framingham Heart Study. *Circulation, 107*, 1486–1491.

[67]   Krabbe, K.S., Pedersen, M., Bruunsgaard, H. (2004). Inflammatory mediators in the elderly. *Experimental Gerontology, 39*, 687-699.

[68]   von Haehling, S., Jankowska, E.A., Anker, S.D. (2004). Tumor necrosis factor-α and the failing heart: pathophysiology and therapeutic implications. *Basic Research in Cardiology, 99*, 18-28.

[69]   Ridker, P.M., Rifai, N., Pfeffer, M., Sacks, F., Lepage, S., Braunwald, E. (2000). Elevation of tumor necrosis factor-α and increased risk of recurrent coronary events after myocardial infarction. *Circulation, 101*, 2149–2153.

[70]   Deswal, A., Petersen, N.J., Feldman, A.M., Young, J.B., White, B.G., Mann, D.L. (2001). Cytokines and cytokine receptors in advanced heart failure: an analysis of the cytokine database from the Vesnarinone trial (VEST). *Circulation, 103*, 2055-2059.

[71]   Dibbs, Z., Thornby, J., White, B.G., Mann, D.L. (1999). Natural variability of circulating levels of cytokines and cytokine receptors in patients with heart failure: implications for clinical trials. *Journal of the American College of Cardiology, 33*, 1935–1942.

[72]   Valgimigli, M., Ceconi, C., Malagutti, P., Merli, E., Soukhomovskaia, O., Francolini, G., Cicchitelli, G., Olivares, A., Parrinello, G., Percoco, G., Guardigli, G., Mele, D., Pirani, R., Ferrari, R. (2005). Tumor necrosis factor-alpha receptor 1 is a major predictor of mortality and new-onset heart failure in patients with acute myocardial infarction: the Cytokine-Activation and Long-Term Prognosis in Myocardial Infarction (C-ALPHA) study. *Circulation, 111*, 863-870.

[73]   Kop, W.J. (2003). The integration of cardiovascular behavioral medicine and psychoneuro-immunology: new developments based on converging research fields. *Brain, Behavior and Immunity, 17*, 233-237.

[74]   Cohen, S., Tyrrell, D.A., Smith A.P. (1991). sychological stress and susceptibility to the common cold. *New England Journal of Medicine, 325*, 606-612.

[75]   Denollet, J., Conraads, V. M., Brutsaert, D. L., De Clerck, L. S., Stevens, W. J., & Vrints, C. J. (2003). Cytokines and immune activation in systolic heart failure: The role of type D personality. *Brain, Behavior, and Immunity, 17*, 304-309.

[76]   Parissis, J.T., Adamopoulos, S., Rigas, A., Kostakis, G., Karatzas, D., Venetsanou, K., Kremastinos, D.T. (2004). Comparison of circulating proinflammatory cytokines and soluble apoptosis mediators in patients with chronic heart failure with versus without symptoms of depression. *American Journal of Cardiology, 94*, 1326-1328.

[77] Andrei, A.M., Fraguas, R. Jr., Telles, R.M., Alves, T.C., Strunz, C.M., Nussbacher, A., Rays, J., Iosifescu, D.V., Wajngarten, M. (2007). Major depressive disorder and inflammatory markers in elderly patients with heart failure. *Psychosomatics*, *48*, 319-324.

[78] Conraads, V. M., Denollet, J., De Clerck, L. S., Stevens, W. J., Bridts, C., & Vrints, C. J. (2006). Type D personality is associated with increased levels of tumour necrosis factor (TNF)-alpha and TNF-alpha receptors in chronic heart failure. *International Journal of Cardiology*, *113*, 34-38.

[79] von Haehling, S., Genth-Zotz, S., Sharma, R., Bolger, A.P., Doehner, W., Barnes, P.J., Coats, A.J., Anker, S.D. (2003). The relationship between age and production of tumour necrosis factor-alpha in healthy volunteers and patients with chronic heart failure. *International Journal of Cardiology*, *90*, 197-204.

[80] Graham, J.E,. Christian, L.M., Kiecolt-Glaser, J.K. (2006). Stress, age, and immune function: toward a lifespan approach. *Journal of Behavioral Medicine*, *29*, 389-400.

[81] Sorrells, S.F. & Sapolsky, R.M. (2007). An inflammatory review of glucocorticoid actions in the CNS. *Brain, Behavior and Immunity*, *21*, 259–272.

[82] Williams, L., O'Connor, R.C., Howard, S., Hughes, B.M., Johnston, D.W., Hay, J.L., O'Connor, D.B., Lewis, C.A., Ferguson, E., Sheehy, N., Grealy, M.A., O'Carroll, R.E. (2008b). Type D personality mechanisms of effect: The role of health-related behavior and social support. *Journal of Psychosomatic Research*, *64*, 63-69.

[83] Haskell, W.L., Alderman, E.L., Fair, J.M., et al. (1994). Effects of intensive multiple risk factor reduction on coronary atherosclerosis and clinical cardiac events in men and women with coronary artery disease: The Stanford Coronary Risk Intervention Project (SCRIP). *Circulation*, *89*, 975-990.

[84] Horwitz RI, Viscoli CM, Berkman L, et al. (1990). Treatment adherence and risk of death after a myocardial infarction. *Lancet*, *336*, 542-545.

[85] Kirkcaldy, B.D., Shephard, R.J., Siefen, R.F. (2002). The relationship between physical activity and self-image and problem behaviour among adolescents. *Social Psychiatry and Psychiatric Epidemiology*, *37*, 544-550.

[86] Ziegelstein, R.C., Bush, D.E., Fauerbach, J.A. (1998). Depression, adherence behavior, and coronary disease outcomes. *Archives of Internal Medicine*, *158*, 808-809.

[87] Broström A., Strömberg A., Mårtensson J., Ulander M., Harder L., Svanborg, E. (2007). Association of Type D personality to perceived side effects and adherence in CPAP-treated patients with OSAS. *Journal of Sleep Research*, *16*, 439-447.

[88] Simon, A., Tringer, I., Berényi, I., Veress, G. (2007). Psychological factors considerably influence the results of 6-min walk test after coronary bypass surgery [Article in Hungarian]. *Orv Hetil.*, *148*, 2087-2094.

[89] Stulemeijer, M., Andriessen, T.M., Brauer, J.M., Vos, P.E., Van Der Werf, S. (2007). Cognitive performance after mild traumatic brain injury: the impact of poor effort on test results and its relation to distress, personality and litigation. *Brain Injury*, *21*, 309-318.

[90]   Hershberger, P.J., Robertson, K.B., Markert, R.J. (1999). Personality and appointment-keeping adherence in cardiac rehabilitation. *Journal of Cardiopulmonary Rehabilitation, 19*, 106-111.

[91]   Pereira, D.B., Antoni, M.H., Danielson, A., Simon, T., Efantis-Potter, J., O'Sullivan, M.J. (2004). Inhibited interpersonal coping style predicts poorer adherence to scheduled clinic visits in human immunodeficiency virus infected women at risk for cervical cancer. *Annals of Behavioral Medicine, 28*, 195-202.

[92]   Roter, D.L. & Ewart, C.K. (1992). Emotional inhibition in essential hypertension: Obstacle to communication during medical visits. *Health Psychology, 11,* 163-169.

[93]   Schiffer, A.A, Denollet, J., Widdershoven, J.W., Hendriks, E.H., Smith, O.R. (2007). Failure to consult for symptoms of heart failure in patients with a Type D personality. *Heart, 93*, 814-818.

[94]   Thomas G., de Jong, F.I., Kooijman, P.G., Cremers, C.W. (2006). Utility of the Type D Scale 16 and Voice Handicap Index to assist voice care in student teachers and teachers. *Folia Phoniatrica et Logopaedica, 58*, 250-263.

[95]   Steptoe, A. & Molloy, G.J. (2007). Personality and heart disease. *Heart, 93*, 783-784.

[96]   de Jonge, P., Denollet, J., van Melle, J.P., Kuyper, A., Honig, A., Schene, A.H., Ormel, J. (2007). Associations of Type D personality and depression with somatic health in myocardial infarction patients. *Journal of Psychosomatic Research, 63*, 477-482.

[97]   Kupper, N., Denollet, J., de Geus, E.J., Boomsma, D.I., Willemsen, G. (2007). Heritability of Type D personality. *Psychosomatic Medicine, 69*, 675-681.

[98]   Denollet, J. (2005). DS14: Standard assessment of negative affectivity, social inhibition, and type D personality. *Psychosomatic Medicine, 67*, 89-97.

[99]   Emons, W.H., Meijer, R.R., Denollet J. (2007). Negative affectivity and social inhibition in cardiovascular disease: Evaluating type-D personality and its assessment using item response theory. *Journal of Psychosomatic Research, 63*, 27-39.

[100]   Albus, C., Jordan, J., & Herrmann-Lingen, C. (2004). Screening for psychosocial risk factors in patients with coronary heart disease-recommendations for clinical practice. *European Journal of Cardiovascular Prevention and Rehabilitation, 11*(1), 75-79.

In: Psychological Factors and Cardiovascular Disorders   ISBN: 978-1-60456-871-4
Editor: Leo Sher   © 2008 Nova Science Publishers, Inc.

Chapter XVII

HOSTILITY AS A RISK FACTOR FOR CORONARY HEART DISEASE

Paola Gremigni

Department of Psychology, University of Bologna, Italy.

ABSTRACT

Hostility has been viewed as a "toxic" psychological dimension related to coronary heart disease (CHD) since the late 1980s. Reviews and meta-analyses have confirmed its association with adverse health outcomes and CHD risk factors, although the direct link with CHD is controversial. Hostility is a broad concept which still needs to be clarified as regards definition, measurements, and underlying physiological mechanisms of its association with CHD. This chapter tries to give a brief review of the state of the art of the studies that address these issues.

INTRODUCTION

Hostility is a multidimensional construct which is assumed to include cognitive, affective, and behavioral components characterized by negative beliefs about and attitudes toward others [1].

High levels of hostility have been traditionally associated with adverse health outcomes, especially cardiovascular diseases (CVD), and a meta-analytic review published in 1996 concluded that it was an independent risk factor for coronary heart disease (CHD) and all-cause mortality [2]. Hostility has been also associated with a variety of health behaviors, including smoking, alcohol consumption, and weight [3]. Moreover, a recent meta-analysis provides cross-sectional evidence for an association between hostility, together with other psychological characteristics, and the metabolic syndrome [4]. Taken together, the available evidence indicates that hostility plays a complex role in the aetiology of heart disease, and it does increase the risk of CVD in healthy populations [5], although it does not appear to be a strong predictor of recurrent events or mortality in coronary patients [6].

Understanding the relationship between hostility and health behaviours and outcomes may aid the development of psychosocial interventions designed to prevent and decrease risk of CHD.

This chapter will attempt to give a brief review of the association between hostility and the risk of developing CHD by tracing its historical aspects; illustrating the definitional complexity of its concept; describing the instruments used to measure such trait; examining the mechanisms linking hostility and coronary disease, and reporting on current data regarding its impact on heart diseases.

HISTORY

Modern research on the association between psychological factors and the risk of developing CHD has been based on the work of Friedman and Rosenman [7] on the role of the Type A behavior pattern (TABP).

The TABP is defined as an action–emotion complex stimulated by certain environmental events. It is characterized by a) predispositions such as impatience, aggressiveness, competitiveness, a sense of time urgency, and the desire to achieve recognition and advancement; b) specific behaviors and physical manifestations such as muscle tenseness, alertness, rapid speech, interruption of others' speech, and accelerated pace of activities; c) emotional responses such as irritation, hostility, and increased anger [8].

This concept was studied extensively from the 1960s to the 1980s [9], and initial population studies offered enough evidence for the National Heart, Lung, and Blood Institute in 1981 to conclude that TABP was associated with an increased risk of clinically apparent CHD in middle aged citizens in industrialized areas [10].

Subsequent studies challenged the independent predictive value of the global TABP with respect to CHD [11]. In a large meta-analysis published in 1987, Booth-Kewley and Friedman [12] suggested that only certain elements of this complex may be related to CHD. Other researchers [13] stressed the potential importance of hostility, in particular, as a risk factor for CHD.

Inasmuch as ensuing large epidemiological studies failed to confirm the pathological effects of TABP on CHD [14], the inconclusive evidence was attributed in part to the complexity of measuring the global behavioral pattern. In efforts to manage the complexity of this construct, researchers broke down the TABP to study its many sub components; thus, gradually the emphasis moved to hostility. Since then, hostility has been generally viewed as the most "toxic" component of the global TABP related to CHD [15,16].

A meta-analysis by Myrtek [17] confirms that there is no significant association between TABP and heart disease, while hostility yields a significant association with CHD, although the effect size of this relationship is modest.

A question that the researchers have tried to answer since the 1990s is which component of hostility is most strongly and consistently associated with CHD [18,19].

Any attempt to advance our understanding of this relationship needs to pay attention to definitions, measurements, and underlying physiological mechanisms.

DEFINITION

Hostility is a broad and complex concept which has been defined in different ways by different investigators. It is not simple to measure, is influenced by other traits, and occurs in different personal and social contexts [20].

Hostility has been treated either as part of a general personality construct or as an independent personality trait. For example, it has been considered as a part of the factor L (suspiciousness) of Cattell's 16-PF personality measure [21] or as related to the global psychoticism factor of Eysencks' personality dimensions [22].

On the other hand, potential for hostility has been conceptualized as an independent pre-disposition to respond to a broad range of frustrating circumstances with anger, irritation, and arrogance, sometimes associated with overt behavior directed against the source of the frustration [23]. Smith [1] summarized hostility as a general personality trait that involves a devaluation of the worth of others and a desire to inflict harm or see others harmed. Hostility has been found relatively stable across time, with some evidence for a heritable component [24].

The most widely accepted definition of hostility has been presented by Barefoot in 1992 [25] and it is based on the division of experience into three components: cognitive, affective, and behavioral. The cognitive component consists of negative beliefs about others, who are viewed as untrustworthy, undeserving, and selfish. These beliefs produce interpretation of the behavior of others as antagonistic or threatening, and reactive aggression in the hostile person. The affective component includes anger, resentment, and contempt. Affective arousal is accompanied by cardiovascular reactivity that may play a role in the pathogenesis of CHD [26]. The main aspect of the behavioral component of hostility is aggression, in particular verbal aggression and other forms of antagonistic behavior. A distinction has been also drawn between the experience of hostility and its expression [10]. The experience of hostility is subjective and includes angry feelings, suspicious and cynical thoughts. Expressive or behavioral hostility implies observable acts of aggression, which may be verbal or physical.

Hostility is viewed as a multidimensional construct including three components that not necessarily occur together, although they are correlated. For that reason, it has been hypothesized that some dimensions may be more predictive of disease than others. Accordingly attempts have been made to identify and assess the sub components of hostility most predictive of CHD [27,28]. Among the cognitive components, those involving thoughts and attitudes, cynicism or mistrust received the most attention [29,30].

Though the different components of hostility are conceptually distinct, they are difficult to distinguish clearly at an operational level, partly because the various aspects have an influence on each other. This difficulty is reflected in the assessment of hostility: instruments do vary in their emphasis on particular components; this is a reason for the great dispersion of hostility scales observed by Miller and colleague in their meta-analytic review [2]. Furthermore, such instruments often assess different but overlapping aspects of the trait and this may easily lead to inconsistent findings in the studies on the relationship between hostility and health [19]. Thus the choice of measurement instruments plays a key role in interpreting empirical findings.

ASSESSMENT

Miller and colleagues [2] found 63 different measures of hostility, but some of them lacked sufficient information regarding psychometric characteristics, especially construct validity [31]. Among these either various versions of the observed Type A Structured Interview (SI; [32]) or self-report methods can be found. Since the most reliable observational method, the Videotaped Structured Interview, requires extensive training in recognizing overt signs of hostility traits, the self-report questionnaire has been the most frequently used approach. It has the main advantages of being reliable, ease of administration, and cost-effectiveness, although the disadvantage of being influenced by social desirability.

The most widely used self-reported measures are the 50-item Cook–Medley Hostility Inventory (Ho; [33]), which was taken from the Minnesota Multiphasic Personality Inventory. It's more predictive version developed by Barefoot and colleagues [25] classified the items composing the Ho into five categories (cynicism, hostile attribution, aggressive responding, hostile affect, and social avoidance) based on item content. The Ho became popular since Williams and colleagues [34] found it to be related to coronary artery disease severity in cardiac patients. In prospective studies, Ho successfully predicted CHD events, total mortality, and overall risk profiles, although in other studies it failed to predict the same outcomes [3]. A similar 33-item hostility scale was developed from the California Psychological Inventory [35] and serves as an alternative for the Ho, as it either duplicated or was close equivalent of the MMPI derived scale as regards the five hostility categories identified by Barefoot [25].

Another comprehensive self-report instrument to assess hostility is the 76-item Buss–Durkee Hostility Inventory (BDHI; [36]), which includes eight sub scales to tap different aspects of the cognitive, affective and behavioral components of hostility. The expressive component of the BDHI was positively correlated with an index of coronary artery disease severity [27], although the strength of this relation was age dependent. Experiential hostility, comprised of the sub scales Resentment and Suspicion, was significantly associated with myocardial infarction in adult males [37]. High hostile subjects exhibited increased salt-intake and cardiovascular hyper-reactivity to stress [38].

To identify more specific factors involved in the relation between hostility and health outcomes, several other measurement instruments have been developed.

The most used specific sub scale was the 8-item Cynical Distrust Scale derived from the Ho to assess the cognitive component of hostility [39]. Cynicism is the belief that others are motivated primarily by selfish concerns and distrust is the expectation that people are frequent sources of mistreatment. This scale has been shown to predict 2-year progression of carotid atherosclerosis [29] and incident myocardial infarction and mortality [40]. It also showed a positive relationship with body mass index [40], waist-to-hip ratio [41] and the metabolic syndrome [42], suggesting that more cynical-hostile persons engage in adverse health behaviors that constitute relevant CVD risk factors.

Few studies have examined the underlying structural relations between the different measures of hostility that typically predict CHD. Results of these studies, that factor analyzed several common used self-report measures, identified different patterns: a three-factor model of Aggressive Acting-Out, Poorly Controlled Anger, and Anger Suppression [43]; eight separate factors including Hostile Anger Expression, Hostile Outlook, Cynicism, and others [44]; a three-factor model of Overt Hostility, Covert Hostility, and Hostile Beliefs [45]; five factors including Neuroticism, Aggressive Hostility, Suspicious Hostility, Introversion, and Impulse Control Avoidance [46], and a four-factor solution of Anger-out, Negative Affect, Coping, and Anger-in [19]. Suggestions coming from such studies were that researchers examining the role of hostility patterns in health should recognize the distinct nature of the different measures, the interrelations between them, the links of different measures to different underlying psychological constructs, and the influence of a variety of socio-psychological mediating circumstances and variables on how individuals interact or cope with their situation [19]. In keeping with these suggestions, researchers should also address at least four basic constructs: (a) aggressive overt hostility, (b) cynical alienation, (c) introversion, and (d) neuroticism [46].

In conclusion, studies have yet to fully investigate the relationship of these different hostility sub components to negative health outcomes and their cardiovascular correlates.

MECHANISMS LINKING HOSTILITY AND CORONARY DISEASE

An essential approach to the association of hostility and increase risk of CHD is to understand the physiologic mechanisms that could produce or exacerbate CHD, although the underlying neurogenic mechanisms due to emotional reactions in general remain unclear. Nevertheless, it is generally believed that hostility may increase cardiovascular risk either through neuroendocrine risk factors or risk-related behaviors.

Four principal underlying models have been identified which conceptualized these two alternatives: a stress moderation model, a constitutional vulnerability model, a transactional model that attempts to integrate and extend the first two, and a health behavior model [31].

The Physiological Reactivity Model is included in the stress moderation models which suggest that hostile individuals may be constitutionally more reactive to stress, with their exaggerated stress response leading to an increased risk of disease [34]. Frequent episodes of anger and increased levels of hostility have been reported to produce elevated levels of cardiovascular and neuroendocrine responses that may contribute to CHD [47]. A recent study has found ambulatory heart rate and blood pressure to be higher for individuals high but not low in hostility when they experienced negative affect or social stress [48]. Another study has found an interactive effect of hostility and perceived social support on systolic and diastolic blood pressure reactivity to laboratory stressors; in particular higher hostility scores were associated with greater blood pressure reactivity for participants who were high in perceived social support [49]. Hostile individuals have been shown to display both larger and longer lasting blood pressure responses to anger provoking situations [50], as well as greater post-stressor elevations in heart rate and systolic blood pressure following the cold pressor task [51]. Delayed CV recovery to stress may be a risk factor for hypertension as well as a critical factor in the hostility-CHD link [52]. Empirical evidence of the link between cardiovascular reactivity and CHD has contributed to establish the Physiological Reactivity Model as the most frequently applied.

The Psychosocial Vulnerability Model implies fundamental differences for hostile individuals, perhaps at the genetic level, that place them at increased risk for disease. That people with high hostility are also characterized by relevant risk factors for CHD such as low social support, high level of stress, and depression. Cross-sectional studies have provided evidence to this model, indicating that hostile individuals typically have higher levels of interpersonal distress, avoid seeking social support, tend to feel isolated and frustrated and develop depressive symptoms [53]. Recent research confirms the explicative role of the Psychosocial Vulnerability Model reporting that hostility is significantly associated with life stress and loneliness [54]. As regards social support, results are controversial, as they report either a lack of association with hostility, after controlling for the effect of negative affectivity, or a role of cynicism in predicting inferior social support, in terms of both quality and amount [55]. Thus the link between psychosocial vulnerability and CHD has yet to be established firmly.

The Transactional Model attempts to integrate and extend the physiological reactivity and psychosocial vulnerability models [1]. This model suggests that hostility influences health in part through its effects on social relationships and on the patterns of cardiovascular reactivity associated with interpersonal stressors. Negative thoughts and actions toward others induce a hostile individual to over-react to non-threatening events and engender hostility from others. Over-reacting causes an increasing in the number of heightened cardiovascular reactivity responses. The cumulative effects of these stress-related episodes of heightened cardiovascular reactivity may contribute to the development of CHD [56]. Furthermore, the nature of hostile individuals' social interactions produce interpersonal conflict that lead to a reduction in social support, and consequently create a more stressful social environment that confirms the negative expectations of others' behaviours [57]. A recent study [58] found a positive association between trait hostility, the frequency and intensity of negative interactions, and increases in diastolic blood pressure. The magnitude of the increase in blood pressure was associated with perception of the interaction as negative. Findings of this study confirmed those of retrospective, self-report, and laboratory studies that provided support for the Transactional Model of hostility and health [59].

The Health Behavior Model suggests that hostility produces poor physical health through the adoption of high-risk behaviors [61].

Several studies have found hostility to be associated with other risk factors for CVD such as smoking, greater alcohol consumption, higher lipid ratios, greater body mass, high higher fat and caloric intake, physical inactivity and non adherence to medical regimens [62,3]. Most of these factors occur together to constitute the metabolic syndrome, a cluster of anthropometric, metabolic, and hemodynamic perturbations that increase the risk for type II diabetes and cardiovascular morbidity and mortality [63]. A recent review concluded that available research data suggest that hostility, as well as its components cynicism and aggression, predicts the presence and development of the metabolic syndrome over time [4].

A recent cross-sectional study not included in the review has confirmed this association, reporting a prevalence of hostile cynicism among patients with the metabolic syndrome [42].

In addition to the above models, hostility also appears to be associated with demographic variables that are associated with CHD such as male sex, greater age, not being married, lower social status, occupation, and income [2]. Recent studies [64] have found a significant interaction between age and hostility in a large sample of patients with documented coronary artery disease (CAD), after controlling for disease severity. Findings indicate that hostility predicts poorer survival only in people younger than 61 years. Other studies have found a significant relationship between anger/hostility and reporting increased cardiovascular symptoms also among women [65]. Although results of the association between hostility patterns and socio-demographic variables are not univocal, Matthews' hypothesis [66] that hostility mediates the relationship between socio-demographic indices and health is still valid today.

EVIDENCE OF AN IMPACT OF HOSTILITY ON HEART DISEASES

At the time of earlier reviews of the literature, most studies of hostility and subsequent health found that both behavioral ratings and self-reports of hostility were significantly associated with CHD [1], despite several inconsistencies across studies were also found by other authors. For example, Myrtek's meta-analysis [67] on TABP or hostility and CHD, which only used prospective studies, concluded that the weighted mean effect size for anger/hostility was both minimal and non-significant. He found similar results in another meta-analysis [68] where he found a reliable and significant relationship between hostility and CHD, but still with a so law effect size as to be unimportant.

A meta-analysis by Miller and colleagues, [2] reported evidence from 41 both cross-sectional and prospective studies supporting the hypothesis that hostility is an independent risk factor for the development of CHD and premature mortality. This meta-analysis was criticized by Petticrew et al. [69]; adjusting the effect sizes for confounding variables, they found no significant correlation between hostility and CHD.

Subsequent reviews also found mixed results. Rozanski and colleague [70] found that 5 of 11 examined publications on the impact of hostility on the pathogenesis of CVD in healthy populations and all 4 examined studies on patients with CAD reported positive results. In a more recent review, Rozanski and colleagues [71] has indicated that hostility is one of the many factors associated with more rapid progression of atherosclerosis and CHD processes.

In 1999 Kop [72] concluded from the examined literature that hostility can be construed as a chronic psychological risk factor that may have adverse cardiovascular consequences by promoting atherosclerosis or by increasing the risk of more proximate psychological risk factors, such exhaustion and acute psychological arousal.

In 1999, Hemingway and Marmot [6] published a systematic review of large prospective cohort studies, which they and Kuper updated in 2002 [73], on the relationship of psychosocial factors and CVD. They found that only 6 of the 18 examined studies on the relationship of TABP or hostility to the development of cardiac events in healthy subjects and 2 of 15 prognostic studies conducted in patients with cardiac disease reported a strong to moderate association. Thus they concluded that studies did not support any evidence of hostility as a predictor of CVD.

Smith and Ruiz in 2002 [74] reported evidence from the literature supporting the effects of anger and hostility as associated with mechanisms that potentially influence CAD and CHD. However, they advised that prospective studies of initially healthy persons produced some negative findings and that there was little, although existing, evidence that individual differences in hostility were consistent risk factors among patients with established disease. After reviewing the limited direct evidence between negative emotions and physical health, Gallo and Matthews [75] examined indirect evidence showing that low socioeconomic status (SES) environments are stressful and reduce individuals' capacity to manage stress, thereby increasing vulnerability to negative emotions and cognition. Actually, SES appeared to be associated with hostility in most of the reviewed studies; furthermore, hostility was stronger in ethnic minorities, and it was likely to begin in childhood. In a subsequent updated review Smith and colleagues [76] stressed the relevance of large, well-controlled prospective studies replicating the association between hostility and CHD. The reported studies suggest that anger, hostility, and aggressiveness may contribute to CHD by both promoting the development of CAD and the emergence of manifestations of CHD later in the course of disease. Although not all the studies produced positive result, and some used insufficiently validated measures, these authors suggest that the A large body of supportive evidence encouraged continued research.

More recently, Everson and colleagues [5] confirmed the available evidence, especially from methodologically strong population-based studies, of the relevant role of anger and hostility in increasing the risk of CVD in healthy populations. Suls and Bunde [77] reported that in healthy populations, 7 of 11 reviewed studies resulted in statistically significant positive results for cynical hostility; another 2 of 9 studies were positive for sub-samples of women and younger people (aged 48 to 59 years), while in populations with known CHD, only 1 of 6 showed positive results. They concluded that the effects of hostility were very weak and inconsistent. Given this weak direct relationship, these authors, in subsequent reviews [3], examined the available meta-analyses on the relationship between hostility and CAD risk factors. They reported strong evidence from the literature of a relationship between hostility and body mass index, waist-to-hip ratio, insulin resistance, lipid ratio, triglycerides, glucose, alcohol consumption, smoking, and socioeconomic status (SES). Evidence that hostile persons also have elevations on CAD risk factors was assumed as one possible explanation for the association between hostility and premature CAD morbidity and mortality. This conclusion has been supported by another recent meta-analysis on the positive association between hostility and the metabolic syndrome [4].

The most recent review by Schulman and Stromberg [78] identified 7 meta-analyses and 5 qualitative reviews on Type A behavior, anger, and hostility as psychosocial risk factors for CVD. The authors concluded that the existing data do not support a meaningful clinical relationship between current measurements of these traits and the development of CVD. Thus, they suggest being careful to state that hostility is a potential psychosocial risk factor, although they found that the effect sizes of the reported association were in some cases clinically significant. In the opinion of these authors "currently, the issue of whether or not some form of hostility is a psychosocial risk factor for CVD is still in the realm of epidemiology and research" Schulman and Stromberg [78] (p. 131). They especially recommend cardiologists to pay attention to their patients' treatable risk factors other than hostility as there is such a variety of tests used to measure this personality style that it is not clear, at this point, how to screen patients.

I searched the Medline and PsychLit databases for studies involving the relationship of hostility to CVD since 2006. Of the 6 studies encountered, selected findings are noted below. Recent research examining associations of psychosocial factors with the presence of sub clinical coronary atherosclerosis have reported contrasting results. Hostility, as rated by spouse, has been associated with concurrent asymptomatic CAD assessed with computed tomography scans of coronary artery calcification [79], independent of other psychosocial and demographic factors (e.g., socioeconomic status, marital satisfaction, age, gender), behavioral risk factors (e.g., smoking, exercise, alcohol use), and biomedical risk factors. This association was significant among older but not middle-aged participants. Authors of the study suggest that hostile personality may contribute to early stages of CAD. However, another study on a large multiethnic population has reported inconsistent results of an association between a number of psychosocial factors, including anger, and coronary calcium in healthy adults [80].

A qualitative study conducted in a sample of Korean patients with CAD [81] has reported that serum homocysteine, a risk factor for ischemic heart disease, increased in a statistically consistent pattern with the level of cynical hostility. A cross-sectional study [65] on a large sample of women with suspected CAD referred for diagnostic angiography has found that anger and hostility were higher among women without angiographic CAD reporting increased cardiovascular symptoms, particularly non-anginal chest pain. A qualitative cross-sectional study [82] estimating the level of hostility in CAD patients and in health care workers showed high level of hostility in both groups, with no difference between them.

A laboratory study [83] has confirmed previous research showing that hostility exerts significant influences on diastolic blood pressure (DBD) in reactivity to a cognitive stressor task, although not on systolic blood pressure (SBP) or heart rate. As DBP, independently of SBP, is a risk factor for disease outcomes (e.g. stroke, ischemic heart disease) in the general population, findings which have implicated hostility in irregular patterns of DBP responding are consistent with the hypothesis of an association between hostile style and increased risk for CHD. However, another laboratory study [84] has presented mixed findings regarding the relationship of defensive hostility to cardiovascular stress reactivity and recovery. Defensive men did display significantly larger heart rate reactivity to the stressor, consistently with previous research, but no reactivity differences related to defensive hostility were found on any cardiovascular variable other than heart rate, and no differences were found at baseline or in response to the active task, in conflict with previous studies.

In sum, a large number of studies investigating hostility and incident CVD have been published since the late 1980s; although findings are not univocal, some of them reported positive associations. Thus, further investigation is needed to clarify this association and limitations and inconsistencies in the literature could be taken as the outlines of an agenda for future research.

CONCLUSION

The research has tried to improve clinicians' ability to predict who is most vulnerable to CHD, thus to identify people who are most likely to benefit from prevention programs. Although not unequivocal, available evidence indicates that hostility is a potential psychosocial factor associated with increased risk of CVD. Actually, many problems are far from being resolved and many questions remain to be answered. Some of the most important challenges facing future research in this area include identifying valid and reliable instruments of measurement; clarifying the pathophysiological mechanisms linking hostility to CHD, that are multi-factorial and act in a synergistic fashion; developing appropriate models to explore the complexity of the relationship between this personality trait, situational factors and other psychosocial and behavioral determinants of cardiovascular health.

REFERENCES

[1]   Smith TW. Concepts and methods in the study of anger, hostility, and health. In AW Siegman, TW Smith (Eds.), *Anger, Hostility, and the Heart*. Hillsdale, NJ: Lawrence Erlbaum Associates, 1994, 23–42.

[2]   Miller TQ, Smith TW, Turner CW, Guijarro ML, Hallet AJ. A meta-analytic review of research on hostility and physical health. *Psychological Bulletin* 1996;119:322–48.

[3]   Bunde J, Suls J. A quantitative analysis of the relationship between the Cook–Medley Hostility Scale and traditional coronary artery disease risk factors. *Health Psychology* 2006;25:493–500.

[4]   Goldbacher EM, Matthews KA. Are Psychological Characteristics Related to Risk of the Metabolic Syndrome? A Review of the Literature. *Annals of Behavioral Medicine* 2007, 34(3):240–252.

[5]   Everson-Rose SA, Lewis TT. Psychosocial factors and cardiovascular diseases. *Annual Review of Public Health* 2005;26:469–500.

[6]   Hemingway H, Marmot M. Evidence based cardiology: psychosocial factors in the aetiology and prognosis of coronary heart disease. Systematic review of prospective cohort studies. *British Medical Journal* 1999;318:1460–67.

[7]   Friedman M, Rosenman R. Association of specific overt behavior pattern with blood and cardiovascular findings. *JAMA* 1959;12:1286-96.

[8]   Rosenman RH. Type A behavior pattern and coronary heart disease: The hostility factor? *Stress Medicine* 1991;7:245–253.

[9]   Siegman AW. From type A to hostility to anger: reflections on the history of coronary-prone behavior. In AW Siegman, TW Smith (Eds.), *Anger, hostility and the heart*. Hillsdale, NJ: Erlbaum, 1994.

[10]   Review panel on coronary-prone behavior and coronary heart disease Coronary-prone behavior and coronary heart disease: a critical review. The review panel on coronary-prone behavior and coronary heart disease. *Circulation* 1981;63;1199-1215.

[11] Shekelle RB, Hulley SB, Neaton JD, et al. The MRFIT behavior pattern study. Type A behavior and incidence of coronary heart disease. *American Journal of Epidemiology* 1985;122:559-70.

[12] Booth-Kewley S, Friedman HS. Psychological predictors of heart disease: A quantitative review. *Psychological Bulletin* 1987;101:343-62.

[13] Dembroski TM, Costa PT. Coronary-prone behavior: components of the Type A pattern and hostility. *Journal of Personality* 1987; 55:211-35.

[14] Shekelle RB, Gale M, Norusis M. Type A score (JAS) and risk of recurrent coronary heart disease in the Aspirin Myocardial Infarction Study. *American Journal of Cardiology* 1985; 56: 221-5.

[15] Ricci Bitti PE, Gremigni P, Bertolotti G, Zotti AM. Dimensions of anger and hostility in cardiac patients, hypertensive patients, and controls. *Psychotherapy and Psychosomatics* 1995;64(3-4):162-72.

[16] Williams RB, Barefoot JC, Shekelle RB: The health consequences of hostility. In MA Chesney, RH Rosenman (Eds.). *Anger and Hostility in Cardiovascular and Behavioral Disorders*, New York: Hemisphere, 1985.

[17] Myrtek M. Type A Behavior and Hostility as Independent Risk Factors for Coronary Heart Disease. In J Jordan, B Bardé, AM Zeiher (Eds.). *Contributions toward Evidence-Based Psycho cardiology: A Systematic Review of the Literature* Washington, DC: American Psychological Association, 2007.

[18] Dembroski TM, MacDougall JM, Costa PT, Grandits GA. Components of hostility as predictors of sudden death and myocardial infarction in the multiple risk factor intervention trial. *Psychosomatic Medicine* 1989;51(5):514–22.

[19] Donker FJS, Breteler MHM, van der Staak CPF. Assessment of Hostility in Patients with Coronary Heart Disease. *Journal of Personality Assessment* 2000;75(1):158–177.

[20] Friedman HS (Ed.). *Hostility, coping and health*, Washington DC: APA, 1992.

[21] Bouchard TJ, Loehlin JC. Genes, evolution, and personality. *Behavior Genetics* 2001;31:243-273.

[22] Aldwin CM, Spiro III A, Levenson MR, Cupertino AP. Longitudinal findings from the Normative Aging Study, III. Personality, health trajectories, and mortality. *Psychology and Aging* 2001;16:450–465.

[23] Zuckerman M, Cloninger CR. Relationships between Cloninger's, Zuckerman's, and Eysenck's dimensions of personality. *Personality and Individual Differences* 1996;21, 283-285.

[24] Iwata N, Suzuki T, Ikeda M, Kitajima T, Yamanouchi Y, Inada T, Ozaki N. A genome scan for hostility: the national heart, lung, and blood institute family heart study. *Molecular Psychiatry* 2004;9:124–127.

[25] Barefoot JC. Developments in the measurements of hostility. In HS Friedman (Ed.). *Hostility, coping and health*. Washington DC: APA, 1992.

[26] Suarez EC, Williams RB Jr. Situational determinants of cardiovascular and emotional reactivity in high and low hostile me. *Psychosomatic Medicine* 1989;51:404-418.

[27] Siegman AW, Dembroski TM, Ringel N. Components of hostility and the severity of coronary artery disease. *Psychosomatic Medicine* 1987;49:27-130.

[28] Arthur HM. Cynical hostility was associated with increased risk of mortality and MI. *Evidence Based Cardiovascular Medicine* 1998;2(1):8-9.

[29] Julkunen J, Salonen R, Kaplan GA, Chesney MA, Salonen JT. Hostility and the progression of carotid atherosclerosis. *Psychosomatic Medicine* 1994;56:519–25.

[30] Rosenberg EL, Ekman P, Blumenthal JA. Facial expression and the affective component of cynical hostility in male coronary heart disease patients. *Health Psychology* 1998;17(4):376-80.

[31] Smith TW, Gallo LC: Personality traits as risk factors for physical illness. In A Baum, TA Revenson, JE Singer (Eds.). *Mahwah, Handbook of Health Psychology*. NJ: Lawrence Erlbaum Associates, 2001.

[32] Rosenman RH. The interview method of assessment of the coronary-prone behaviors in the Western Collaborative Group Study. In TM Dembroski, SM Weiss, JL Shields, M Feinleib (Eds.). *Coronary prone behaviour*. New York: Springer-Verlag, 1978.

[33] Cook W, Medley D. Proposed hostility and pharisaic-virtue scales for the MMPI. *Journal of Applied Psychology* 1954;38:414-8.

[34] Williams RB Jr. Refining the Type A hypothesis: emergence of the hostility complex. *American Journal of Cardiology* 1987;60(18):27J-32J.

[35] Adams S, John OP. A Hostility Scale for the California Psychological Inventory: MMPI, Observer Q-Sort, and Big-Five Correlates. *Journal of Personality Assessment* 1997;69(2):408-424.

[36] Buss AH, Durkee A. An inventory for assessing different kinds of hostility. *Journal of Consulting Psychology* 1957;21:343-349.

[37] Meesters CM., Muris P, Backus IP. Dimensions of hostility and myocardial infarction in adult males. *Journal of Psychosomatic Research* 1996;40(1):21-28.

[38] Miller SB, Friese M, Dolgoy L, Sita A, Lavoie K, Campbell T. Hostility, sodium consumption, and cardiovascular response to interpersonal stress. *Psychosomatic Medicine* 1998;60(1):71-7.

[39] Greenglass ER, Julkunen J. Construct validity and sex differences in Cook-Medley hostility. *Personality and Individual Differences* 1989;10:209– 18.

[40] Everson SA, Kauhanen J, Kaplan GA, Goldberg DE, Julkunen J, Tuomilehto J, Salonen JT. Hostility and increased risk of mortality and acute myocardial infarction: the mediating role of behavioral risk factors. *American Journal of Epidemiology* 1997;146:142–52.

[41] Haukkala A, Uutela A. Cynical Hostility, Depression, and Obesity: The Moderating Role of Education and Gender. *International Journal of Eating Disorders* 2000;27:106–109.

[42] Gremigni P. Cynical hostility and the metabolic syndrome: a case-control study. *Monaldi Archives of Chest Diseases* 2006;66(3):224-9.

[43] Kopper BA, Epperson DL. The experience and expression of anger: Relationship with gender, gender role socialization, depression, and mental health functioning. *Journal of Consulting Psychology* 1996;43:158-165.

[44] Miller TQ, Jenkins CD, Kaplan GA, Salonen JT. Are all hostility scales alike? Factor structure and covariation among measures of hostility. *Journal of Applied Social Psychology* 1995;25:1142-1168.

[45] Barefoot JC, Lipkus IM. The assessment of anger and hostility. In A W Siegman, TW Smith (Eds.). *Anger, Hostility, and the Heart*. Hillsdale, NJ: Lawrence Erlbaum, 1994.

[46] Friedman HS, Tucker JS, Reise SP. Personality dimensions and measures potentially relevant to health: A focus on hostility. *Annals of Behavioral Medicine* 1995;17(3):245-253.

[47] Houston BK. Anger, hostility and psycho physiological reactivity. In A W Siegman, TW Smith (Eds.), *Anger, Hostility and the Heart*. Hillsdale, NJ: Lawrence Erlbaum and Associates, 1994.

[48] Gallo LC, Smith TW, Kircher JC. Cardiovascular and electro dermal responses to support and provocation: Interpersonal methods in the study of psycho physiological reactivity. *Psychophysiology* 2000;37(3):289-301.

[49] Chen YY, Gilligan S, Coups EJ, Contrada RJ. Hostility and perceived social support: interactive effects on cardiovascular reactivity to laboratory stressors. *Annals of Behavioral Medicine* 2005;29(1):37-43.

[50] Fredrickson BL, Maynard KE, Helens MJ, Haney TL, Siegler IC, Barefoot JC... Hostility predicts magnitude and duration of blood pressure response to anger. *Journal of Behavioral Medicine* 2000;23:229–243.

[51] Demaree HA, Harrison DW, Rhodes RD. Quantitative electroencephalographic analyses of cardiovascular regulation in low- and high hostile men. *Psychobiology* 2000;28(3):420–431.

[52] Brosschot JF, Thayer JF. Anger inhibition, cardiovascular recovery, and vagal function: a model of the link between hostility and cardiovascular disease. *Annals of Behavioral Medicine* 1998;20(4):326–332.

[53] Smith TW, Pope MK, Sanders JD, et al: Cynical hostility at home and work: Psychosocial vulnerability across domains. *Journal of Research in Personality* 1988;22:525-548.

[54] Hart KE, Hope C. Cynical Hostility and the Psychosocial Vulnerability Model of Disease Risk: Confounding Effects of Neuroticism Bias. *Personality & Individual Differences* 2004;36:1571-1582.

[55] Kaplan SA, Bradley JC, Ruscher JB. The inhibitory role of cynical disposition in the provision and receipt of social support: the case of the September 11th terrorist attacks. *Personality and Individual Differences* 2004;37(6):1221-1232.

[56] Sloan RP, Shapiro PA, Bagiella E, et al. Cardiac autonomic control buffers blood pressure variability responses to challenge: A psycho physiologic model of coronary artery disease. *Psychosomatic Medicine* 1999;61:58–68.

[57] Lee DJ, Markides KS. Irritability and physical symptoms in a three-generations study of Mexican Americans. *Stress Medicine* 1989;5:253-242.

[58] Brondolo E, Rieppi R, Erickson SA, Bagiella E, Shapiro PA, McKinley P, et Al. Hostility, interpersonal interactions, and ambulatory blood pressure. *Psychosomatic Medicine* 2003;65:1003–1011.

[59] Hardy JD, Smith TW. Cynical hostility and vulnerability to disease: Social support, life stress, and physiological response to conflict. *Health Psychology* 1988;7:447–459.

[60] Houston BK, Kelly KE. Hostility in employed women: Relation to work and marital experience, social support, stress, and anger expression. *Personality and Social Psychological Bulletin* 1989;15:175–182.

[61] Leiker M, Hailey BJ. A link between hostility and disease: Poor health habits? *Behavioral Medicine* 1988;3:129-133.

[62] Boyle SH, Mortensen L, Grønbæk M, Barefoot JC. Hostility, drinking pattern and mortality. *Addiction* 2008;103: 54–59.

[63] Alberti KG, Zimmet P, Shaw J. The metabolic syndrome— A new worldwide definition. *Lancet* 2005;366:1059–1062.

[64] Boyle SH, Williams RB, Mark DB, Brummett BH, Siegler IC, Barefoot JC, Hostility. Age and Mortality in a Sample of Cardiac Patients. *American Journal of Cardiology* 2005;96:64–66.

[65] Krantz DS. Olson MB, Francis JL, et al. Anger, Hostility, and Cardiac Symptoms in Women with Suspected Coronary Artery Disease: The Women's Ischemia Syndrome Evaluation (WISE) Study. *Journal of Women's Health* 2006;15(10):1214-1223.

[66] Matthews KA. Are socio-demographic variables markers for psychological determinants of health? *Health Psychology* 1989;8:641-648.

[67] Myrtek M. Type-A behavior pattern, personality factors, disease, and physiological reactivity: a meta-analytic update. *Personality and Individual Differences* 1995;18:491–502.

[68] Myrtek M. Meta-analyses of prospective studies on coronary heart disease, Type A personality, and hostility. *International Journal of Cardiology* 2001;79:245– 51.

[69] Petticrew M, Gilbody S, Sheldon TA. Relation between hostility and coronary heart disease. Evidence does not support link. *BMJ* 1999;319:917–918.

[70] Rozanski, A., Blumenthal, J. A., & Kaplan, J. (1999). Impact of psychological factors on the pathogenesis of cardiovascular disease and implications for therapy. *Circulation, 99*, 2192–2217.

[71] Rozanski A, Blumenthal JA, Davidson KW, Saab PG, Kubzansky L. The epidemiology, pathophysiology, and management of psychosocial risk factors in cardiac practice: The emerging field of behavioral cardiology. *Journal of the American College of Cardiology.* 2005;45,637–651.

[72] Kop WJ. Chronic and acute psychological risk factors for clinical manifestations of coronary artery disease. *Psychosomatic Medicine* 1999;61:476–487.

[73] Kuper H, Marmot M, Hemingway H. Systematic review of prospective cohort studies of psychosocial factors in the etiology and prognosis of coronary heart disease. *Seminars in Vascular Medicine* 2002;2:267–314.

[74] Smith TW, Ruiz JM. Psychosocial influences on the development and course of coronary heart disease: Current status and implications for research and practice. *Journal of Consulting and Clinical Psychology* 2002;7:548–568.

[75] Gallo LC, Matthews KA. Understanding the Association Between Socioeconomic Status and Physical Health: Do Negative Emotions Play a Role? *Psychological Bulletin* 2003;129(1):10–51.

[76] Smith TW, Glazer K, Ruiz JM, Gallo LC. Hostility, Anger, Aggressiveness, and Coronary Heart Disease: An Interpersonal Perspective on Personality, Emotion, and Health. *Journal of Personality* 2004;72(6): 1217-70.

[77] Suls J, Bunde J. Anger, anxiety, and depression as risk factors for cardiovascular disease: the problems and implications of overlapping affective dispositions. *Psychological Bulletin* 2005;131:260 –300.

[78] Schulman JK, Stromberg S. On the Value of Doing Nothing Anger and Cardiovascular Disease. *Clinical Practice Cardiology in Review* 2007;15:123–132.

[79] Smith TW, Uchino BN, Berg CA, Florsheim P, Pearce G, Hawkins M, Hopkins PN, Yoon HC. Hostile Personality Traits and Coronary Artery Calcification in Middle-Aged and Older Married Couples: Different Effects for Self-Reports Versus Spouse Ratings. *Psychosomatic Medicine* 2007;69:441–448.

[80] Diez Roux AV, Ranjit N, Powell L, Jackson S, Lewis TT, Shea S, Wu C. Psychosocial factors and coronary calcium in adults without clinical cardiovascular disease. *Annals of Internal Medicine* 2006;144:822–31.

[81] Son YJ. Hostility and serum homocysteine as cardiovascular risk factors in Korean patients with coronary artery disease. *Journal of Clinical Nurses* 2007;16(4):672-8.

[82] Selko D, Bacharova L, Rusnakova V, Katina S, Liska B Hostility in coronary artery disease patients and health care workers in Slovakia. *Journal of Health Organ Management* 2007;21(1):79-91.

[83] Hughes BM. Individual differences in hostility and habituation of cardiovascular reactivity to stress. *Stress and Health* 2007;23:37–42.

[84] Vella EJ, Friedman BH. Autonomic characteristics of defensive hostility: Reactivity and recovery to active and passive stressors. *International Journal of Psychophysiology* 2007;66:95–101.

In: Psychological Factors and Cardiovascular Disorders   ISBN: 978-1-60456-871-4
Editor: Leo Sher   © 2008 Nova Science Publishers, Inc.

Chapter XVIII

HOSTILITY AND BRAIN FUNCTION: THE IMPACT OF HOSTILITY ON BRAIN ACTIVITY DURING AFFECTIVE VERBAL LEARNING

D. Erik Everhart[1-2], Heath A. Demaree[3] and David W. Harrison[4]

[1]Department of Psychology, East Carolina University, Greenville, North Carolina, USA;
[2]Pitt County Memorial Hospital Sleep Center, Greenville, North Carolina, USA;
[3]Department of Psychology, Case Western Reserve University, Cleveland, Ohio, USA;
[4]Department of Psychology, Virginia Polytechnic Institute and State University, Blacksburg, Virginia, USA.

ABSTRACT

The relationship between hostility and coronary artery disease and the effects of hostility on physiological reactivity to mental/emotional stressors is well known. Yet, precise understanding of the underlying neurophysiological mechanisms and neuroanatomical systems associated with emotional processing in hostility remains a target for further understanding. This chapter provides brief review of the neuropsychological theories that are pertinent to hostility and focuses on an area of research that holds promise in advancing current understanding of the impact of hostility on brain function. Specifically, this chapter examines the relationship between hostility, affective verbal learning, and regional brain activity using quantified electroencephalography (qEEG). The chapter concludes with discussion of the limitations in previous research and targets for future direction.

INTRODUCTION

The relationship between hostility and coronary artery disease [1-5] is well known, as are the effects of hostility on physiological reactivity to mental/emotional stressors [6-12]. It is now important to develop an understanding of the underlying neurophysiological mechanisms and neuroanatomical systems associated with emotional processing in hostility. This chapter provides a brief review of the neuropsychological theories that are pertinent to hostility as well as supportive evidence. Following this review, discussion focuses on one relatively new area of research that holds promise in advancing current understanding of the impact of hostility on brain function. Specifically, findings from studies that examine regional brain activity among hostile individuals during an affective verbal learning task are described and the implications are discussed. The last portion of the chapter describes future directions in research as they pertain to hostility and brain function.

DEFINING HOSTILITY

Hostility has been defined in a myriad of ways, with many of the descriptors contained in a description by Smith [13]:

> . . . hostility entails a negative attitude toward others, consisting of enmity, denigration, and ill will... a devaluation of the worth and motives of others, an expectation that others are likely sources of wrong doing, a relational view of being in opposition toward others, and a desire to inflict harm or see others harmed (p. 26).

Likewise, hostile individuals have been suggested to show elevated levels of angerability and cynicism [14], more antagonistic behavior [15] and greater physiological reactivity to stress relative to low-hostile people [16]. Behaviorally, hostility is described as an attitude that motivates aggressive behavior towards objects and people [17] and physiologically, hostility has been associated with the chronic over activation of the sympathetic nervous system leading to heightened arousal levels [18].

Within our research, the construct of hostility has been defined and measured via use of the Cook Medley Hostility Scale (CMHO) [19]. The CMHO is a 50-item true/false questionnaire that predicts poor medical, psychological, and interpersonal outcomes [20]. Although several scales measuring "hostility" exist, the CMHO is used primarily because of its inclusion in the Minnesota Multiphasic Personality Inventory (MMPI) and because the instrument has been found to have good convergent and discriminant validities [21]. For instance, high correlations with other MMPI-2 scales suggest that the CMHO is related to general psychopathology and negative affectivity [20]. Moreover, Smith and Frohm [22] found that the CMHO correlates significantly higher with trait anger than with self-reported trait anxiety or depression. Factor analysis of the CMHO reveals a general factor involving "cynicism" and "distrust" [23]. The internal-consistency reliability of the CMHO has been reported as .86 [19] and, in our samples of undergraduates, we have reliably found median splits of around 17 or 18 (defined as low and high-hostiles).

THE APPLICATION OF NEUROPSYCHOLOGICAL THEORIES OF EMOTION TO THE STUDY OF HOSTILITY

Several prominent general models of emotion and cerebral function suggest that individuals with characterologic negative affect experience relative right hemisphere activity in comparison to the left hemisphere. A variety of other negative affective responses such as sadness and anxiety have also been implicated [24-27]. A similar model makes predictions regarding asymmetrical cortical activity within the left and right frontal lobes. For instance, Davidson and colleagues [28], as well as other laboratories [29] have frequently reported that increased left frontal activity is associated with positive affect, while increased right frontal activity is associated with negative affect [27]. A derivative of this model suggests that these differences may be contingent upon approach versus withdrawal-related behavior [30]. Regardless of the specific neuropsychological theory, a consistent theme is observed in that activity in the right hemisphere is associated with negative affect. This holds important implications for understanding of hostility, which by definition is largely associated with negative affect.

In following neuropsychological theory, hostility has been theorized to be central to right hemisphere activity [7,32,32]. Activation of the right anterior temporal region has been found to yield heightened anger or rage behaviors, while activation of the right orbital-frontal region has been found to reduce anger or rage behaviors. It has been hypothesized that the anterior temporal region and the orbital-frontal cortex interact to form a constant, conservative aggression level among normal individuals [33].

A variety of behavioral studies that examine bilateral processing support the notion that individuals with hostility experience relative right hemisphere activity. For example, studies of hostility and its effects on the recognition of stimuli have shown faster facial affect perception by the right hemisphere than the left hemisphere, and that there are hemispheric differences related to affective valence. Specifically, hostile participants perceive neutral faces presented to the right hemisphere as angry. This bias is restricted to the left visual field, suggesting increased activity within right cerebral systems among high-hostiles [34,35]. Likewise, Herridge et al [36] found evidence that hostile participants are more accurate at assessing angry and happy affective faces and less accurate at assessing a neutral affective face in their left visual field than low-hostile participants. The effects of hostility on the auditory system have also been examined via the use of the dichotic listening tasks. Demaree and Harrison [7] utilized a cold pressor method and dichotic listening procedures to evaluate laterality in response to painful stress. This study found that high-hostile participants evidence greater right hemisphere activity to cold pressor stress as indicated by enhanced performance when stimuli are presented to the left ear (right hemisphere). Opposite effects are demonstrated among low-hostile participants (i.e., enhanced performance observed with the right ear). Asymmetry within the motor system has also been observed among high versus low hostiles. For example, Demaree, Higgins, Williamson, and Harrison [37] found that high hostiles display greater grip strength in the left hand compared to low hostiles. With regard to prefrontal function, a relative increase in perseverative errors on nonverbal fluency tasks has been observed among individuals with high levels of hostility [38]. Finally, differences in hemispheric activity as a function of hostility (also favoring the right hemisphere) have also been observed during the performance of affective learning tasks, though detailed review of these findings is saved for a latter portion of this chapter [39,40].

As indicated previously, inherent within the definition of hostility is the notion of the overactive sympathetic nervous system (or a relative decrease in parasympathetic nervous system activity) [18]. A relationship between hemispheric processing, hostility, and the cardiovascular system has also been demonstrated in previous studies. For example, previous studies have demonstrated that in general, high hostile individuals display increased heart rate (HR) and systolic blood pressure (SBP) [7,31,36,38,41]. Also relative to hostility, a differential rate of right hemisphere activation occurring with increases in HR and SBP has been observed in other studies [42], and Whittling et al demonstrated an increase in SBP during presentation of emotional stimuli to the right hemisphere [43]. Taken together, the studies described above are indicative of relative right hemisphere activity among high versus low hostiles. Moreover, a complex relationship exists between patterns of laterality and the cardiovascular system, as some studies have demonstrated a relationship between hostility, the right hemisphere, and sympathetic output.

Some have suggested that increased (or chronic) levels of physiological arousal exist among high hostiles at baseline and as such these individuals are less physiologically reactive during certain cognitively challenging tasks [41]. This same effect has been observed with other negative emotional states such as trait anxiety [44]. It is also plausible that the long-term levels of physiological arousal observed in hostility lead to diminished reactivity during cognitive challenge and thus decrease cerebral arousal. If this is indeed the case, this phenomenon should be observable via recording of electrical brain activity during the performance of cognitively challenging tasks. The next sections of this chapter detail the examination of patterns of brain activity during the performance of affective (or emotional) learning tasks. Prior to discussion of these findings and implications, however, it is important to introduce and describe a task that has now been used in multiple studies, the Affective Auditory Verbal Learning Test (AAVL) [45].

DEVELOPMENT OF THE AFFECTIVE AUDITORY VERBAL LEARNING TEST

As previously discussed, many studies have examined the performance of hostile individuals on various bilateral sensory and motor tasks. Less is known about how hostility interacts with affective learning and cognition. The original purpose of creating the *Affective Auditory Verbal Learning Test* (AAVL) was to provide data on the effects of positive and negative verbal stimuli on acquisition patterns [45]. The AAVL provides an important interface between cognitive and affective processing. It was thought that the AAVL would be useful in the examination of patients with hemispheric dysfunction, as previous studies reported that left hemisphere activity is associated with the processing of positive valence, while right hemisphere activity is associated with negative valence [46,47].

The AAVL, as originally developed by Snyder & Harrison [45], consists of two 15-item word lists. One word list is comprised of positive affective words, while the other is comprised of negative affective words. The word lists were developed using an index of word norms [48]. Within this index of word norms, a total of 2854 words were initially evaluated using a seven point Likert Scale for concreteness, imagery, categorizability, meaningfulness, familiarity (FAM), number of attributes, and pleasantness (PLS). The positive affective words selected for the AAVL were the 15 words that had the highest mean PLS rating, while the negative affective words selected for the AAVL were the 15 words that had the lowest mean PLS rating. An additional criterion for word selection included a FAM rating of at least 5.0 or better. Of note, the words from the original English translation of the Auditory Verbal Learning Test (AAVL) are considered neutral, as the PLS ratings for all of the words fall near the middle of the seven point Likert scale in Toglia and Battig's index. In administering the AAVL, five successive learning trials are used. However, interference and recognition components have not been included to date; these components remain a target for future study. More details about the history and development of the AAVL are available in another writing [49] and within Snyder's original article [45].

In the initial study, Snyder and Harrison [45] reported that the acquisition patterns of the positive and negative word lists produce similar patterns as observed during the learning of neutral words. Specifically, a "typical" learning curve was reported during acquisition, with the total number of words recalled increasing with each successive trial. In contrast, however, differential primacy and recency effects were reported for the positive and negative word lists. The words within both the positive and negative AAVL lists have been broken down into three categories – primacy, middle, and recency – by their serial position within each list. Specifically, primacy and recency words were defined as those words in serial positions 1-5 and 11-15, respectively, with the remaining words comprising the "middle" category. These serial positions were selected because they have been commonly used in memory research investigating primacy and recency effects [45,50-52]. In their original research using the AAVL, Snyder and Harrison [45] found a heightened primacy effect for participants learning the negative list and a heightened recency effect for participants learning the positive list. These findings have been replicated in other studies [53,54].

There is some evidence that recency effects are associated with short-term or working memory processes (e.g., "anterior circuits"), while primacy effects reflect encoding into long-term memory [49,55-57] which is reflective of hippocampal processes [56,58]. In previous research, we have suggested that negative affective information may be incorporated into long-term memory stores more quickly than positive affective information. The rapid consolidation of negative information could be related to the necessary ability of rapid threat identification and reaction for survival [49,53]. As such, the AAVL is thought as a useful tool for study of hostility and associated function. The findings from studies that have examined the performance of hostile participants on the AAVL are reviewed below.

PRIMACY AND RECENCY EFFECTS WITH HOSTILE PARTICIPANTS

In one experiment [53], we expected that high- relative to low-hostiles would recall more words from the negative version of the AAVL. This prediction was made because it has been well documented that negative and positive mood states aid in the acquisition and recall of mood congruent stimuli [e.g., 59]. Participants were administered the CMHO and parsed into low- and high-hostile groups using the median split (low-hostiles < 17.5; high-hostiles > 17.5). The results of the experiment did not support our hypothesis in that hostility level did not impact learning and memory of affective material. These data appear to conflict with the mood congruence model of learning and memory, but may be attributable to our use of a highly-functioning (participants were recruited from an academically competitive University) healthy population generally showing normal variability with regard to hostility level. Of course, while it is well established that mood states affect mood congruent affective learning and memory, it is also possible that more stable mood traits, such as hostility, do not have the same robust effect on memory. A more recent study has demonstrated differences in learning patterns on the AAVL in high versus low hostile individuals. Mollet et al [60] found that high hostiles learned negative emotional words significantly better than they learned positive words. Additionally, high hostiles evidenced diminished acquisition of verbal material relative to low hostile participants. A primary difference between the two studies is the mean level of hostility (as defined by CMHO score [19]). In first study, the mean was 23.3 compared to the second study, where the mean was 34.0. This may indicate that higher levels of hostility are associated with altered patterns of learning on the AAVL.

QUANTITATIVE EEG AND HOSTILITY

In an attempt to understand the complicated relationship between affective learning, emotional experience, and brain activity, our laboratory examined changes across various bandwidths of the EEG spectrum during administration of the AAVL using quantitative electroencephalographic (qEEG) recording techniques [54]. Previous studies found that qEEG is a sensitive measure during presentation of verbal stimuli [61-63], and other groups have used QEEG for examination of regional brain activity correlates during emotional states [47,64,65].

Comprehensive review of qEEG technique and methodology is beyond the scope of this manuscript. In brief, previous studies have demonstrated that the alpha bandwidth (8-13 Hz) yields reliable differences in scalp topography during the performance of emotional tasks and cognitive tasks. Early findings indicated that alpha power was inversely associated with brain activity and as such, a decrease in alpha power is associated with an increase in brain activity. Conversely, increased alpha power is associated with a decrease in brain activity [47,66]. Recently, however, some laboratories have recommended separating the alpha bandwidths (as well as other bandwidths) into smaller components [67]. Further study of small bandwidths within the alpha power spectrum has demonstrated that the inverse relationship between alpha power and brain metabolic activity (as measured by PET) is fairly restricted to the low alpha bandwidth (~7.5 – 10.0 Hz) [68,69]. Although more in depth study is required, it is also plausible that high alpha power (~11.0 – 13.0 Hz) is positively associated with brain activity and is sensitive to cognitive load [70-72]. Regarding other bandwidths, Crawford [67] also commented on the importance of separating low and high theta bands, and other laboratories have indicated a preference for separating beta bandwidths (Cole, 1985; Stenberg, 1992). Specific to hostility, more recent findings indicate the need to separate high and low beta bandwidths as well as separate regional scalp sites such as frontal versus temporal [73].

In the initial study of the AAVL that utilized qEEG, hostility levels were not examined [54]. Thirty-seven healthy undergraduate men and women underwent electrophysiological recording from multiple scalp electrode sites during the presentation of the positive and negative AAVL word lists. Initially, seven EEG frequency bandwidths were considered for analyses. However, only the alpha bandwidth (8-13 Hz) yielded significant effects associated with affective learning. As recommended by Crawford et al [67], the alpha bandwidth was separated into three components including low-alpha (7.5-9.5 Hz), mid alpha (9.5-11.5 Hz), and high alpha (11.5-13.0 Hz). Further analyses revealed that significant interactions or main effects involving valence (positive or negative) were observed for only the low alpha band. More specifically, participants who completed the negative word list evidenced a decline in low alpha power over bilateral parietal scalp site locations in comparison to baseline recordings. Significant changes were not observed among participants who completed the positive word list. As indicated previously, the decrements in low alpha power are thought to be inversely correlated with brain activity [68,69]. Thus, the observed decline in low alpha power during the negative word list was interpreted as evidence for increased brain activity within the parietal regions. Of additional interest is the self-reported "mood state" ratings that were recorded prior to completion of the positive and negative word lists of the AAVL. Participants who completed the negative word list reported significantly greater negative affect, as measured using a 10-point Likert scale. In contrast, no significant differences in mood state were reported for participants who completed the positive word list (although it is acknowledged by the authors of this study that experimenter demand characteristics may be at play here).

The results of the study reviewed above, as well as the previous studies that have examined primacy and recency effects indicate that a complex relationship exists between learning and encoding strategies, affect, mood state, and regional brain activity. Although this relationship is complex, the studies do indicate that the positive and negative words lists are associated with differences in self-reported mood and regional brain activity. Of particular interest is the potential relationship between increased parietal lobe activity [54] during the negative word lists, and increased heart rate and blood pressure, as previously reported by Snyder et al [74] (1998). In considering potential neuroanatomical mechanisms to explain this relationship, Heller and colleagues [27,75] proposed that the posterior right hemisphere is important for regulation of autonomic and physiological arousal (see Heller's original article for more detailed information). Negative affective states (which are accompanied by increased physiological arousal) are associated with increased activity within the posterior aspects of the right hemisphere. The original qEEG study with the AAVL did find increased activity within the parietal lobes during presentation of the negative word list; this finding is possibly reflective of brain mechanisms that are associated with modulation of physiological arousal. However, asymmetry was not observed, as activity increased within right and left parietal regions. In explaining this finding, prior studies that have observed alterations in right hemisphere activity or function have typically utilized nonverbal stimuli, whereas the Everhart & Demaree [54] study utilized an emotional verbal learning paradigm (i.e., the

AAVL). In our discussion, we speculated that the verbal (left hemisphere) and emotional (right hemisphere) nature of the stimuli invoked bilateral changes in brain activity.

Two qEEG studies have examined the relationship between hostility and emotional learning [39,40]. In the first study 48 undergraduate men and women were separated into low and high hostile groups using the CMHO. Electrophysiological recording over various scalp sites occurred before testing, as well as after the third and fifth learning trials of the AAVL. Half of the participants received the positive word list, while the other half received the negative word list. As observed in the original qEEG study with the AAVL [54], significant effects were isolated within the low alpha bandwidth (7.5-9.5 Hz). Low alpha power was significantly diminished over all left hemisphere scalp sites, which suggests increased brain activity over the left hemisphere during the AAVL, regardless of which list is presented. It is posited that this asymmetry is reflective of the verbal nature of the task. Specific to hostility, however, low-alpha power was greater for high hostiles at every site during presentation of the negative word list; though the difference reached statistical significance for only the occipital sites. In noting the inverse relationship between low alpha power and brain activity, these results suggest that, within posterior regions high hostiles evidence less brain activity during the learning trials of the negative affective word list. These findings remained unchanged when the data were reanalyzed using hostility as a continuous measure rather than as a dichotomy.

In explaining these group differences we initially speculated that low-hostiles may have a reduced number of associations with negative words in comparison to high hostiles. While the psychometric data (i.e., word recall patterns) do not seem to reflect differences in task difficulty, it is plausible that low hostiles evidence increased posterior arousal when modulating sympathovagal balance, whereas high-hostiles do not. As discussed previously, it is also plausible that high hostiles experience cortical underarousal during this cognition-emotional task, as a form of "habituation" or diminished responsivity may occur when high hostiles are challenged in this paradigm.

This particular study suffered from several shortcomings in that the design did not allow for examination of within group differences (e.g., low and high hostiles) of EEG changes that occur to the positive versus negative word list. Relatedly, the study design did not permit comprehensive examination of narrow bandwidths. In order to remedy the problems of the previous research, which presented only the positive or negative word lists of the AAVL, a second study entailed presentation of both the positive and negative wordlists to high and low hostile participants in a counterbalanced fashion [40]. In effect, this increased the overall task demands, but also allowed for examination of within group differences across the EEG spectrum. Likewise, the research design of the second study allowed for more comprehensive examination of specific narrow bandwidths. Specifically, seven separate bandwidths were examined, including low alpha (7.5 to 9.5Hz), mid alpha (9.5 to 11.5Hz) high alpha (11.5 to 13.0Hz), low beta (13 to 21Hz), high beta (21 to 32Hz), low theta (4 to 5.4 Hz), and high theta (5.5 to 7.5z).

Consistent with previous studies using the same word lists [39,45,53,54,74], primacy effects were demonstrated with the negative version of the AAVL, whereas recency effects were observed with the positive version of the AAVL. Of note, regardless of word list, a group difference emerged when considering recency items. Second, and consistent with previous studies [39,54], participants reported significantly greater negative affect following presentation of the negative AAVL (no change in mood following the positive AAVL was revealed).

With regard to group (i.e., high versus low hostile) differences in bandwidths, multiple differences were observed, regardless of word list. Specifically, low hostiles evidenced greater high alpha power (11.5 to 13.0Hz) than did high hostiles. In addition, while high alpha power was symmetrically distributed across left and right hemisphere scalp sites for low hostiles, high hostiles evidenced greater high alpha power over right versus left hemisphere scalp sites.

Several thoughts can be gleaned from these findings. As previously described, it is thought that high alpha may be positively associated with brain metabolism [69]. Likewise, other laboratories have found positive associations between high alpha activity and memory performance or cognitive load [70,76]. If this is indeed the case, then low hostiles experience greater brain activity during affective learning. This is consistent with the notion that high hostiles may experience relative decrements in arousal during this cognitive task. This finding is also consistent with the first qEEG study involving high hostiles [39], in that increased in low alpha power (i.e., decreased brain activity) was observed among high hostiles.

Also, as previously discussed, asymmetrical patterns in alpha power have not been observed among individuals with low hostility (as found in previous studies). We interpreted the lack of asymmetry as a function of the infusion of verbal (left hemisphere) requirements into an affective (right hemisphere) task. In contrast to low hostiles, however, high hostiles evidence greater right versus left hemisphere high alpha power during the AAVL. Thus, it is plausible that high hostiles utilize more right hemisphere resources for completion of this task. This is consistent with the neuropsychological theories of emotion that were presented earlier in this manuscript. For example, Heller and colleagues [27,75,77], Davidson and colleagues [28,78,79] and researchers from our laboratories [7,32,80,81] have presented strong evidence that withdrawal-related (or "brooding") negative affect (such as anxiety and and chronic characterologic traits such as hostility) is associated with relative right hemisphere activity.

With regard to other bandwidths, low hostiles evidenced greater low beta power (13 to 21 Hz) than did high hostiles. Although previously implicated as an important component of the EEG spectra with emotion processing [82], less is known about the relationship between beta activity and emotional processes [67], and in particular how this relationship may be altered during the processing of emotional words. One potentially promising line of research entails examination of the relationship between beta power and other physiological variables such as heart rate and blood pressure, as high hostiles are known to experience elevations on these physiological markers. One recent experiment did find a negative correlation between low beta power and systolic blood pressure when participants were asked to remember an event from the past that invoked anger [73]. As previously discussed, we have found that high-hostiles evidence reduced sympathovagal reactivity to the negative AAVL [83], which we speculate to be a sign of autonomic "inflexibility." Understanding the cerebral mechanisms that underlie these autonomic reactions is important because reduced autonomic flexibility and decreased parasympathetic arousal may be an important predictor of coronary artery disease (CAD) [84,85].

Summary and Future Directions

The theories and studies reviewed in this chapter highlight several key issues that pertain to hostility and brain function. First, it is thought that relative right hemisphere activity exists among high hostiles; a variety of studies exist within the literature that are supportive of this notion. Second, this pattern of differences holds important implications for overall brain function, as evidenced by the performance of hostile individuals on various sensory and motor tasks, as well as on tasks that require emotional learning. There is also a link between hostility, cortical arousal during cognitive and affective challenges, and cardiovascular arousal. The precise relationship between these variables is not well understood, although based on the literature reviewed it is thought that high hostiles experience chronic sympathetic arousal and reductions in cortical arousal during cognitive tasks.

While the experiments discussed are enlightening, there are some shortcomings that must be remedied in future research. First, one limitation exists in that previous qEEG studies have focused on discrete time-locked recordings during the administration of various portions of the AAVL. This limitation was necessary because of technological limitations at the time the data were collected. As a result, it is possible the regional brain differences as a function of trial were missed. That is, is regional brain activity during the first learning trial of the AAVL different than the fifth trial? With advances in technology, we are now capable of continuous recording and as such, potential habituation effects can now be examined. This opens up new doors, as it is possible that high hostiles habituate differently to positive or negative stimuli than do low hostiles. This groundwork has already been laid, as our previous studies have demonstrated lower levels of high alpha activity during the AAVL for high hostiles.

Also related to technological limitations, previous methods have not permitted another very important analysis, source localization. In the past, the number of active channels during electrophysiological recording have been limited, which has minimized utilization of source localization techniques. Advances in technology have remedied this issue, and efforts to disentangle the relationships between various brain regions and functional cerebral systems are now underway. Review of source localization techniques with electrophysiology is beyond the scope of this chapter. For more information, the reader is referred to Oakes et al [69].

One additional area for future research entails examination of potentially meaningful sex-related differences as a function of hostility. It is well known that men and women process emotional stimuli differently [86,87]. Sex-related differences in EEG bandwidths in our analyses were not observed. However, these studies were not specifically designed to detect differences among the sexes, as in some cases sample sizes were not equivalent. One recent study using the AAVL has examined the impact of hostility on women. Results indicate that high hostile women learn fewer words across conditions [88].

Finally, the present discussion has focused on high hostiles individuals who are currently in good medical condition. While it is known that some of these individuals will go on to suffer from cardiovascular disease and related illness, the relationship between brain function and high hostile cardiac patients is not well understood. This too remains an area for future study.

REFERENCES

[1]   Siegman, A.W., et al., Antagonistic behavior, dominance, hostility, and coronary heart disease. *Psychosomatic Medicine*, 2000. 62(2): p. 248-57.

[2]   Miller, T.Q., et al., A meta-analytic review of research on hostility and physical health. *Psychological Bulletin*, 1996. 119(2): p. 322-48.

[3]   Hecker, M.H., et al., Coronary prone behaviors in the Western Collaborative Study. *Psychosomatic Medicine*, 1988. 50: p. 153-164.

[4]   Dembroski, T.M., et al., Components of hostility as predictors of sudden death and myocardial infarction in the Multiple Risk Factor Intervention Trial. *Psychosomatic Medicine*, 1989. 51(5): p. 514-22.

[5]   Littman, A.B., Review of psychosomatic aspects of cardiovascular disease. *Psychotherapy and Psychosomatics*, 1993. 60(3-4): p. 148-67.

[6]   Vogele, C., Serum lipid concentrations, hostility and cardiovascular reactions to mental stress. *International Journal of Psychophysiology*, 1998. 28(2): p. 167-79.

[7]   Demaree, H.A. and D.W. Harrison, Physiological and neuropsychological correlates of hostility. *Neuropsychologia*, 1997. 35(10): p. 1405-11.

[8]   Demaree, H.A., D.W. Harrison, and R.D. Rhodes, Quantitative electroencephalographic analyses of cardiovascular regulation in low- and high-hostile men. *Psychobiology*, 2000. 28(3): p. 420-431.

[9]   Fredrickson, B.L., et al., Hostility predicts magnitude and duration of blood pressure response to anger. *Journal of Behavioral Medicine*, 2000. 23(3): p. 229-43.

[10] Everson, S.A., B.S. McKey, and W.R. Lovallo, Effect of trait hostility on cardiovascular responses to harrassment in young men. *International Journal of Behavioral Medicine*, 1995. 2(2): p. 172-191.

[11] Rhodes, R.D., D.W. Harrison, and H.A. Demaree, Hostility as a moderator of physiological reactivity and recovery to stress. *International Journal of Neuroscience*, 2002. 112: p. 167-186.

[12] Smith, T.W. and L.C. Gallo, Hostility and cardiovascular reactivity during marital interaction. *Psychosomatic Medicine*, 1999. 61(4): p. 436-45.

[13] Smith, T.W., *Concepts and methods in the study of anger, hostility, and health, in Anger, hostility, and the heart*, A.W. Siegman and T.W. Smith, Editors. 1994, Lawrence Erlbaum Associates: Hillsdale, NJ. p. 23-42.

[14] Houston, B.K., *Personality characteristics, reactivity, and cardiovascular disease, in Individual differences in cardiovascular response to stress*, J.R. Turner, A. Sherwood, and K.C. Light, Editors. 1992, Plenum Press: New York. p. 103-123.

[15] Williams Jr., R.B. and V.W. Williams, *Anger Kills*. 1993, New York: McGraw-Hill.

[16] Smith, T.W. and K.D. Allred, Blood-pressure during social interaction in high and low cynically hostile males. *Journal of Behavioral Medicine*, 1989. 12: p. 135-143.

[17] Spielberger, C., et al., *The experience and expression of anger: construction and validation of an anger expression scale, in Anger and hostility in cardiovascular and behavioral disorders*, M.A. Chesney and R.H. Roseman, Editors. 1985, Hemisphere: Washington.

[18] Keefe, F., P. Castell, and J.A. Blumenthal, Angina pectoris in Type A and Type B cardiac patients. *Pain*, 1985. 27: p. 211-218.

[19] Cook, W.W. and D.M. Medley, Proposed hostility and paraphaisic-virtue scales for the MMPI. *The Journal of Applied Psychology*, 1954. 38(6): p. 414-418.

[20] Han, K., et al., Psychometric characteristics of the MMPI-2 Cook-Medley Hostility Scale. *Journal of Personality Assessment*, 1995. 65(3): p. 567-585.

[21] Barefoot, J.C., et al., The Cook-Medley Hostility Scale: Iten content and ability to predict survival. *Psychosomatic Medicine*, 1989. 51: p. 219-233.

[22] Smith, T.W. and K.D. Frohm, What's so unhealthy about hostility? Construct validity and psychosocial correlates of the Cook and Medley Ho scale. *Health Psychology*, 1985. 4(6): p. 503-520.

[23] Greenglass, E.R. and J. Julkunen, Construct validity and sex differences in Cook-Medley Hostility. *Personality and Individual Differences*, 1989. 10(2): p. 209-218.

[24] Borod, J.C., Cerebral mechanisms underlying facial, prosodic, and lexical emotional expression: A review of neuropsychological studies and methodological issues. *Neuropsychology*, 1993. 7(4): p. 445-463.

[25] Borod, J.C., et al., Right hemisphere emotional perception: evidence across multiple channels. *Neuropsychology*, 1998. 12(3): p. 446-558.

[26] Demaree, H.A., et al., Brain lateralization of emotional processing:Historical roots and a future incorporating "Dominance." *Behavioral and Cognitive Neuroscience Reviews*, 2005. 4(1): p. 3-20.

[27] Heller, W., Neuropsychological mechanisms of individual differences in emotion, personality, and arousal. *Neuropsychology*, 1993. 7(4): p. 476-489.

[28] Davidson, R.J., Anterior electrophysiological asymmetries, emotion, and depression: Conceptual and methodological conundrums. *Psychophysiology*, 1998. 35: p. 607-614.

[29] Harmon-Jones, E., Clarifying the emotive functions of asymmetrical frontal cortical activity. *Psychophysiology*, 2003. 40: p. 838-848.

[30] Harmon-Jones, E. and J.J.B. Allen, Anger and frontal brain activity: EEG asymmetry with approach motivation despite negative affective valence. *Journal of Personality and Social Psychology*, 1998. 74(5): p. 1310-1316.

[31] Herridge, M.L. and D.W. Harrison, The effects of hostility and arousal affect perception: A test of a neuropsychological model of hostility [abstract]. *Archives of Clinical Neuropsychology*, 1998. 13(1): p. 58.

[32] Demaree, H.A. and D.W. Harrison, A neuropsychological model relating self-awareness to hostility. *Neuropsychology Review*, 1997. 7(4): p. 171-85.

[33] Heilman, K.M., D. Bowers, and E. Valenstein, *Emotional disorders associated with neurological diseases, in Clinical neuropsychology*, K.M. Heilman and E. Valenstein, Editors. 1993, Oxford University Press: New York. p. 461-498.

[34]   Harrison, D.W. and P.O. Gorelczenko, Functional asymmetry for facial affect perception in high and low hostile men and women. *International Journal of Neuroscience*, 1990. 55: p. 89-97.

[35]   Harrison, D.W., P.O. Gorelczenko, and J. Cook, Functional asymmetry for facial affect perception. *International Journal of Neuroscience*, 1990. 52: p. 11-16.

[36]   Herridge, M.L., D.W. Harrison, and H.A. Demaree, Hostility, facial configuration, and bilateral asymmetry on galvanic skin response. *Psychobiology*, 1997. 25(1): p. 71-76.

[37]   Demaree, H.A., et al., Asymmetry in hand grip strength and fatigue in low and high hostile men. *International Journal of Neuroscience*, 2002. 112: p. 415-428.

[38]   Williamson, J.B. and D.W. Harrison, Functional cerebral asymmetry in hostility: A dual task approach with fluency and cardiovascular regulation. *Brain and Cognition*, 2003. 52(2): p. 167-174.

[39]   Everhart, D.E., H.A. Demaree, and K.L. Wuensch, Healthy high-hostiles evidence low-alpha power (7.5-9.5Hz) changes during negative affective learning. *Brain and Cognition*, 2003. 52(3): p. 334-342.

[40]   Everhart, D.E., H.A. Demaree, and D.W. Harrison, The influence of hostility on electroencephalographic activity and memory functioning during an affective memory task. *Clinical Neurophysiology*, 2008. 119(1): p. 134-143.

[41]   Herridge, M.L., et al., Hostility and facial affect recognition: Effects of a cold pressor stressor on accuracy and cardiovascular reactivity. *Brain and Cognition*, 2004. 55(3): p. 564-571.

[42]   Oppenheimer, S.M., G. Kedem, and W.M. Martin, Left-insular cortex lesions perturb cardiac autonomic tone in humans. *Clinical Autonomic Research*, 1996. 6: p. 131-140.

[43]   Whittling, W., et al., Hemisphere asymmetry in sympathetic control of the human myocardium. *Brain and Cognition*, 1998. 38: p. 17-35.

[44]   Everhart, D.E. and D.W. Harrison, Heart rate responsivity and fluency performance in anxious and nonanxious men following a painful stimulus. *International Journal of Neuroscience*, 2002. 112: p. 1049-1071.

[45]   Snyder, K.A. and D.W. Harrison, The Affective Auditory Verbal Learning Test. *Archives of Clinical Neuropsychology*, 1997. 12(5): p. 477-482.

[46]   Bryden, M.P. and L. MacRae, Dichotic laterality effects obtained with emotional words. *Neuropsychiatry, Neuropsychology, and Behavioral Neurology*, 1989. 1: p. 171-176.

[47]   Davidson, R.J. and J.B. Henriques, *Regional brain function in sadness and depression, in The Neuropsychology of Emotion*, J.C. Borod, Editor. 2000, Oxford Press: New York. p. 269-297.

[48]   Toglia, M.P. and W.F. Battig, *Handbook of word norms*. 1978, Hillsdale, NJ: Lawrence Erlbaum.

[49]   Everhart, D.E., H.A. Demaree, and D.W. Harrison, *The merging of cognitive and affective neuroscience: Studies of the Affective Auditory Verbal Learning Test, in Causes, Role, and Influence of Mood States*, F. Columbus, Editor. 2005, Nova Science: Haupagge. p. 75-90.

[50]   Fox, M.A., R.S. Chen, and C.S. Holmes, Gender differences in memory and learning in children with insulin-dependent diabetes mellitus (IDDM) over a 4-year follow-up interval. *Journal of Pediatric Psychology*, 2003. 28(8): p. 569-578.

[51]   Godoy, J.F., et al., Recency effect in multiple sclerosis. *Applied Neuropsychology*, 1996. 3(2): p. 93-96.

[52]   Stefanova, E.D., et al., Serial position learning effects in patients with aneurysms of the anterior communicating artery. *Journal of Clinical and Experimental Neuropsychology*, 2002. 24(5): p. 687-694.

[53]   Demaree, H.A., et al., Primacy and recency effects found using affective word lists. *Cognitive and Behavioral Neurology*, 2004. 17(2): p. 102-108.

[54]   Everhart, D.E. and H.A. Demaree, Low alpha power (7.5-9.5Hz) changes during positive and negative affective learning. *Cognitive, Affective, and Behavioral Neuroscience*, 2003. 3(1): p. 39-45.

[55]   Baddeley, A.D. and G. Hitch, The recency effect: Implicit learning with explicit retrieval? *Memory & Cognition*, 1993. 21(2): p. 146-155.

[56]   Tops, M., et al., Free recall of pleasant words from recency positions is especially sensitive to acute administration of cortisol. *Psychoneuroendocrinology*, 2004. 29(3): p. 327-338.

[57]   Tops, M., et al., Acute cortisol efects on immediate free recall and recognition of nouns depend on stimulus valence. *Psychophysiology*, 2003. 40: p. 167-173.

[58]   Lupien, S.J., et al., The modulatory effects of corticosteroids on cognition: studies in young human populations. *Psychoneuroendocrinology*, 2002. 27(3): p. 401-416.

[59]   Yang, J.A. and L.P. Rehm, A study of autobiographical memories in depressed and nondepressed elderly individuals. *International Journal of Aging and Human Development*, 1993. 36: p. 39-55.

[60]   Mollet, G.A. and D.W. Harrison, Affective verbal learning in hostility: An increased primacy effect and bias for negative emotional material. *Archives of Clinical Neuropsychology*, 2007. 22(1): p. 53-61.

[61]   Dolce, G. and H. Waldeier, Spectral and multivariate analysis of EEG changes during mental activity in man. *Electroencephalography and Clinical Neurophysiology*, 1974. 36(6): p. 577-584.

[62]   Glass, A., Comparison of the effect of hard and arithmetic upon blocking of the occipital alpha rhythm. *Quarterly Journal of Experimental Psychology*, 1966. 18: p. 142-152.

[63]   Osaka, M., Peak alpha frequency of EEG during a mental task: Task difficulty and hemispheric differences. *Psychophysiology*, 1984. 21(1): p. 101-105.

[64]   Davidson, R.J., *Cerebral asymmetry, emotion, and affective style, in Brain asymmetry*, R.J. Davidson and K. Hugdahl, Editors. 1995, MIT Press: Cambridge. p. 361-388.

[65]   Henriques, J.B. and R.J. Davidson, Decreased responsiveness to reward in depression. *Cognition and Emotion*, 2000. 14(5): p. 711-724.

[66]   Fox, N.A. and R.J. Davidson, Patterns of brain electrical activity during facial signs of emotion in 10-month-old infants. *Developmental Psychology*, 1988. 24(2): p. 230-236.

[67]   Crawford, H.J., S.W. Clarke, and M. Kitner-Triolo, Self-generated happy and sad emotions in low and highly hypnotizable persons during waking and hypnosis:

laterality and regional EEG activity differences. *International Journal of Psychophysiology*, 1996. 24(3): p. 239-266.

[68] Cook, I.A., et al., Assessing the accuracy of topographic EEG mapping for determining local brain function. *Electroencephalography and Clinical Neurophysiology*, 1998. 107(6): p. 408-414.

[69] Oakes, T., et al., Functional coupling of simultaneous electrical and metabolic activity in the human brain. *Human Brain Mapping*, 2004. 21(4): p. 257-270.

[70] Klimesch, W., EEG alpha and theta oscillations reflect cognitive and memory performance: a review and analysis. *Brain Research Reviews*, 1999. 29(2-3): p. 169-195.

[71] Klimesch, W., et al., 'Paradoxical' alpha synchronization in a memory task. Cognitive *Brain Research*, 1999. 7(4): p. 493-501.

[72] Sterman, M.B., et al., Multiband topographic EEG analysis of a simulated visuomotor aviation task. *International Journal of Psychophysiology*, 1994. 16(49-56).

[73] Foster, P.S. and D.W. Harrison, The covariation of cortical electrical activity and cardiovascular responding. *International Journal of Psychophysiology*, 2004. 52(3): p. 239-255.

[74] Snyder, K.A., D.W. Harrison, and B.V. Shenal, The Affective Auditory Verbal Learning Test: Peripheral arousal correlates. *Archives of Clinical Neuropsychology*, 1998. 13(3): p. 251-258.

[75] Heller, W. and J.B. Nitschke, Regional brain activity in emotion: A framework for understanding cognition in depression. *Cognition and Emotion*, 1997. 11: p. 637-661.

[76] Vogt, F., W. Klimesch, and M. Doppelmayr, High frequency components in the alpha band and memory performance. *Journal of Clinical Neurophysiology*, 1997. 16: p. 167-172.

[77] Heller, W., M.A. Etienne, and G.A. Miller, Patterns of perceptual asymmetry in depression and anxiety: Implications for neuropsychological models of emotion and psychopathology. *Journal of Abnormal Psychology*, 1995. 104(2): p. 327-333.

[78] Davidson, R.J., Cognitive neuroscience needs affective neuroscience (and vice versa). *Brain and Cognition*, 2000. 42(1): p. 89-92.

[79] Davidson, R.J., Affective style, psychopathology, and resilience: Brain mechanisms and plasticity. *American Psychologist*, 2000. 55: p. 1196-1214.

[80] Everhart, D.E. and D.W. Harrison, Hostility following right CVA: Support for right orbital frontal deactivation and right temporal activation. *Journal of Neurotherapy*, 1995. 1(2): p. 55-59.

[81] Williamson, J.B. and D.W. Harrison, Functional cerebral asymmetry in hostility: A dual task approach with fluency and cardiovascular regulation. *Brain and Cognition*, 2003. 52: p. 167-174.

[82] Cole, H.W. and W.J. Ray, EEG correlates of emotional tasks related to attentional demands. *International Journal of Psychophysiology*, 1985. 3: p. 33-41.

[83] Demaree, H.A. and D.E. Everhart, Healthy high-hostiles: Reduced parasympathetic activity and decreased sympathovagal flexibility during emotional processing. *Personality and Individual Differences*, 2004. 36(2): p. 457-469.

[84] Brosschot, J.F. and J.F. Thayer, Anger inhibition, cardiovascular recovery, and vagal function: A model of the link between hostility and cardiovascular disease. *Annals of Behavioral Medicine*, 1998. 20(4): p. 326-332.

[85] Stein, P.K. and R.E. Kleiger, Insights from the study of heart rate variability. *Annual Review of Medicine*, 1999. 50: p. 249-61.

[86] Everhart, D.E., et al., Sex-related differences in event-related potentials, face recognition, and facial affect processing in prepubertal children. *Neuropsychology*, 2001. 15(3): p. 329-341.

[87] Everhart, D.E., H.A. Demaree, and A.J. Shipley, Perception of Emotional Prosody: Moving Toward a Model That Incorporates Sex-Related Differences 10.1177/1534582306289665. *Behav Cogn Neurosci Rev*, 2006. 5(2): p. 92-102.

[88] Mollet, G.A. and D.W. Harrison, Effects of hostility and stress on affective verbal learning in women. *International Journal of Neuroscience*, 2007. 117: p. 63-83.

In: Psychological Factors and Cardiovascular Disorders   ISBN: 978-1-60456-871-4
Editor: Leo Sher   © 2008 Nova Science Publishers, Inc.

Chapter XIX

NEGATIVE AFFECTIVE STATES AND ARRHYTHMOGENESIS

Lephuong Ong and Jane Irvine

Department of Psychology, York University, Toronto, Ontario, Canada;
Behavioural Health Sciences Division, Toronto General Hospital, Canada.

ABSTRACT

Sudden cardiac death (SCD) is defined as unexpected death due to cardiac causes within one hour of symptom onset. The majority of these are attributable to ventricular tachycardia (VT) or ventricular fibrillation (VF). The purpose of this chapter is to review the empirical evidence linking psychological stress and negative affective states (i.e., depression, anxiety, and anger) to the development of life-threatening ventricular arrhythmias. Laboratory and population-based prospective studies of healthy individuals, coronary heart disease (CHD) patients, and implantable cardioverter defibrillator (ICD) patients will be reviewed. Pathophysiological mechanisms underlying these relationships and intervention studies aimed at reducing arrhythmia risk will be discussed.

INTRODUCTION

Sudden cardiac death (SCD) is defined as unexpected death due to cardiac causes within one hour of symptom onset [1]. In industrialized nations, SCD accounts for approximately one-half of all deaths due to cardiovascular disease [1-3]. The majority of the estimated yearly 400,000 SCD's in North America are attributable to ventricular tachycardia (VT) or ventricular fibrillation (VF) [4-7].

Potential pathophysiological mechanisms underlying ventricular arrhythmias include: 1) myocardial changes which enhance inhomogeneity of excitability and repolarization [8,9]; 2) transient myocardial ischemia [10]; and 3) disparity in the responsiveness of different myocardial regions to sympathetic neural activity and to circulating catecholamines [11]. Since sympathetic neural activity can influence each of these mechanisms [12], it has been postulated that stimuli that increase sympathetic tone, such as psychological stress [13,14] or negative affective states [15-17], may precipitate ventricular arrhythmias and SCD. The purpose of this chapter is to review the empirical evidence linking psychological stress and negative affective states (i.e., depression, anxiety, and anger) to the development of life-threatening ventricular arrhythmias.

HISTORICAL PERSPECTIVE

Folklore provides colourful accounts of individuals dying suddenly when psychologically stressed, hence the expression, "scared to death" [18]. In 1971, George Engel [18] reported on 170 cases of sudden death presumed to be linked to psychological stress or emotional upheaval, such as intense grief or personal threat. In 1942, Walter Cannon postulated that sympatho-adrenal activation was the primary pathophysiological mechanism underlying the phenomenon of sudden, unexplained deaths following a voodoo curse [19]. Contemporary research has since integrated and provided empirical support for Engel and Cannon's early speculations about sudden death.

ANIMAL STUDIES

Animal studies indicate that diverse behavioural stressors (e.g., repeated delivery of electric shocks, prolonged suspension in a Pavlovian sling, restraint stress) predispose the acutely ischemic heart to arrhythmias [20] and VF [21], and reduce the threshold needed to provoke arrhythmias [22-27]. Anger-like behavioural states have also been shown to increase cardiac instability in canines [28]. Additionally, stress-induced anhedonia in rodents is associated with a reduced threshold for premature ventricular complexes and VT [29].

Research evidence suggests that these acute stress-induced changes in cardiac vulnerability may be mediated by activation of the sympathetic nervous system. For instance, hypothalamic stimulation, which increases sympathetic activity on the myocardium, has been shown to create a 40% decrease in VF threshold [30]. Subsequent administration of beta-adrenergic blocking agents was shown to completely eliminate this decrease in arrhythmic threshold.

CASE REPORTS IN HUMANS

Human case studies suggest that intense psychological distress, such as anger, despair, fear, and grief-related depression may have triggered or predisposed individuals to SCD in some cases [31-37]. Stress-induced VF has been shown to occur, even in the absence of organic heart disease and impairments in cardiac function [36]. However, these retrospective accounts are subject to reporting biases and may be influenced by patients' and observers' own causal explanations for heart disease and sudden death [38,39]. None of these reports included a comparison group of sudden, noncardiac death victims or an appropriate control time period.

Human Experimental Studies

The direct study of SCD and ventricular arrhythmias is impeded by their low incidence, thus many studies rely on proxy measures of arrhythmic risk (e.g., T-wave alternans, QT interval variability, ventricular premature beats). With the advent of the implantable cardioverter defibrillator (ICD), a first-line treatment for terminating malignant ventricular arrhythmias, the study of the relationship between psychological factors and ventricular arrhythmias has been greatly facilitated. The ICD's intracardiac electrogram documents electrophysiological activity and arrhythmic episodes, thus permitting a more precise examination of the association between psychological factors and arrhythmic events.

This section will review the experimental evidence linking psychological stress, depression, anxiety, and anger to ventricular arrhythmias and SCD. Laboratory and population-based prospective studies of healthy individuals, coronary heart disease (CHD) patients, and ICD patients will be reviewed.

Psychological Stress

Retrospective Studies

Based on the reports of family members and bystanders, Myers and Dewar [37] reported that acute psychological stress was significantly related to SCD in 100 males. Lane et al. [40] assessed perceived chronic (i.e., 6 months pre-cardiac event) and acute stress (i.e., 24 hours pre-cardiac event) in 25 patients with idiopathic VF and 25 matched CHD controls. Cardiac events of interest were cardiac arrest for the VF patients and myocardial infarction or unstable angina for the CHD patients. They found that idiopathic VF patients reported experiencing moderate to severe chronic and acute psychological stress more frequently before their cardiac event than did the CHD controls. In two independent samples of ICD recipients [41,42], ICD shocks were found to be more prevalent in the month after the World Trade Centre attack relative to the month before the attack.

Experimental Studies in Healthy Subjects

Experimental studies in healthy individuals suggest that acute psychological stress is associated with increased arrhythmia risk despite the absence of structural heart disease and impaired cardiac function. Toivonen et al. [43] examined ventricular polarization via ambulatory electrocardiography in 30 healthy physicians during emergency calls while they were on duty in the hospital. QT intervals were significantly longer during arousal compared to similar heart rates during stable conditions. Similarly, Andrassy et al. [44] studied 30 healthy males and observed significant QT prolongation during the performance of mental arithmetic. The extent to which these transient electrophysiological changes translate into increased arrhythmic risk requires further study.

Experimental Studies in CHD Patients

Psychological stress has been shown to provoke ventricular arrhythmias and proarrhythmic electrophysiologic changes in patients with established heart disease. Tavazzi and colleagues [45] showed that the performance of mental arithmetic during electrophysiologic programmed stimulation (EPS) was associated with a reduction in the ventricular refractory period and increased incidence of nonsustained VT or VF in post myocardial infarction patients compared with observations made during the EPS control trial. In this study, VF only occurred during the EPS-mental arithmetic trial. James et al. [46] found that psychological stress induced by cognitive stress tasks increased inhomogenous myocardial repolarization (assessed via QT dispersion) in patients with coronary disease (n = 17), but not in controls (n = 7). These changes were found to be mediated by ischemia-related changes in action potential. Recent work by Smith et al. [47] demonstrated that diary-reported stress correlated with total ventricular ectopic beats in acute postinfarct patients (N = 80). Temporal analysis of the association between diary-reported stress and ventricular ectopy showed a positive link between stress and increased ectopic beats in the following hour.

Experimental Studies in ICD Patients

Experimental studies have shown mental stress to increase inhomogeneity of electrical repolarization, which in turn increases arrhythmia susceptibility in ICD patients [48,49]. For instance, Kop and colleagues [49] found stress-induced increases in T-wave alternans (i.e., a marker of cardiac instability characterized by temporal and spatial heterogeneity of repolarization) in ICD patients with documented CAD (n = 23) but not in age-matched controls (n = 17). Lampert et al. [48] reported similar findings in their sample of ICD patients (N = 33) and noted that a greater increase in epinephrine was associated with a greater increase in T-wave alternans, which provides support for the hypothesis that sympathetic activation underlies the development of ventricular arrhythmias. Additionally, Lampert et al. [50] found that acute psychological stress shortens VT cycle length. This alteration was associated with increases in norepinephrine and occurred in the absence of ischemia. In this study, stress-induced VT was faster and more difficult to terminate, as evidenced by decreased effectiveness of antitachycardia pacing and increased failure rate of initial shocks in ICD patients.

Depression

Prospective Population-based Studies

Several large population-based studies have shown depression to be an independent risk factor for cardiac arrest and SCD. In a large (N = 915), prospective, population-based Finnish study, Luukinen et al. [51] showed that the presence of depressive symptoms conferred a 2.7-fold increased risk of SCD among elderly individuals over an eight-year follow-up period.

This effect was specific to SCD and not non-SCD cardiac mortality. More recently, Empana et al. [52] found that clinical depression conferred a 1.4-fold increased risk of out-of-hospital cardiac arrest in their population-based, case-control study, after adjusting for clinical and behavioural covariates (cases, n = 2228; controls, n = 4164). Unexpectedly, those without heart disease were at higher risk for cardiac arrest relative to those with heart disease (odds ratio: 1.71 versus 1.27) and stratification of cases by severity of depression showed that risk for cardiac arrest was higher in more severely depressed participants relative to less depressed participants (odds ratio: 1.77 versus 1.30).

Prospective Studies in CHD Patients

Depression has been implicated to be a significant risk factor for SCD and ventricular events in CHD patients. In the Montreal Heart Attack Readjustment Trial (N = 896), depression symptoms assessed in-hospital after a myocardial infarction, conferred a 3.1-fold increased risk for arrhythmic events during the initial year post myocardial infarction [53]. In the Canadian Amiodarone Myocardial Infarction Arrhythmia Trial (N = 671) that consisted of survivors of recent myocardial infarction, depression symptoms were associated with significantly greater risk of SCD (defined as arrhythmic death or resuscitated VF) over the two-year follow-up period (relative risk = 2.5) [54]. However, this association was diluted (relative risk = 1.1) when cognitive-affective symptoms of depression were examined apart from somatic symptoms of depression and the confounding effects of fatigue were statistically controlled. Recently, Watkins et al. [55] showed that symptoms of depression predicted the occurrence of ventricular arrhythmias in 940 CHD patients over a 3-year follow-up, after controlling for known demographic and clinical covariates (odds ratio = 1.40). There is also evidence that VF is more common in clinically depressed patients with myocardial infarction or unstable MI than in nondepressed patients [56].

Prospective/Longitudinal Studies in ICD Patients

Depression has also been found to be an independent risk factor for arrhythmic events in ICD patients. For instance, Herrmann et al. [57] reported that depression independently predicted the incidence of VT during the initial year post-implantation (n = 105, odds ratio = 3.1). In a multi-center study in the United States (N = 645), Whang et al. [58] found that ICD recipients with moderate to severe levels of depression at the time of study entry had a 3.2-fold increased risk for appropriate shocks for VT and/or VF (median follow-up = 359 days), after controlling for potential demographic (e.g., age, gender), cardiovascular (e.g., prior ICD discharges, history of cardiac arrest), and behavioral confounds (e.g., smoking, alcohol use). The majority of Whang et al.'s [58] sample had their ICDs implanted more than 6 months prior to study entry, suggesting that the observed depressed mood is not an acute, transient reaction to ICD implantation, but may represent a more persistant or chronic dysphoria.

Electrophysiological Evidence from Laboratory Studies

Laboratory studies have demonstrated a relationship between depression and arrhythmia events or electrophysiological markers of arrhythmic risk. A frequently studied marker is QT interval variability, which is an indicator of abnormalities in ventricular repolarization time and has been shown to predict arrhythmia events and SCD in CHD patients [59-61]. Rainey et al. [62] examined the QT intervals of drug-fee depressed patients (n = 21), substance disorder patients, and healthy controls and reported more frequent and severe QT prolongation in the depressed patients relative to the controls. Carney et al. [63] studied 103 patients with coronary artery disease and found that patients who met diagnostic criteria for major or minor depression (n = 21) were significantly more likely (relative risk = 8.2) to have one or more documented episodes of VT on Holter monitoring than nondepressed controls. This association was found despite between-group similarities in heart disease severity and ventricular function. In a subsequent study, Carney et al [64] demonstrated that depressed postmyocardial infarction patients had higher QT interval variability relative to gender- and age-matched controls.

Anxiety

Prospective Population-based Studies

As with depression, anxiety has been shown to be an independent risk factor for SCD in large prospective studies. Research evidence indicates that phobic anxiety is an especially potent risk factor. In a large cohort of 72 359 healthy women followed for a mean of twelve years, higher levels of phobic anxiety was identified as a risk factor for SCD in multivariate analyses adjusting for age and behavioral risk factors (e.g., smoking, alcohol intake, physical activity levels) [65]. Albert and colleagues [65] also found that women with the highest phobic anxiety scores had a 1.5-fold elevated risk for SCD relative to women who scored lower on phobic anxiety. Likewise, in the US Health Professionals Follow-up Study of 33 999 men free of CHD, Kawachi et al. [17] found that men who reported the highest levels of phobic anxiety had a 6.1-fold elevated risk of SCD during the two-year follow-up period. They also found no relationship between phobic anxiety and non-fatal cardiac events, which suggests a specific relationship between phobic anxiety and SCD. It is unclear whether other forms of anxiety (generalized anxiety, panic, or social anxiety) confer a similar degree of arrhythmic risk.

Prospective Studies in CHD Patients

Phobic anxiety has also been found to be a predictor of arrhythmic events in patients with documented coronary disease. A recent study (N = 940) by Watkins et al. [55] demonstrated that that ventricular arrhythmia occurrence was independently related to higher phobic anxiety scores in CHD patients (odds ratio = 1.4).

Prospective Studies in ICD Patients

Anxiety symptoms have been found to be independent predictors of arrhythmic events in ICD recipients. In a sample of 176 ICD recipients, Dunbar et al. [66] reported that post-implant anxiety levels, assessed at 1- and 3- months post-implant, predicted arrhythmic events at the 3- and 6-month follow-up periods, respectively. After finding that anxiety levels remained unchanged before and after the arrhythmic events, Dunbar et al. [66] argued that anxiety was the cause, rather than the consequence of the arrhythmic events. Similarly, Herrmann et al. [57] assessed the association between anxiety symptoms and arrhythmic events in 105 defibrillator patients and found that anxiety symptoms predicted the incidence of VF over a 12-month follow-up period, after controlling for age, sex, and cardiac severity (odds ratio = 3.7).

Electrophysiological Evidence from Laboratory Studies

Electrophysiological studies have documented an association between anxiety symptoms and markers of arrhythmia events. Ambulatory studies have documented relationships between increased QT dispersion and the following: state and trait anxiety in healthy males (N = 726) [67], state anxiety in hypertensive patients (N = 105) [68], and social anxiety in individuals with social phobia [69]. In a sample of 80 acute postinfarct patients, higher state anxiety was found to be related to greater total 24-hour ventricular ectopic beats, after adjusting for the effects of age, sex, ventricular function, and coronary artery disease severity [47]. These studies provide important insights into the potential pathophysiological mechanisms that underlie the relationship between anxiety and increased risk for ventricular arrhythmias and SCD.

Anger

Prospective evidence indicates that anger can independently trigger ventricular arrhythmias in ICD patients [70,71]. Using a case-crossover design, Lampert et al. [70] examined whether anger could trigger ventricular arrthythmias in 42 ICD patients who had 107 documented arrhythmic events requiring shock. Levels of predefined mood states were recorded in diaries for time periods preceding shock and for control time periods one week post-shock. They found that increased anger was more likely during the preshock period than the control periods. Follow-up analyses of this sample indicated that VT associated with anger-triggered episodes were more likely to be polymorphic, pause-dependent, and initiated by premature ventricular contractions [72].

NEGATIVE AFFECT AND ARRHYTHOMOGENESIS: POTENTIAL PATHOPHYSIOLOGICAL MECHANISMS

Autonomic Dysregulation

Investigators studying the associations between anxiety, depression, and arrhythmic events generally emphasize the mediating role of the autonomic nervous system in the pathogenesis of cardiac arrhythmias. Cardiac instability is thought to be driven by dysregulation of the autonomic nervous system at the level of its two component systems, the sympathetic and parasympathetic nervous systems. Specifically, it is a reduction in parasympathetic tone and increased sympathetic tone, or a change in overall sympathetic/parasympathetic balance, that is believed to be the arrhythmogenic mechanism [73,74]. For instance, depression has been linked to elevated levels of plasma and urinary catecholamines, such as norepinephrine [15,16,75,76], increased urinary cortisol [75], higher resting heart rates [77-79], and lower parasympathetic tone [78-80]. Likewise, anxiety has been associated with increased urinary norepinephrine excretion [75], elevated urinary cortisol [75], decreased parasympathetic tone [68,81,82], and alterations in sympathovagal balance [83]. Altogether, these alterations suggest a bias towards sympathetic neural activation and a reduction in parasympathetic activity, which can provoke myocardial ischemia and malignant ventricular arrhythmias particularly in the context of occluded coronary arteries [26,84-86].

Myocardial Ischemia

The relationship between psychological stress and increased arrhythmic risk may be mediated by myocardial ischemia [10,46]. Acute psychological stress has been observed to induce myocardial ischemia as evidenced by ST segment depression [87-94] or myocardial wall-motion abnormalities [92,95]. The experience of intense anger has also been shown to be a strong trigger of ischemia in CHD patients [93]. Structurally diseased hearts may be especially reactive and may be more vulnerable to stress-induced arrhythmias via increased susceptibility to myocardial ischemia, however, arrhythmias can be triggered even in the absence of ischemia, particularly in those with a history of ventricular arrhythmias [50].

Asymmetric Cerebral Activity

Psychological stress, anxiety, and depression have also been shown to trigger instability in myocardial repolarization [46,48,49,62,64,68], which increases arrhythmia susceptibility [96,97]. This process may be driven centrally, through stress-triggering of asymmetric cerebral activity [9,98]. Lateralization of cerebral activity during stress may result in asymmetric sympathetic stimulation of the heart, produce areas of inhomogenous repolarization and lead to electrical instability, thereby facilitating the development of VT and VF [98].

HUMAN INTERVENTION STUDIES

The observed link between negative affective states, psychological stress, and increased arrhythmia susceptibility suggests that interventions aimed at stress reduction or improving affective status may reduce the incidence of arrhythmic events in vulnerable individuals. Given the connection between increased sympathetic tone and lowered arrhythmic threshold, the potential for psychosocial interventions to reduce arrhythmic events may depend on the extent to which alleviation of stress and negative affect simultaneously dampens sympathetic drive [99]. Interventions that concurrently enhance vagal tone may also prove beneficial [100].

To date, the benefit of psychosocial intervention studies on reducing arrhythmic events in individuals at risk for ventricular arrhythmias (i.e., ICD patients) have yielded mixed findings. Dougherty et al. [101,102] studied 168 ICD patients and evaluated the effect of a telephone-based nursing intervention on the number of shocks received at 1-, 3-, 6-, and 12-months postimplantation. The intervention consisted of education about the ICD, psychological support, and counseling, which aimed to improve physical and psychological functioning, improve self-management skills, and lower health care consumption. They examined the effect of the intervention and found no reliable differences between the intervention and usual care groups with respect to shocks at any of the time points. Kohn et al. [103] reported similar findings in their prospective study of cognitive behavioral intervention involving 25 ICD patients randomized to treatment and 24 patients to usual care. The intervention consisted of psychoeducation about fear and anxiety, avoidance behaviors, fear of shocks, stress management, cognitive restructuring, and resumption of normal activities. At the 9-month follow-up, the mean number of shocks did not differ between the intervention and usual care group; however, when the shock variable was converted into a categorical variable (i.e., 0, 1, 2-5, 6-10, or 11 or more shocks), there was a trend for more shocks in the intervention versus usual care group (61% with ≥ 1 shocks versus 33%, $p = 0.07$). However, these findings are difficult to interpret and are limited by the lack of statistical adjustment for clinical covariates (e.g., ejection fraction, antiarrhythmic medications). Nonetheless, subsequent analyses indicated that those who were shocked benefited most from the intervention from a psychological standpoint, suggesting that the intervention itself did not *trigger* arrhythmic episodes, but facilitated coping in response to ICD shocks.

In a pilot study of ICD recipients randomized to six sessions of cognitive behavioral therapy (N = 70), Chevalier et al. [104] reported that patients in the intervention group received fewer shocks compared to patients in the usual care group at the 12-month follow-up, but this difference was not statistically reliable. Further subgroup analyses involving patients without antiarrhythmic drugs revealed that none of the subjects randomized to cognitive behavioral therapy had experienced arrhythmic events requiring ICD therapy at the 3-month follow-up, as compared to 4 events in the control group ($p = .04$). The results of 24-hour Holter monitoring data suggest that this difference may be due to improved sympathovagal balance, as daytime pNN50 and nocturnal SDNN increased significantly in the intervention group, but not in the control group.

In summary, none of the reviewed studies demonstrated a reliable reduction in shocks among ICD patients randomized to a psychosocial intervention following implantation. However, these studies are limited by a modest sample sizes, short follow-up periods, and a very low incidence of arrhythmic events necessitating ICD therapy, resulting in low statistical power for hypothesis testing and increasing the probability of Type II error. Null findings may also be explained by the fact that the ICD patients included these studies reported fewer symptoms of anxiety and depression compared to other cardiac patients in studies demonstrating a link between affective symptoms and mortality [53,105,106]. Studies with larger sample sizes and longer follow-up periods are needed to examine these relationships.

SUMMARY

Prospective studies and laboratory investigations in animals and humans support an association between negative affective states, such as acute psychological stress, depression, anxiety, and anger, and increased risk of ventricular arrhythmias and SCD. Autonomic dysregulation, myocardial ischemia, and asymmetric cerebral activity have been implicated as important pathophysiological mechanisms underlying these relationships. While these associations suggest that psychosocial interventions aimed at improving negative affect might produce a reduction in arrhythmic events, studies to date have yielded mixed findings and thus further research is required to better understand these relationships.

REFERENCES

[1]   Fox CS, Evans JC, Larson MG, Kannel WB, Levy DL: Temporal trends in coronary heart disease mortality and sudden cardiac death from 1950 to 1999: The Framingham Heart Study. *Circulation* 2004; 110:522-527.

[2]   Zipes DP, Wellens HJJ: Sudden cardiac death. *Circulation* 1998; 98(21):2334-2351.

[3]   Tang AS, Ross H, Simpson CS, Mitchell LB, Dorian P, Goeree R, Hoffmaster B, Arnold M, Talajic M: Canadian Cardiovascular Society/Canadian Heart Rhythm Society position paper on implantable cardioverter defibrillator use in Canada. *Can J Cardiol* 2005; 21(Suppl A):11A-18A.

[4]   Olsson G, Rehnqvist N: Sudden death precipitated by psychological stress. *A case report. Acta Med Scand* 1982; 212(6):437-41.

[5]   Roelandt J, Klootwijk P, Lubsen J, Janse MJ: Sudden death during longterm ambulatory monitoring. *Eur Heart J* 1984; 5(1):7-20.

[6]   Schmidinger H, Weber H: Sudden death during ambulatory Holter monitoring. *Int J Cardiol* 1987; 16(2):169-76.

[7]   Verrier RL: Mechanisms of behaviorally induced arrhythmias. *Circulation* 1987; 76(1 Pt 2):I48-56.

[8]   Taggart P, Sutton PM, Treasure T, Lab M, O'Brien W, Runnalls M, Swanton RH, Emanuel RW: Monophasic action potentials at discontinuation of cardiopulmonary bypass: evidence for contraction-excitation feedback in man. *Circulation* 1988; 77(6):1266-75.

[9]   Kuo CS, Munakata K, Reddy CP, Surawicz B: Characteristics and possible mechanism of ventricular arrhythmia dependent on the dispersion of action potential durations. *Circulation* 1983; 67(6):1356-67.

[10]   Lazzara R, Scherlag BJ: Generation of arrhythmias in myocardial ischemia and infarction. *Am J Cardiol* 1988; 61(2):20A-26A.

[11]   Randall WC, Kaye MP, Hageman GR, Jacobs HK, Euler DE, Wehrmacher W: Cardiac dysrhythmias in the conscious dog after surgically induced autonomic imbalance. *Am J Cardiol* 1976; 38(2):178-83.

[12]   Zipes DP, Levy MN, Cobb LA, Julius S, Kaufman PG, Miller NE, Verrier RL:
         Sudden cardiac death. Neural-cardiac interactions. *Circulation* 1987; 76(1 Pt
         2):I202-7.

[13]   Dimsdale J, Young D, Moore R, Strauss H: Do plasma norepinephrine levels reflect
         behavioral stress? *Psychosom Med* 1987; 49:375-382.

[14]   Dimsdale J, Moss J: Plasma catecholamines in stress and exercise. *JAMA* 1980;
         243:340-342.

[15]   Veith R, Lewis N, Linares O, Barnes R, Raskind M, Villacres E, Murburg M,
         Ashleigh E, Castillo S, Peskind E, Pascualy M, Halter J: Sympathetic nervous
         system activity in major depression: Basal and desipramine-induced alterations in
         plasma norepinephrine kinetics. *Arch Gen Psychiatry* 1994; 51(5):411-22.

[16]   Esler M, Turbott J, Schwarz R, Leonard P, Bobik A, Skews H, Jackman G: The
         peripheral kinetics of norepinephrine in depressive illness. *Arch Gen Psychiatry*
         1982; 39(3):295-300.

[17]   Kawachi I, Colditz GA, Ascherio A, Rimm EB, Giovannucci E, Stampfer MJ,
         Willett WC: Prospective study of phobic anxiety and risk of coronary heart disease
         in men. *Circulation* 1994; 89(5):1992-7.

[18]   Engel GL: Sudden and rapid death during psychological stress. Folklore or folk
         wisdom? *Ann Intern Med* 1971; 74(5):771-82.

[19]   Cannon W: "Voodoo" death. *Am J Public Health* 2002; 92(10):1593-1596.

[20]   Rosenfeld J, Rosen M, Hoffman B: Pharmacologic and behavioral effects on
         arrhythmias that immediately follow abrupt coronary occlusion: A canine model of
         sudden coronary death. *Am J Cardiol* 1978; 41:1075-1082.

[21]   Skinner J, Lie J, Entman E: Modification of ventricular fibrillation latency following
         coronary artery occlusion in the conscious pig. The effects of psychological stress
         and beta adrenergic blockade. *Circulation* 1975; 51:656-667.

[22]   Matta R, Lawler J, B L: Ventricular electrical instability in the conscious dog.
         Effects of psychological stress and beta adrenergic blockade. *Am J Cardiol* 1976;
         38:594-598.

[23]   Lown B, Verrier R, Corbalan R: Psychologic stress and threshold for repetitive
         ventricular response. *Science* 1973; 182(114):834-6.

[24]   Lown B, Verrier R: Neural activity and ventricular fibrillation. *N Engl J Med* 1976;
         294:1165-1170.

[25]   Corbalan R, Verrier R, Lown B: Psychological stress and ventricular arrhythmias
         during myocardial infarction in the conscious dog. *Am J Cardiol* 1974; 34:692 696.

[26]   Lown B, Verrier R, Rabinowitz S: Neural and psychologic mechanisms and the
         problem of sudden cardiac death. *Am J Cardiol* 1977; 39:890-902.

[27]   Natelson B, Cagin N: Stress-induced ventricular arrhythmias. *Psychosom Med* 1979;
         41:259-262.

[28]   Kovach J, Nearing B, Verrier R: Angerlike behavioral state potentiates myocardial
         ischemia-induced T-wave alternans in canines. *J Am Coll Cardiol* 2001;
         2001(37):1719-1725.

[29]   Grippo A, Santos C, Johnson R, Beltz T, Martins J, Felder R, Johnson A: Increased susceptibility to ventricular arrhythmias in a rodent model of experimental depression. *Am J Physiol Heart Circ Physiol* 2004; 286:H619-26.

[30]   Verrier RL, Calvert A, Lown B: Effect of posterior hypothalamic stimulation on ventricular fibrillation threshold. *Am J Physiol* 1975; 228(3):923-7.

[31]   Kuller L: Sudden death in arteriosclerotic heart disease; the case for preventive medicine. *Am J Cardiol* 1969; 24(5):617-28.

[32]   Reich P, DeSilva RA, Lown B, Murawski BJ: Acute psychological disturbances preceding life-threatening ventricular arrhythmias. *JAMA* 1981; 246(3):233-5.

[33]   Greene WA, Goldstein S, Moss AJ: Psychosocial aspects of sudden death. A preliminary report. *Arch Intern Med* 1972; 129(5):725-31.

[34]   Rissanen V, Romo M, Siltanen P: Premonitory symptoms and stress factors preceding sudden death from ischaemic heart disease. *Acta Med Scand* 1978; 204(5):389-96.

[35]   Ziegelstein RC: Acute emotional stress and cardiac arrhythmias. *JAMA* 2007; 298(3):324-9.

[36]   Lown B, Temte J, Reich P, Gaughan C, Regestein Q, Hal H: Basis for recurring ventricular fibrillation in the absence of coronary heart disease and its management. *N Engl J Med* 1976; 294:623-629.

[37]   Myers A, Dewar HA: Circumstances attending 100 sudden deaths from coronary artery disease with coroner's necropsies. *Br Heart J* 1975; 37(11):1133-43.

[38]   Strike P, Steptoe A: Behavioral and emotional triggers of acute coronary syndromes: A systematic review and critique. *Psychosom Med* 2005; 67:179-186.

[39]   French D, Senior V, Weinman J, Marteau T: Causal attributions for heart disease: A systematic review. *Psychological Health* 2001; 16:77-98.

[40]   Lane RD, Laukes C, Marcus FI, Chesney MA, Sechrest L, Gear K, Fort CL, Priori SG, Schwartz PJ, Steptoe A: Psychological stress preceding idiopathic ventricular fibrillation. *Psychosom Med* 2005; 67(3):359-65.

[41]   Steinberg JS, Arshad A, Kowalski M, Kukar A, Suma V, Vloka M, Ehlert F, Herweg B, Donnelly J, Philip J, Reed G, Rozanski A: Increased incidence of life-threatening arrhythmias in implantable defibrillator patients after the World Trade Center attack. *J Am Coll Cardiol* 2004; 44(6):1261-1264.

[42]   Shedd OL, Sears SF, Jr., Harvill JL, Arshad A, Conti JB, Steinberg JS, Curtis AB: The World Trade Center attack: increased frequency of defibrillator shocks for ventricular arrhythmias in patients living remotely from New York City. *J Am Coll Cardiol* 2004; 44(6):1265-7.

[43]   Toivonen L, Helenius K, Viitasalo M: Electrocardiographic repolarization during stress from awakening on alarm call. *J Am Coll Cardiol* 1997; 30:774-9.

[44]   Andrassy G, Szabo A, Ferencz G, Trummer Z, Simon E, Tahy A: Mental stress may induce QT-interval prolongation and T-wave notching. *Ann Noninvasive Electrocardiol* 2007; 12(3):251-259.

[45]   Tavazzi L, Zotti AM, Rondanelli R: The role of psychologic stress in the genesis of lethal arrhythmias in patients with coronary artery disease. *Eur Heart J* 1986; 7(Suppl A):99-106.

[46] James P, Taggart P, McNally S, Newman S, Sporton S, Hardman S: Acute psychological stress and the propensity to ventricular arrhythmias. *Eur Heart J* 1999; 21:1023-1028.

[47] Smith P, Blumenthal J, Babyak M, Georgiades A, Sherwood A, Sketch M, Jr., Watkins L: Ventricular ectopy: Impact of self-reported stress after myocardial infarction. *Am Heart J* 2007; 153:133-9.

[48] Lampert R, Shusterman V, Burg MM, Lee FA, Earley C, Goldberg A, McPherson CA, Batsford WP, Soufer R: Effects of psychological stress on repolarization and relationship to autonomic and hemodynamic factors. *J Cardiovasc Electrophysiol* 2005; 16:372-377.

[49] Kop WJ, Krantz DS, Nearing BD, Gottdiener JS, Quigley JF, O'Callahan M, DelNegro AA, Friehling TD, Karasik P, Suchday S, Levine J, Verrier RL: Effects of acute mental stress and exercise on T-wave alternans in patients with implantable cardioverter defibrillators and controls. *Circulation* 2004; 109(15):1864-9.

[50] Lampert R, Jain D, Burg MM, Batsford WP, McPherson CA: Destabilizing effects of mental stress on ventricular arrhythmias in patients with implantable cardioverter-defibrillators. *Circulation* 2000; 101(2):158-64.

[51] Luukinen H, Laippala P, Huikuri H: Depressive symptoms and the risk of sudden cardiac death among the elderly. *Eur Heart J* 2003; 24:2021-2026.

[52] Empana J, Jouven X, Lemaitre R, Sotoodehnia N, Rea T, Raghunathan T, Simon G, Siscovick D: Clinical depresison and risk of out-of-hospital cardiac arrest. *Arch Intern Med* 2006; 166:195-200.

[53] Frasure-Smith N, Lesperance F, Juneau M, Talajic M, Bourassa MG: Gender, depression, and one-year prognosis after myocardial infarction. *Psychosom Med* 1999; 61:26-37.

[54] Irvine J, Basinski A, Baker B, Jandciu S, Paquette M, Cairns J, Connolly S, Roberts R, Gent M, Dorian P: Depression and risk of sudden cardiac death after acute myocardial infarction: Testing for the confounding effects of fatigue. *Psychosom Med* 1999; 61:729-737.

[55] Watkins L, Blumenthal J, Davidson J, Babyak M, McCants C, Jr., Sketch M, Jr.: Phobic anxiety, depression, and risk of ventricular arrhythmias in patients with coronary heart disease. *Psychosom Med* 2006; 68:651-656.

[56] Catipovic-Veselica K, Galic A, Jelic K, Baraban-Glavas V, Saric S, Prlic N, Catipovic B: Relation between major and minor depression and heart rate, heart-rate variability, and clinical characteristics of acute coronary syndrome. *Psychol Rep* 2007; 100:1245-54.

[57] Herrmann C, Bergmann G, Drinkmann A, Dumn K, Fritzsche H, Kanwischer B, Smeritschnig P: Anxiety and depression in patients awaiting ICD implantation predict one-year incidence of malignant arrhythmias. *Psychosom Med* 1999; 61:114.

[58] Whang W, Albert CM, Sears Jr. SF, Lampert R, Conti JB, Wang PJ, Singh JP, Ruskin JN, Muller JE, Mittleman MA: Depression as a predictor for appropriate shocks among patients with implantable cardioverter-defibrillators. *J Am Coll Cardiol* 2005; 45:1090-1095.

[59]   Atiga W, Calkins H, Lawrence J, Tomaselli G, Smith J, Berger R: Beat-to-beat repolarization lability identifies patients at risk for sudden cardiac death. *J Cardiovasc Electrophysiol* 1998; 9:899-908.

[60]   Maison-Blanche P, Coumel P: Changes in repolarization dynamicity and the assessment of arrhythmic risk. *Pacing Clin Electrophysiol* 1997; 20:2614-2624.

[61]   Haigney M, Zareba W, Gentlesk P, Goldstein R, Illovsky M, McNitt S, Andrews M, Moss A: QT interval variability and spontaneous ventricular tachycardia or fibrillation in the Multicenter Automatic Defibrillator Implantation Trial (MADIT) II patients. *J Am Coll Cardiol* 2004; 44:1481-1487.

[62]   Rainey J, Jr., Pohl R, Bilolikar S: The QT interval in drug-free depressed patients. *J Clin Psychiatr* 1982; 5(2):39-40.

[63]   Carney RM, Freedland KE, Rich MW, Smith LJ, Jaffe AS: Ventricular tachycardia and psychiatric depression in patients with coronary artery disease. *Am J Med* 1993; 95(1):23-8.

[64]   Carney R, Freedland K, Stein P, Watkins L, Catellier D, Jaffe A, Yergani V: Effects of depression on QT interval variability after myocardial infarction. *Psychosom Med* 2003; 65(177-80)

[65]   Albert CM, Chae CU, Rexrode KM, Manson JE, Kawachi I: Phobic anxiety and risk of coronary heart disease and sudden cardiac death among women. *Circulation* 2005; 111(4):480-7.

[66]   Dunbar SB, Kimble LP, Jenkins LS, Hawthorne M, Dudley W, Slemmons M, Langberg JJ: Association of mood disturbance and arrhythmia events in patients after cardioverter defibrillator implantation. *Depress Anxiety* 1999; 9:163-168.

[67]   Uyarel H, Okmen E, Cobanolu N, Karabulut A, Cam N: Effects of anxiety on QT dispersion in healthy young men. *Acta Cardiol* 2006; 61:83-87.

[68]   Piccirillo G, Viola E, Nocco M, Santagada E, Durante M, Bucca C, Marigliano V: Autonomic modulation and QT interval dispersion in hypertensive subjects with anxiety. *Hypertension* 1999; 34:242-246.

[69]   Nahshoni E, Gur S, Marom S, Levin J, Weizman A, Hermesh H: QT dispersion in patients with social phobia. *J Affect Disord* 2004; 78:21-26.

[70]   Lampert R, Joska T, Burg MM, Batsford WP, McPherson CA, Jain D: Emotional and physical precipitants of ventricular arrhythmia. *Circulation* 2002; 106(14):1800-5.

[71]   Stopper M, Joska T, Burg MM, Batsford WP, McPherson CA, Jain D, Lampert R: Electrophysiologic characteristics of anger-triggered arrhythmias. *Heart Rhythm* 2006; 4:268-273.

[72]   Stopper M, Joska T, Burg MM, Batsford WP, McPherson CA, Jain D, Lampert R: Electrophysiologic characteristics of anger-triggered arrhythmias. *Heart Rhythm* 2007; 4:268-273.

[73]   Albert CM, Ruskin JN: Risk stratifiers for sudden cardiac death (SCD) in the community: primary prevention of SCD. *Cardiovasc Res* 2001; 50(2):186-96.

[74]   Meredith IT, Broughton A, Jennings GL, Esler MD: Evidence of a selective increase in cardiac sympathetic activity in patients with sustained ventricular arrhythmias. *N Engl J Med* 1991; 325(9):618-24.

[75] Hughes J, Watkins L, Blumenthal J, Kuhn C, Sherwood A: Depression and anxiety symptoms are related to 24-hour urinary norepinephrine excretion among healthy middle-aged women. *J Psychosom Res* 2004; 57:353-58.

[76] Otte C, Neylan T, Pipkin S, Browner W, Whooley M: Depressive symptoms and 24-hour urinary norepinephrine excretion levels in patients with coronary disease: Findings from the Heart and Soul Study. *Am J Psychiatry* 2005; 162(11):2139-2145.

[77] Carney R, Freedland K, Veith R, Cryer P, Skala J, Lynch T, Jaffe A: Major depression, heart rate, and plasma norepinephrine in patients with coronary heart disease. *Biol Psychiatry* 1999; 45(458-63)

[78] Lehofer M, Moser M, Hoehn-Saric R, McLeod D, Liebmann P, Drnovsek B, Egner S, Hildebrandt G, Zapotoczky H: Major depression and cardiac autonomic control. *Biol Psychiatry* 1997; 42:914-19.

[79] Agelink M, Boz C, Ullrich H, Andrich J: Relationship between major depression and heart rate variability: Clinical consequences and implications for antidepressive treatment. *Psychiatry Res* 2002; 113:139-49.

[80] Carney R, Blumenthal J, Stein P, Watkins L, Catellier D, Berkman L, Czajkowski S, O'Connor C, Stone P, Freedland K: Depression, heart rate variability, and acute myocardial infarction. *Circulation* 2001; 104(17):2024-8.

[81] Watkins L, Grossman P, Krishnan R, Sherwood A: Anxiety and vagal control of heart rate. *Psychosom Med* 1998; 60:498-502.

[82] Thayer J, Friedman B, Borkovec: Autonomic characteristics of generalized anxiety disorder and worry. *Biol Psychiatry* 1996; 39:255-66.

[83] Piccirillo G, Bucca C, Tarantini S, Santagada E, Viola, E, Durante M, Raganato P, Mariano A, Cacciafesta M, Marigliano V: Sympathetic activity and anxiety in hypertensive and normotensive subjects. *Arch Gerontol Geriatr* 1998; 26(Suppl. 1):399-406.

[84] Gantenberg N, Hageman G: Enhanced induction of ventricular arrhythmias during sympathetic stimulation before and during coronary artery occlusion. *Int J Cardiol* 1992; 34(1):75-83.

[85] Kliks B, Burgess M, Abildskov J: Influence of sympathetic tone on ventricular fibrillation threshold during experimental coronary occlusion. *Am J Cardiol* 1975; 36:45-9.

[86] Podrid P, Fuchs T, Candinas R: Role of the sympathetic nervous system in the genesis of ventricular arrhythmia. *Circulation* 1990; 82(Suppl. 2):I103-13.

[87] Barry J, Schoyn A, Nabel E, Rocco M, Mead K, Campbell S, Rebecca G: Frequency of ST segment depression produced by mental stress in stable angina pectoris from coronary artery disease. *Am J Cardiol* 1988; 61:989-993.

[88] Schiffer F, Hartley L, Schulman C, Abelman W: Evidence for emotionally induced coronary arterial spasm in patients with angina pectoris. *Br Heart J* 1980; 44:62-66.

[89] Deanfield J, Shea M, Kenselt M, Horlock P, Wilson R, DeLandsheere C, Selwyn A: Silent myocardial ischemia due to mental stress. *Lancet* 1984; 2(8410):1001-1004.

[90] Jennings J, Follansbee W: Task-induced ST segment depression, ectopic beats, and autonomic responses in coronary heart disease patients. *Psychosom Med* 1985; 47:415-430.

[91]   Specchia G, deServi S, Falcone C, Gavazzi A, Angoli L, Bramucei E, Ardissimo P, Mussini A: Mental arithmetic stress testing in patients with coronary artery disease. *Am Heart J* 1984; 108:56-63.

[92]   Rozanski A, Bairey C, Krantz D, Friedman J, Risser K, Morell M, Hilton-Chalfen S, Hestrin L, Bietendorf J, Berman D: Mental stress and the induction of silent myocardial ischemia in patients with coronary artery disease. *N Engl J Med* 1988; 318:1005-1012.

[93]   Gabbay F, Krantz D, Kop W, Hedges S, Klein J, Gottdiener JS, Rozanski A: Triggers of myocardial ischemia during daily life in patients with coronary artery disease: Physical and mental activities, anger and smoking. *J Am Coll Cardiol* 1996; 27(3):585-92.

[94]   Stone P, Krantz DS, McMahon R, Goldberg A, Becker L, Chaitman B, Taylor H, Cohen J, Freedland K, Bertolet B, Coughlan C, Pepine C, Kaufmann P, Sheps D: Relationship among mental stress-induced ischemia and ischemia during daily life and during exercise: the Psychophysiologic Investigations of Myocardial Ischemia (PIMI) Study. *J Am Coll Cardiol* 1999; 33(6):1476-84.

[95]   Gottdiener JS, Krantz DS, Howell RH, Hecht GM, Klein J, Flalconer JJ, Rozanski A: Induction of silent myocardial ischemia with mental stress testing: Relation to the triggers of ischemia during daily life activities and to ischemic functional severity. *J Am Coll Cardiol* 1994; 24(7):1645-51.

[96]   Hohnloser S, Klingenheben T, Li Y, Zabel M, Peetermans J, Cohen R: T wave alternans as a predictor of recurrent ventricular tachyarrhythmias in ICD recipients: Prospective comparison with conventional risk markers. *J Cardiovasc Electrophysiol* 1998; 9(12):1258-68.

[97]   Shusterman V, Goldberg A, London B: Upsurge in T-wave alternans and nonalternating repolarization instability precedes spontaneous initiation of ventricular tachyarrhythmias in humans. *Circulation* 2006; 113(25):2880-7.

[98]   Critchley HD, Taggart P, Sutton PM, Holdright DR, Batchvarov V, Hnatkova K, Malik M, Dolan RJ: Mental stress and sudden cardiac death: asymmetric midbrain activity as a linking mechanism. *Brain* 2005; 128(Pt 1):75-85.

[99]   Cruess D, Antoni M, McGregor B, Kilbourn K, Boyers A, Alferi S, Carver C, Kumar M: Cognitive-behavioral stress management reduces serum cortisol by enhancing benefit finding among women being treated for early stage breast cancer. *Psychosom Med* 2000; 62:304-308.

[100]   Nolan R, Kamath M, Floras J, Stanley J, Pang C, Picton P, Young Q: Heart rate variability biofeedback as a behavioral neurocardiac intervention to enhance vagal heart rate control. *Am Heart J* 2005; 149:1137.

[101]   Dougherty CM, Lewis FM, Thompson EA, Baer JD, Kim W: Short-term efficacy of a telephone intervention by expert nurses after an implantable cardioverter defibrillator. *Pacing Clin Electrophysiol* 2004; 27:1594-1602.

[102]   Dougherty CM, Thompson EA, Lewis FM: Long-term outcomes of a telephone intervention after an ICD. *Pacing Clin Electrophysiol* 2005; 28:1157-1167.

[103] Kohn C, Petrucci R, Baessler C, Soto D, Movsowitz C: The effect of psychological intervention on patients' long-term adjustment to the ICD: A prospective study. *Pacing Clin Electrophysiol* 2000; 23:450-56.

[104] Chevalier P, Cottraux J, Mollard E, Sai N, Brun S, Burri H, Restier L, Adeleine P: Prevention of implantable defibrillator shocks by cognitive behavioral therapy: A pilot trial. *Am Heart J* 2006; 151:191.e1-191.e6.

[105] Frasure-Smith N, Lesperance F, Talajic M: Depression and 18-month prognosis after myocardial infarction. *Circulation* 1995; 91:999-1005.

[106] Szekely A, Balog P, Benko E, Breuer T, Szekely J, Kertai M, Horkay F, Kopp M, Thayer J: Anxiety predicts mortality and morbidity after coronary artery and valve surgery: A 4-year follow-up study. *Psychosom Med* 2007; 69:625-31.

In: Psychological Factors and Cardiovascular Disorders   ISBN: 978-1-60456-871-4
Editor: Leo Sher   © 2008 Nova Science Publishers, Inc.

Chapter XX

Mental Health Comorbidity in Cardiovascular Heart Disease: Implications for Interdisciplinary Intervention

Amy L. Ai
University of Pittsburgh, Pittsburgh, Pennsylvania, USA.
Hoa Appel and Jagoda Pasic
University of Washington, Seattle, Washington, USA.

Abstract

Population aging will inevitably increase the incidence of cardiovascular disease (CVD), a major chronic condition among adults in the United States (U.S.). This chapter begins by setting out the historical relationship between the heart and mind and then focuses on the role of mental health comorbidity in cardiac conditions. Current research suggests that depression and anxiety play a significant role in coronary heart disease, involving related personality traits, critical behavioral elements, and psychoneuroimmunological mechanisms. Next, it addresses factors that seem to protect against CVD and mental health issues, including positive attitudes, coping, social support, and spirituality. Finally, the chapter delineates implications for an interdisciplinary intervention. In particular, issues in clinical assessment of the above symptoms and beyond are highlighted.

Introduction

About nine years ago, the first author was asked to assist Dr. Hart (not his real name), a senior psychiatrist and former faculty member at a prestigious medical school, and, then, a cardiac patient. He maintained a private practice and also owned a computer business. His wife was a physician, leading a large group practice. Their children were all successful adults. At a time when his life could not have been happier, it was turned completely upside down by his heart attack and three subsequent hospitalizations. The first hospitalization was for a triple coronary artery bypass graft surgery (CABG) and valve replacement. A week later, a stroke brought "executive dysfunction," which he first assumed himself, leading to re-hospitalization. A month later, major depression resulted in his being placed on suicide watch in a locked psychiatric unit. At the first meeting, the pale doctor spoke only of impending mortality and the end of a successful scientific career. Yet after a year-long psychosocial and existential intervention, he survived and thrived. The retired doctor has found new meaning in his life, gained physical fitness, and has become a mentor of youths at his Unitarian church.

Cardiovascular disease (CVD) includes coronary artery disease (CAD), rheumatic heart disease, cardiomyopathy, pulmonary heart disease, congestive heart failure (CHF), ischemic attack in the brain (stroke), myocardial infarction (MI or heart attack), irregular heart beat (arrhythmia), and hypertension (high blood pressure), to name a few [1]. The study of depression and CVD, particularly the effect of depression on prognosis, remains to be further examined due to its complexity, especially when incorporating various fields such as psychiatry, cardiology, nursing, epidemiology, and health psychology [2]. For this important subject, recently the National Heart, Lung and Blood Institute initiated a work group to address issues related to the diagnosis and measurement of depression in patients with CAD, to review the treatment for patients with CAD and depression, and to make recommendations for further research [3].

The burden of CVD goes beyond its physical manifestations. Psychological distress is a significant comorbidity of CVD and many studies have documented this [4,5]. The results from the 2002 National Health Interview Survey showed that only 31%-35% of patients with heart disease and psychological distress visited a mental health professional [4]. Dr. Hart's true story is an example of psychological stress brought on by CVD. The challenges that he faced were not limited to his heart damage, cognitive decline, and major depression, but extended also to his loss of personal and professional identity which had supplied purpose and meaning to his life. In this regard, additional psychosocial and existential intervention may help rebuild the disrupted internal world and provide the motivation for a new journey.

To enhance cardiac care, it is important that medical, health, and mental health professionals be cognizant of the mind-heart association and the need of interdisciplinary intervention for a whole person, rather than simply for impaired organs. Therefore, this chapter will discuss the heart's historical philosophical role with a brief overview of the heart-mind link, especially with regard to mental health issues and CVD, and discuss the gap in the current CVD practice. It will further focus on depression and anxiety as major cardiac risk factors, the role of personality traits and negative emotion, and pathogenic mechanisms. Then, it comments on evidence of some factors which may protect against CVD mental health comorbidity, including positive attitudes, coping, social support, and spirituality. Lastly, it delineates implications for interdisciplinary intervention, including clinical assessment and practice for mental health comorbidity in CVD.

A MYSTIFIED, MEANINGFUL ORGAN IN HUMAN HISTORY

Throughout human history, the heart has played a role of much more significance than that of a mere pump, its purpose according to science. The operative philosophy of science is embodied in Aristotelian empirical materialism. The formulation of a Cartesian mind/matter dualism in the 17th century helped bring about the birth of modern sciences, including modern medicine [6]. In the scientific paradigm, observable indices of radionucleotide studies, coronary arteriography, electrocardiograms, echocardiograms, laboratory tests, and imaging technology have shown the physical side of the heart and the circulation system with precision. Indeed, CVDs are mostly classified with structural and physiological changes, as mentioned above [1], unlike the physical and biophysiological mind, the *psyche* and *soul*, which are mostly untouchable by the surgical knife and invisible in the high technological arena, though closely related to the health and diseases of the heart.

Yet, in the world's great many legacies, the heart has been mythologized, linked with various aspects of mind, and located at the core of life, deep emotions, and human relationships [6]. In various languages, people seem to share the meaning of heart-related expressions. For example, a "stolen" or "broken heart" appears to be a universal idiom that crosses linguistic boundaries to indicate a crisis in a profound relationship, a romantic tie, or strong commitment. Most cultural traditions do not honor the liver, kidneys, or lungs in the same way. In Western history, Seneca, teacher to the roman Emperor Nero, wrote that the place of spiritual belief is seated in the heart. In Christian tradition, the heart is a symbol for devotion, as in the writing of Saint Teresa of Avila, and the flaming heart is a symbol of both devotion and charity. English medical doctor William Harvey (1578-1657) was the first to correctly describe, in exact detail, the systemic circulation and the physical function of the heart. In 1628, he assumed a link between the mind (e.g., a sense of pleasure, hope, or fear) and the heart. Likewise, French mathematician, physicist, and religious philosopher Blaise Pascal (1623-1662) in his classic *Pensées* stated: "The heart has its reasons which reason does not know." In the German language, the term heart, *herzzentrum*, symbolizes emotional warmth, and its famous writer Johann Wolfgang von Goethe (1749-1832) used the heart in a romantic sense throughout his poems. Further, the American poet, Henry Wadsworth Longfellow (1807-1882), wrote:

> "The heart hath its own memory like the mind,
> And in it are enshrined
> The precious keepsakes, into which is wrought

The giver's loving thought." In short, we see a dichotomy between the heart as seen mostly by the scientist or medical professional, and the heart in literature and even in daily speech. This mind/body dichotomy does not apply in traditional Oriental medicine, which primarily follows a "psychosomatic" model [6,7,8]. This paradigm associates each organ with a pattern of emotion and symbolic element, so that each illness possesses psychosocial components. The heart is sometimes mistaken as *an organ of the mind*, because it is highly sensitive to abrupt emotional stress. It is classified as the "fire" element – an "emperor" organ which houses the individual's *Shen* or mental energy [6,7]. As such, the heart is considered equivalent to the mind which is involved in many neuroendrocrine activities in contemporary medical science today. When this function, or the *Shen* of the heart, is impaired, Oriental medicine dictates that disharmony may become manifest as insomnia, anxiety, irritability, excessive dreaming, poor concentration, or forgetfulness. Even more seriously, the patient may experience depression, insanity, hysteria, or delirium [6,7].

A brief review of some historical accounts of the heart is not meant to ask medicine to follow mythology. Rather, acknowledging the cultural context of cardiac patients will help health professionals to understand the meaning of CVD with respect to individuals' lives, to be better related to their patients, and to thereby enhance the quality of their health care services and disease management. Modern health care recognizes the importance of mental health care within individuals' social context. At the first International Conference on Health Promotion held in Ottawa, Canada 20 years ago, the World Health Organization (WHO) Regional Office for Europe made a milestone commitment to health promotion world wide [8]. According to the Ottawa Charter, health, including cardiac health, is not created solely in medical clinics. Rather, "Health is created where people live, love, work, and play." Unlike the places where people live, work, and play, however, the place of *love* is deeply inside people's hearts. This implies that cardiac health care should move beyond the physician's clinic to improving people's real life situations and to healing of the mind and soul.

COMORBID MENTAL HEALTH ISSUES AND CVD

In the United States (U.S.), the National Comorbidity Survey-Replication (NCS-R) study includes anxiety, mood, impulse-control, and substance abuse disorders, defined by the Diagnostic and Statistical Manual for Psychiatric Disorders-IV (DSM-IV), 4th edition [9]. According to the NCS-R study, more than one in four adults in the U.S. have suffered from some form of mental illness in the past 12 months [10]. Among these, 22% have experienced serious mental illness [10]. The NCS-R defined serious mental illness as a mental disorder that resulted in severe functional disability that may also have included a suicide attempt within the 12 months previous to the study. Another study shows that individuals who have not suffered a mental disorder during the previous year also have a lower risk of CVD and a lower number of chronic physical diseases [11]. In 2003, the direct and indirect yearly economic costs of mental illness were estimated to total $150 billion, not including the costs of research [12]. The challenges resulting from mental illness have been recognized and were the impetus for the President's New Freedom Commission on Mental health in 2002 [13].

Consistent with the historical and cultural wisdoms, contemporary research has found that the burden of CVD goes beyond physical components. The prevalence of comorbid mental health issues (e.g., depression, anxiety, and hostility/anger) in cardiac patients has been well documented [4,5,14,15]. So far, more than 100 studies have evaluated the link between depression and CVDs, presenting a prevalence of 20%-35% in this population [16,17,18]. Over the past decade, evidence has associated depression and anxiety with the poor prognosis of heart diseases, including deadly heart attacks [19,20]. A recent analysis of the United Kingdom's General Practices Research Database suggests those with severe mental illness appear to have an increased risk of death from CVD [21]. A current German prospective study of 1052 CAD patients also shows that symptoms of anxiety seem to be a strong predictor for subsequent adverse cardiovascular events [22]. Both Duits' and Pignay-Demaria's review of psychosocial outcomes following cardiac surgery indicated that anxiety and depressive symptoms predict postoperative maladjustment, including new cardiac events and rehospitalization [15,23].

Depression is commonly encountered in primary care settings, with approximately 10% of patients identified [24,25]. Recognizing symptoms of depression may be difficult, while diagnosis and treatment can be equally challenging [24]. A major gap in current practice with CVD patients lies in the under-assessed and under-treated mental health comorbidities. The results from the 2002 National Health Interview Survey showed that only 31%-35% of patients with heart disease and psychological distress visited a mental health professional [4]. Further, a study of 796 U.S. cardiovascular doctors revealed that 50% of these physicians were unaware of depression as an independent cardiac risk factor, and 79% had no standard screening method to diagnose depression [26]. Moreover, almost half of these physicians stated that they treat the depressive symptoms of their CVD patients in their office instead of referring them out to a mental health professional [26]. These gaps signify the need to educate health providers about psychological and/or mental health issues in CVD patients.

DEPRESSION AND CVD

The World Health Organization (WHO) predicts that by 2020, major depression and CVD will be the two leading contributors to the global burden of disease [27]. Thus far, research has suggested a seemingly bidirectional relationship between these two disease syndromes [2,3]. Current evidence seems not to infer the direction of causality [28]. Earlier, Alexopoulos et al. (1997) proposed the concept of "vascular depression", based on older adults with depression who have evidence of CVD as well as its risk factors [29]. Increasingly, research suggests that CVD plays a significant role in the onset and course of depression, a leading cause of disability [29,30]. One study showed an increase of 30% in the odds of depression among CVD patients [31]. About one-third of MI survivors are depressed [32,33], and approximately one-fourth of patients develop depression after a stroke [34,35]. Neuroimaging research has also associated subcortical white matter ischemic lesion with depressive symptoms and late-onset depression in elderly patients [31].

Conversely, depression has been implicated in the onset and progression of CAD and CHF, and it also predicts poor prognosis and advanced clinical outcomes [3,14,17,18,37,38,39]. Patients with depression and CAD have worse health outcomes than non-depressed patients. Those with post-MI are at greater risk for subsequent reinfarction and rehospitalization than the non-depressed patients [40]. Also, comorbid depression and CAD cause almost twice the social impairment caused by either condition alone [41]. In healthy individuals, depression predicts the onset and the development of CAD [19]. The risk of any CVD was 1.7 times higher among depressed patients compared with non-depressed patients [35]. A recent meta-analysis reveals that depressed mood increased the risk for a wide range of CVDs [42]. The rates of major depression (16% to 23%) and clinically significant depressive symptoms (32%) are both significantly higher among patients with CAD [43].

Cardiologists and interdisciplinary researchers have noted that up to 20% of patients with CVD meet DSM-IV (Diagnostic and Statistical Manual) criteria for major depression [3,44]. These significant rates suggest a need for early assessment.

Depression has been shown to be a risk factor for CVD mortality and for all major disease-related causes of death [45]. A recent meta-analysis has linked depressive symptoms or clinical depression with CAD-related mortality, especially three years after an initial assessment [19]. After an MI, individuals with depression are at greater risk of death compared to those who are not depressed [40,46]. Another meta-analysis links depression with post-MI mortality and cardiovascular events, especially in older adults [20]. Furthermore, depression occurs twice as likely in women as in men [24,47], and mortality from CVD is greater in women than men [36]. Gender differences and physiological, socioeconomic, or psychosocial factors may contribute to varied recovery time from coronary events [48], also reported in noncardiac studies as well [49,50,51]. CVD and its treatment affect women differently compared to men. Women younger than 65 years of age are twice likely to die from MI and CABG surgery than men [52]. Women are also more likely to have non-specific symptoms than typical angina compared with men [53], and about two thirds of women who die suddenly of CAD had no previous symptoms of their illness [52]

For patients undergoing open heart surgery, the incidence of depression varies among studies between 7.5% to 47% and 19% to 61% postoperatively [15], and depressive symptom levels remained stable before and after surgery [15,54]. Even after one year post operation [55], depressive symptoms have been found to predict postoperative cardiac events (unstable angina, acute MI, repeat CABG, angioplasty) and death. Recent studies have documented perioperative depressive symptoms in up to 25% of 963 CABG patients. Such symptoms contributed to impaired functional status 1 year after, especially in women [56], and to short term postoperative global functioning and mental fatigue [57,58]. This fact underscores the importance of preoperative assessment and intervention among cardiac surgery patients [15,18].

ANXIETY, STRESS, AND CVD

Compared to depression, the prevalence and impact of anxiety on heart diseases has been under-recognized and less represented in literature [15,17]. While anxiety as a symptom is very common among the patients in coronary care unit (50%) [59], the vast majority of these patients are undiagnosed or undertreated. Twenty-five percent of patients who present to an Emergency Department with chest pain meet criteria for panic disorder, although 98% are undiagnosed on arrival [60]. What makes it a diagnostic challenge is that patients with chest pain that warrants CAD work-up are as likely to have panic disorder and CAD (22%) as they are to have CAD and no panic disorder (18%) [61]. Panic disorder and generalized anxiety have been associated with recurrent cardiac events among CAD patients [17,48,60], and phobic disorder has been found as a risk factor or predictor of poor prognosis in CAD patients [22].

While the literature on the relationship of anxiety and CAD is conflicting with reports of both positive and negative effects, anxiety has been found to be a risk factor of total mortality in men and women, and CAD and atrial fibrillation in men, but not specifically a risk for cardiac mortality [62]. Epidemiological studies have also associated anxiety with increased carotid atherosclerosis [63]; risk of recurrent cardiac events [22,26,59,64,65], MI, ventricular arrhythmia, and sudden cardiac death [66,67,68,69]. More recently, studies have suggested a relationship between anxiety to both diabetes and CVD in U.S. Latinos [70]. As with depression, anxiety plays a role in CAD prognosis and mortality [17,71]. A recent German study identified anxiety as a much stronger predictor, compared with depression, for long-term subsequent adverse CVD events [22]. Likewise, a US study reported that anxiety predicted poor quality of life at four months after MI and other cardiac events, and health care utilization during a 3.5-year follow-up [72]. This evidence suggests that early assessment and intervention for anxiety may improve the well-being of cardiac patients.

Closely related to anxiety, stress is also known as a cardiac risk factor and is classified into three types: Work-related stress, subacute life stress, and acute stress [17]. Work-related stress and tension has been associated with CAD risk and events [73,74]. Further, research has shown the coexistence of subacute life stress, such as those indicated in the *Recent Life Changes* scores [75], with cardiac events, such as MI and sudden death [17,76]. In addition, there have been reports linking acute stress (eg. bereavement, earthquake, missile attack) with CAD incidence [17,77,78]. Stress can be triggered by poverty that is associated with a cluster of cardiac health risk factors, e.g., unsatisfying living conditions, malnutrition, family disruption, unemployment, hostile neighborhoods, and unhealthy behaviors [79]. Finally, hyperventilation in acute anxiety can promote coronary artery spasm or arrhythmia, as it has been detected by cardio-imaging in experimentally induced panic attack [80], and it may trigger fatal cardiac events in both CAD sufferers and healthy persons [81].

Particularly noteworthy are studies on post-traumatic stress disorder (PTSD) symptoms in patients undergoing cardiac surgery [82,83]. Postoperative PTSD symptoms were related to low mental health scores and poor life satisfaction [83]. These findings have led to a randomized controlled trial on hormonal treatment of PTSD in cardiac surgery patients [82]. Because postoperative patients with PTSD had considerable traumatic memories of an intensive care unit (ICU), even at six-month afterwards, these symptoms were attributable to the ICU care [82]. Another study has associated acute stress two days before cardiac surgery, defined as fitting a symptom criterion for PTSD, with poor adjustment one month after surgery [84]. The latter study assumed that patients may have developed these PTSD symptoms prior to the ICU care for this life-altering surgical event.

PERSONALITY TRAITS, NEGATIVE EMOTION, AND CVD

Over the past fifty years, an anxiety-related personality factor, type A behavior (e.g., time urgency, hostility, achievement-striving), has received much research attention as a CVD-related psychological risk factor [85]. Subsequent studies, however, confirmed that the most harmful contributors are time urgency and hostility within type A personality. Hostility, aggression, and anger have also been linked with carotid atherosclerosis, CAD risk, symptom prognosis and mortality in CAD, angiographic CAD, MI, CHF, and arrhythmias [86-94], especially atrial fibrillation in men [95].

Some studies have found the anger effect on premature CVD [96] and the hostility effect in patients with a CAD history [97,98]. Recent studies have examined hostility and anger in women, demonstrating their relationships with recurrent CAD events [99], ambulatory ischemia [100], and CAD events [101], and angioplasty CAD [93]. Others have associated stroke with anger [102] and depression-related hostility [103]. Yet, there are mixed opinions on the role of such traits [104] and large-scale epidemiological studies are needed to evaluate them in CAD patients [17].

Recently, a new personality construct, the "type D" or "distressed" personality (high negative affect, and high emotional and social inhibition), has received attention in literature after reports of increased cardiac mortality and non-fatal MI in patients with CAD [105-108]. A current 30-year follow-up study finds early evidence that social avoidance, which is associated with depression and hostility, predicted CVD mortality in 2107 initially healthy men [109]. Other personality traits, such as pessimism and hopelessness, were found to increase the risk of developing a fatal CAD or vagal withdrawal [79,110-113] and carotid atherosclerosis [114]. However, these associations need more salient clinical evidence.

MECHANISMS UNDERLYING DEPRESSION IN CVD

Although no conclusive mechanism has been cited, depression has been suggested to have an influence on CVD through both direct (pathophysiological factors) and indirect (heath behaviors and risk factors, such as medical adherence, lifestyle, self-care) pathways [16-18]. Various adverse lifestyle factors may be responsible for the association of depression and CVD, such as smoking, alcohol consumption, low physical activity, medication non-compliance, and risk factors such as obesity, hypertension, and dyslipidemia [39,115,116]. Patients with depression are three times less likely to be compliant with medical treatment regimen compared to non-depressed patients [117].

There are several proposed mechanisms for the contribution of depression to the pathogenesis of CAD: Increased hypothalamic-pituitary-adrenal (HPA) function as demonstrated by elevated corticotrophin-releasing factor, blunting of the adrenocorticotropic hormone response to corticotrophin-releasing factor and elevated serum cortisol levels [118], and increased sympathoadrenal activity, as evidenced by hypersecretion of norepinephrine and an elevated plasma norepinephrine concentration [118]. Depressive disorders may contribute to the pathogenesis of CAD through dysregulation in the autonomic nervous system activity, as shown by reduced heart rate variability that can lead to MI and fatal arrhythmias [115,119,120].

Evidence also suggests other factors underlying pathogenesis of depression and CVD. For example, enhanced platelet activation [121] with elevated plasma factor-4 and β-thromboglobulin [121], and vascular-endothelial damage, which may occur with elevated plasma homocysteine level [31]. This biomarker is of particular interest because it is implicated in the metabolism of the amino acid methionine and folate cycle [17]. On the one hand, homocysteine has been found as an independent marker of vascular risk, and currently effective trial of MI survivors will help answer the question if folate-based homocysteine-lowering therapy would provide cardiac benefits [123]. On the other hand, folate deficiency may lead to increased risk of depression and poorer antidepressant treatment [124], and folate augmentation randomized controlled trial of treatment of depression currently underway in Great Britain will provide information on its benefits [125].

Methionine is the precursor of S-adenosylmethionine (SAMe), which is involved in the synthesis and metabolism of dopamine, norepinephrine, and serotonin in the brain. These neurotransmitters play a significant role in the pathogenesis of depression and anxiety. Some studies, particularly those outside of the U.S., have demonstrated efficacy of SAMe in depression [126], though main-stream clinical practice utility has been limited. The implications of homocysteine, folate and SAMe in depression and CAD seem to be strong, although current literature does not link them as a putative mechanism of comorbidity. Ultimately, the results of the ongoing trial of Omega-3 fatty acids augmentation of sertraline in the treatment of depression in patients following an acute MI or other cardiac events will inform whether there would be reduction of depression and improvement of cardiovascular markers [127].

Last but not least, in the last decade research has pointed to the common underlying factor of dysregulation of immune and inflammatory processes, and the pathophysiology of both depression and heart diseases [128-131]. Cytokines are increasingly considered to be a significant factor in the pathogenesis of CAD [132] and CHF [133], and there is growing evidence of cytokine's importance in major depression [134]. In particular, depressive sympomatology and CAD have been associated with increased levels of IL-1β and IL-6 [132], and IL-1β, IL-2, TNF-α, and IL-6 have been identified as overlapping proinflammatory cytokines in depression and CHF [133]. Recently, C-reactive protein (CRP) and Omega-3 fatty acids have received increased presence in literature on both CAD [135-137] and depression [138-142], as separate conditions, as well as comorbid conditions [143-146].

MECHANISMS UNDERLYING ANXIETY AND STRESS IN CVD

With respect to the mechanism underlying anxiety in CAD, clinical studies have suggested a link between anxiety disorders and autonomic imbalance, such as increased sympathetic stimulation, and impaired vagal control that can cause decreased heart rate variability and fatal ventricular arrhythmia [17,147]. Further, anxiety-related behaviors of some patients (e.g., smoking and alcohol use) may contribute to risk of atherosclerosis progression [148,149]. Psychological stress induces excess homocysteine concentrations, promoting the oxide and therombogenic effects of this amino acid on the vasculature [150,151]. Stress, similar to depression, may also induce inflammation through sympathetic nervous system activation [152,153], such as elevated levels of the transcription factor nuclear factor Kappa B(NF-kB), in circulation, an effect dependent on norepinephrine but diminished by alpha 1-adrenoceptor blockade [154]. Beta-adrenoceptor stimulation may also lead to increased gene expression and protein production of certain cytokines [155].

Some studies have shown a prediction of trait anger and anger-in to carotid intima-media-thickness (IMT) in women [156], including healthy women [157], and the association of anger-out with with dyslipidemia and BMI in women. More recent evidence associated anger-in, but not anger-out or trait anger, with IMT in older men, an effect independent of resting blood pressure and heart rate, suggesting mechanisms beyond sympathetic nervous system activation [158]. One alternative pathway could be inflammation. Excess plasma IL-6 was found in hostile men with depressive symptoms but not those without depression [159]. Another pathway may involve CVD risk factors [160]. Evidence has linked anger-out with dyslipidemia and BMI in women [161] and with progression of angiographic CAD in men. Also, homocysteine has been associated with severity of depression and length of depressive episode in patients with major depression and anger attacks, but not in those with depression alone [162].

PSYCHOLOGICAL PROTECTIVE FACTORS

In the past decade, a few protective factors of human strengths and virtues in health have drawn more research attention in conjunction with positive psychology movement [163]. Behavioral studies have demonstrated the role of optimism and self-efficacy in both better mental health and improved CVD outcomes [164,165]. A U.S. study on cardiac rehabilitation patients found that optimism and social support are independent predictors of posttreatment physical functioning outcomes [166]. Optimism among British patients with recent cardiac disease was related to positive affect [167]. Among elder Dutch patients, dispositional optimism was shown as an independent protective factor and cardiovascular mortality [168]. In MI patients, optimism contributed to fewer hospital readmissions, whereas pessimism predicated subsequent death [165]. Within six months following a first percutaneous transluminal coronary angioplasty, patients who had positive expectations, perceived control over their future, and a positive view of themselves had a lower risk of a new cardiac event [169]. Further, preoperative optimism appears to have a counteracting affect against acute distress and is associated with better adjustment one month following open-heart surgery [84].

Hope, adaptive coping and exercise are positive factors that may improve outcomes and complaints of symptoms after MI, CAGG, and CAD events [170-172]. In a prospective study, hope and social support mediated a favorable influence of positive religious coping styles on depression and anxiety in patients following open-heart surgery [173]. Another study documented a survival advantage after stroke among hopeful patients [174]. Further, self-efficacy was shown as a predictor in health status among patients undergoing cardiac angiography in a six-month follow-up Heart and Soul study [21,175]. Despite emerging evidence, these positive mindsets as protective factors have not yet been rigorously examined in clinical trials as intervention strategies for CVD disease management.

Among cardiac rehabilitation patients, social support contributes to better physical health and coping responses [166]. Perceived social support has been associated with decreased depression in older cardiac surgery patients [176]. Also, many non-cardiac studies have linked religiousness with higher levels of social support [177,178], which often is seen as a mediator of religiousness on health outcomes [179]. Social support is found to mediate a favorable linkage of intrinsic religiousness with trait anxiety in a cross-sectional study of cardiac patients [180]. In 2003, an expert panel organized by the National Institutes of Health suggested that the faith effect on health is more evident among cardiac patients compared with cancer patients [179].

However, this influence may be more complex than previously expected. For example, in a follow-up survey, social participation or religious strength and comfort was a predictor for survival after cardiac surgery [181]. Yet, more recently, stronger religious beliefs were associated with fewer postoperative complications and shorter hospital stay in CABG patients, but religious attendance was related to worse outcomes [182]. A study on open-heart surgery also associated preoperative positive religious coping styles with postoperative vitality and functioning among open-heart patients [57,58].

INTERDISCIPLINARY IMPLICATIONS AND INTERVENTION

An overview of the heart-mind association may help clinicians better understand why cardiac care must go beyond pharmaceutical and operative treatments. Returning to the true case example in the introduction, Dr. Hart had no doubt received the best medical, surgical and psychiatric care. However, all his interventions did not address the fundamental questions about his life after his medical treatment. The very existential questions are whether he wanted to live his life as a physically, functionally, affectively, and cognitively impaired person, and if so, how he could adjusts to that life with his new personal identity. His CVDs deprived his capacity to perform highly demanding professional roles, a source of his self-esteem. Medical intervention can repair Dr. Hart's heart and control his depressive symptoms but may not provide the motivation, meaning, and purpose for an impaired life. Indeed, research evidence has found that many patients desire more for quality of life equally or more than for quantity of life [183].

Although not all CVD patients receive worst results as did Dr Hart, he also had advantages that many others do not. For example, he had access to financial resources, strong social support and a professional network, and timely existential care that helped rebuild his shattered internal world after his MI, surgery and stroke. With all these substantive social and spiritual assistance, Dr. Hart actually reinvented himself on a new journey. This translates to an initiation of a different lifestyle resulting in weight loss, a commitment of life to the future of others in the community, and his courageous combat with cognitive impairment by writing a book on spirituality and interfaith harmony. As suggested by the WHO in 2006, his health has been restored where he "live, love, work and play", drawing strengths from his renewed "self", beloved friends and family, and his faith. This case and contemporary research imply that multidisciplinary interventions are necessary to optimize the health and well-being of CVD patients.

Screening for Mental Health Comorbidity

In order to maximize the benefits of CVD treatment, health care professionals need to be attentive to psychological issues such as mood changes, cognition, and negative emotions as part of treatment [48,184]. Taken into account the time restrictions for physicians, cardiologists, surgeons, and nurses to see patients quickly, two screening questions for depression are suggested:

(a) "During the past month, have you often been bothered by feeling down, depressed, or hopelessness?"; and (b) "During the past month, have you often been bothered by having little interest or pleasure in doing things?" [185]. The Institute of Medicine has taken screening and treatment of depression to be a priority for U.S. medicine in the 21st century [186]. The U.S. Preventive Services Task Force has also recommended that primary care providers regularly screen adult patients for depression in their clinical practices in order to accurately diagnose, effectively treat, and provide follow-up for depression [186]. Moreover, psychiatric disorders and symptoms are ubiquitous in primary care settings, particularly among patients with low socioeconomic status [187]. It has been evident that regular screening in primary care settings yields improved treatment of depressed adults [185]. The screening in CVD patients is crucial since they are mostly seen by primary care providers who make available most of the depression diagnoses [188,189].

Standardized Instruments for Screening

If the responses are positive for both questions above, then standardized instruments such as the Beck Depression Inventory [190], Inventory of Depressive Symptomalogy [3,30], Composite International Diagnostic Intervention [3,5], and Center for Epidemiologic Studies Depression Scale (CES-D) can be further used to assess depression [191]. Other scales include the Geriatric Depression Scale [31], and the Hospital Anxiety and Depression Scale [22,29]. Well-trained individuals should be employed to administer these diagnostic instruments. CVD patients who manifest severe mental health symptoms should be referred to a mental health professional for further diagnosis and intervention.

Assessing Quality of Life (QOL)

Recurrence of clinical depression is common. Screening for mental health comorbidity should include questions pertaining not only to mental illness symptoms, but to related factors such as stressors in life, quality of life, risk behaviors, nutrition, and protective resources [42]. A useful tool for assessing QOL or patients' self-perception of well-being is the Mac New Heart Disease Health-Related Quality of Life [192]. This questionnaire measures three primary components: physical limitations, emotional function, and social functions, as well as the physical symptoms such as chest pains, shortness of breath, fatigue and dizziness [192]. In addition, Hunt's et al.'s (2001) Living with Heart Failure is a measure that evaluates how heart failure interferes with the completion of normal life tasks [193]. Given the special cultural meaning of the heart, health and mental health providers may address the existential issues faced by patients undergoing life-altering cardiovascular events. Psychosocial and pastoral care may be recommended for further assessment of patients' essential needs.

Pharmacotherapy for Cardiac Depression

Pharmacotherapy is one of the acceptable treatments for mild to moderately severe clinical depression. Under surgical or MI circumstances, such treatment may be difficult due to the complex pathophysiology involved, polypharmacy and the potential for drug interactions [15]. The first generation of antidepressants, especially tricyclics may not be for a good choice due to cardiotoxicity despite their benefits in patients with clinical depression [115]. Selective serotonin reuptake inhibitors (SSRIs), have been considered safe for CAD [194,195], and they also have fewer anticholinergic side affects [196]. A recent study suggested SSRIs and clinical management as a first step treatment for patients with coronary artery disease and major depression [197].

SSRIs appear to enhance brain monoaminergic levels and to alter depression-related physiological derangements, evident as normalized urinary cortical excression, improved heart rate variability, decreased platelet activation, reduced inflammatory markers [198-200], and to improve quality of life [201]. In addition, analyses from the Sertraline Antidepressant heart Attack Randomized Trial ([SADHART; 195,199] and the Enhancing Recovery in Coronary Heart Disease [ENRICHD; 202] study have suggested some promising cardiac benefits of SSRIs in patients with more severe depression a history of depression [194]. In the SADHART platelet substudy, patients in sertraline group had significant reduction in platelet activation, which explained by authors, supports the platelet activation in the pathogenesis of depression and CAD [195,203]. In CAD patients, the safety of serotonin-norepinephrine reuptake inhibitors remains unclear [3].

Psychosocial Intervention and Combined Treatment

Psychotherapeutic intervention such as cognitive-behavioral therapy (CBT), interpersonal therapy (IPT), and other behavioral therapies, either alone or combine with SSRIs, have shown to be effective for CVD related depression [195,204]. The ENRICHD trial offered rigorous evaluation in MI patients, and involved licensed and certified mental health professionals, including psychiatrists, psychologists, and social workers [205]. However, this study did not show a difference in survival between patients receiving psychosocial intervention (patients who received CBT) and those in the"usual care" group. The authors attributed these finding to the fact the "usual care" patients did better than expected, which diminished the effect size of the intervention [202]. Despite negative findings, further investigations are recommended to determine whether using CBT or SSRIs will reduce morbidity and mortality in CAD patients [3]. Nevertheless, effective depression intervention should include evaluation, treatment, completion of treatment, and access to health care providers, especially for the disadvantaged population [206], and future trials will likely test the augmentation or sequencing of various treatment strategies [12,13,207].

Multidisciplinary Approach to Rehabilitation and Intervention with Life-induced and Meaningful Stressors

An ideal intervention for CVD patients with mental health comorbidity should reduce mortality risk and morbidity while maintaining social and psychological well-being [208]. However, rehabilitation should not be limited to mental health symptom deduction. The close tie between CVD and mental comorbidity implies that either sides are not an isolated disease but a system involves multi-levels of an individual in his or her sociocultural and ecological context. If stress can trigger both of these pathological responses, the link of CVD and mental illness should reflect the combination of individuals' genetic vulnerability and cognitive-behavioral mal-adaptation. The benefit of standardized cardiac and psychiatric care could be enhanced, if the individual can actively and effectively engage in coping with these diseases and various types of life-induced psychosocial stressors that spiral the illness impact. As the population ages and more patients are seen outside of hospital settings, interdisciplinary management of these diseases will become inevitable and perhaps more cost-effective.

The new form of care should include evaluation of and intervention with various life-induced stressors, coping strategies, and motivation-related meaning-making process. Primary cardiac care should work collaboratively with other providers, such as pharmacists, medical social workers, public health professionals, nutritionists, community service staff members, and pastoral care counselors. A study of 228 patients showed that patients who received collaborative care enjoyed a significant decrease in depressive symptoms, compared with the control group which received no psychiatric visits to monitor their pharmacologic treatment [209]. Another study showed an increase in physical and social functioning of high risk CVD patients visited by home outreach workers [210]. Clearly, more research evidence is needed in this area in order to enhance community care for these patients.

CONCLUSION

The heart has a special position and meaning in many human traditions and in life, and CVD affects both men and women in the U.S. The prevalence of CVD in an aging society, the societal impact of CVD, and the influence of its mental health comorbidity suggest an important role for health and mental health professionals in integrative cardiac care. In this regard, professionals in many areas will need to cross traditional boundaries within the disciplines of clinical medicine, mental health, public health and gerontology to form a collaborative and interdisciplinary approach. Further research needs to examine the precise strategies and effectiveness of mental health promotion and prevention of illness among CVD patients and the public.

REFERENCES

[1]   Rosamond W, Flegal K, Friday G, Furie K, Go A, Greenlund K, et al: Heart Disease and Stroke Statistics 2007. A Report from American Heart Association Statistics

Committee and Stroke Subcommittee. Retrieved September 28, 2007 from http://circ.ahajournals.org/cgi/content/full/115/5/e69

[2] Davidson KW, Kupfer DJ, Kaplan RM: Health psychology and scientific consensus: The case of depression and cardiovascular disease. *Health Psychology* 2007; 26:519-520.

[3] Davidson KW, Kupfer DJ, Bigger JT, Califf RM, Carney RM, Coyne JC et al: Assessment and treatment of depression in patients with cardiovascular disease: National Heart, Lung, and Blood Institute Working Group Report. *Annals Behavioral Med* 2006; 32(2):121-126.

[4] Ferketich AK, Binkley PF: Psychological distress and cardiovascular disease: results from the 2002 National Health Interview Survey. *Eur Heart J* 2005; 26(18):1923-1929.

[5] Carroll D, Phillips AC, Hunt K, Der G: Symptoms of depression and cardiovascular reactions to acute psychological stress: Evidence from a population study. *Biol Psychology* 2007; 75:68-74.

[6] Ai, A L: Psychosocial adjustment and health care practices following coronary artery bypass surgery (CABG). *Dissertation Abstracts International: Section B: The Sciences and Engineering* 1996; 57(6-B):4078.

[7] Ai, A L: Qigong, in Micozzi, MS (Ed.), *Fundamentals of complementary & integrative medicine*, 3rd edition, pp. 418-436, 1996. St Louis, MO: Elsevier Health Sciences.

[8] Ottawa Charter for Health Promotion. First International Conference on Health Promotion 1986. Retrieved November 12, 2007 from http://www.who.int/hpr/NPH/docs/ottawa_charter_hp.pdf

[9] Mental illness as used in the National Comorbidity Survey—Replication (NCS–R) includes anxiety, mood, impulse-control, and substance abuse disorders as defined by the *Diagnostic and Statistical Manual for Psychiatric Disorders-IV* (DSM-IV), 4th ed., American Psychiatric Association, 2000.

[10] Kessler, R.C., et al. Prevalence, severity, and comorbidity of 12-month DSM-IV disorders in the National Comorbidity Survey—Replication (NCS–R). *Arch Gen Psychiatry* 2005; 62(6):617–627.

[11] Keyes CL: Promoting and protecting mental health as flourishing: a complementary strategy for improving national mental health. *American Psychologist* 2007; 62(2):95-108.

[12] Hogan, M.F. The President's New Freedom Commission: Recommendations to transform mental health care in America. *Psychiatric Serv* 2003; 54(11):1467–1474.

[13] Office of the U.S. Surgeon General. Mental Health: A Report of the Surgeon General. Rockville, MD: U.S. Department of Health and Human Services (HHS), *Public Health Service*, 1999.

[14] Hemingway H, Marmot MG. Psychosocial factors in the etiology and prognosis of coronary heart disease: systematic review of prospective cohort studies. *BMJ* 1999; 318:1460-1467

[15]   Pignay-Demaria V, Lespérance F, Demaria RG, et al: Depression and anxiety and outcomes of coronary artery bypass surgery. *Annals Thoracic Surg* 2003; 75, 314–321.

[16]   Lett HS, Blumenthal JA, Babyak MA: Depression as a risk factor for coronary artery disease: evidence, mechanism, and treatment. *Psychosom Med* 2004; 66(3):305-315.

[17]   Rozanski A, Blumenthal JA, Kaplan J: Impact of psychological factors on the pathogenesis of cardiovascular disease and implications for therapy. *Circulation* 1999; 99(16), 2192–2217.

[18]   Rumsfeld RS, Ho PM: Depression and cardiovascular disease: A call for recognition. *Circulation* 2005; 111(3):250-253.

[19]   Barth J, Schumacher M, Herrman-Lingen C: Depression as a risk factor for mortality in patients with coronary heart disease: A meta-analysis. *Psychosomat Med* 2004; 66(6):802-813.

[20]   Van Melle JP, De Jonge P, Spijkerman TA, Tijssen JG, Ormel J, Van Veldhuisen DJ: Prognostic association of depression following myocardial infarction with mortality and cardiovascular events: A meta-analysis. *Psychosomat Med* 2004; 814-822.

[21]   Osborn DP, Levy G, Nazareth I, Petersen I, Islam A, King MB: Relative risk of cardiovascular and cancer mortality in people with severe mental illness from the United Kingdom's General Practice Research Database. *Arch Gen Psychia* 2007; 64(2):242-249.

[22]   Rothenbacher D, Hahmann H, Wusten B, Koenig W, Brenner H: Symptoms of anxiety and depression in patients with stable coronary heart disease: prognostic value and consideration of pathogenetic links. *Eur J Cardiovasc Prev Rehabil* 2007; 14(4):547-554.

[23]   Duits AA, Boeke S, Taamms MA.et al: Prediction of quality of life after coronary artery bypass graft surgery: A review and evaluation of multiple, recent studies. *Psychosomat Med* 1997; 59:257–268.

[24]   Bhatia SC, Bhatia SK: Depression in Women: Diagnostic and treatment considerations. *American Fam Phys* 1999; 60(1):225-240

[25]   Elliott RL: Depression in primary care. *Ethn Dis* 2007; 17(2supp):S2-28-33).

[26]   Feinstein RE, Blumenfield M, Orlowski B, Frishman WH, Ovanessian S: A national survey of cardiovascular physicians' beliefs and clinical care practices when diagnosing and treating depression in patients with cardiovascular disease. *Cardiol Rev* 2006; 14(4):164-169.

[27]   Murray CJ, Lopez AD: *The global burden of disease: summary*. Cambridge: Harvard School of Public Health, 1996.

[28]   Mosovich SA, Boone RT, Reichenberg A et al.: New insights into the link between cardiovascular disease and depression. *Int J Clin Pract* 2007; online article November 20, 2007, 1-10.

[29]   Alexopoulos GS, Meyers BS, Young RC, et al.: 'Vascular depression' hypothesis. *Arch Gen Psychiatry* 1997; 54:915-922.

[30]   Thomas AJ, Kalaria RN, O'Brien JT: Depression and vascular disease: what is the relationship? *J Affect Disord* 2004; 79:81-95.

[31]   Almeida OP, Flicker L, Norman P, et al.: Association of cardiovascular risk factors and disease with depression in later life. *Am J Geriatri Psychiatry* 2007; 15:506-513.

[32]   Lesperance F, Frasure-Smith N, Talajic M. Major depression before and after myocardial infarction: its nature and consequences. *Psychosomatic Medicine* 1996; 58(2): 99-110.

[33]   Regier DA, Narrow WE, Rae DS, et al.: The de facto mental and addictive disorders service system. Epidemiologic Catchment Area prospective 1-year prevalence rates of disorders and services. *Archives of General Psychiatry* 1993; 50(2): 85-94.

[34]   Aben I, Verhey F, Strik J, et al.: A comparative study into the one year cumulative incidence of depression after stroke and myocardial infarction. *J Neurol Neurosurg Psych* 2003; 74(5):581-585.

[35]   Burvill PW, Johnson GA, Jamrozik K, et al: The prevalence of depression following stroke: the Perth community stroke study. *Br J Psychiatry* 1995; 166:320-327.

[36]   McConnell S, Jacka FN, Williams LJ, Dodd S, Berk M: The relationship between depression and cardiovascular disease. *Int J Psychiat Clin Prac* 2005; 9(3):157-167.

[37]   Sherwood A, Blumenthal JA, Trivedi R, Johnson KS, O'Connor CM, Kirkwood FA, et al: Relationship of depression to death or hospitalization in patients with heart failure. *Arch Intern Med* 2007; 167:367-373.

[38]   Westlake C, Dracup K, Fonarow G, Hamilton M. Depression in patients with heart failure. *J Card Fail* 2005; 11:30-35.

[39]   Wulsin LR, Vaillant GE, Wells VE: A systematic review of the mortality of depression. *Psychosomat Med* 1999; 61:6-17.

[40]   Frasure-Smith N, Lesperance F, Talajic M: Depression and 18-month prognosis after myocardial infarction. *Circulation* 1995; 91:999-1005.

[41]   Wells KB, Burnam MA, Rogers W, et al.: The course of depression in adult outpatients. Results from the Medical Outcomes Study. *Arch Gen Psych* 1992; 49:788-794.

[42]   Van der Kooy KG, van Hout HP, van Marjijk HWJ, de Haan M et al: Differences in heart rate variability between depressed and non-depressed elderly. *Int J Geriatr Psychiatry* 2006; 21:147-150.

[43]   Ai, AL, Carrigan, LT: Social-Strata-Related cardiovascular health disparity and comorbidity in an aging society: Implications for professional care. *Health and Soc Work* 2007; 32(2):97-105.

[44]   Sheps DS, Sheffield D: Depression, anxiety, and the cardiovascular system: the cardiologist's perspective. *J Clin Psychiatry* 2001:62(Supp8):12-16.

[45]   Mykletun A, Bjerkeset O, Dewey M, Prince M et al: Anxiety, depression, and cause-specific mortality: the HUNT study. *Psychosom Med* 2007; 69(4):323-331.

[46]   Frasure-Smith N, Lesperance F, Juneau M et al: Gender, depression, and one-year prognosis after myocardial infarction. *Psychosomat Med* 1999; 61:26-37.

[47]   Kornstein SG: Gender differences in depression: implications for treatment. *J Clin Psychiatry* 1997; 58(supp15):12-18.

[48]   Grace SL, Abbey SE, Shnek ZM, Irvine J et al: Cardiac rehabilitation: review of psychosocial factors. *Gen Hosp Psychiatry* 2002; 24(3):121-126

[49]   Maier W, Gansicke M, Gater R, Rezaki M, Tiemens B et al: Gender differences in the prevalence of depression: a survey in primary care. *J Affect Disorders* 1999; 53:241-252.

[50]   Pinninelli M, Wilkinson G: Gender differences in depression: critical review. *British J Psychiatry* 2002; 177:486-492.

[51]   Weissman MM, bland R, Joyce PR, Newman S, Wells JE, Wittchen HU: Sex differences in rates of depression: cross-national perspectives. *J Affect Disorders* 1997; 29:77-84.

[52]   Wenger NK: You've come a long way, baby: Cardiovascular health and disease in women: Problems and prospects. *Circulation* 2004; 109(5):558-560.

[53]   Reis SE, Holubkov R, Smith JC et al: Coronary microvascular dysfunction is highly prevalent in women with chest pain the absence of coronary artery disease: Results from the NHLBI WISE study. *Am Heart J* 2001; 141:735-741.

[54]   Andrew MJ, Baker RA., Kneebone AC, et al.: Mood state as a predictor of neuropsychological deficits following cardiac surgery. *J Psychosomat Res* 2000; 48:537–546.

[55]   Boudrez H., De Backer, G: Psychological status and the role of coping style after coronary artery bypass graft surgery. Results of a prospective study. *Qual Life Res* 2001, 10, 37-47.

[56]   Mallik S, Krumholz HM, Lin ZQ, et al.: Patients with depressive symptoms have lower health status benefits after coronary artery bypass surgery. *Circulation* 2005; 111:271-277.

[57]   Ai, A.L, Peterson C, Bolling SF, Rodgers W: Depression, faith-based coping, and short-term post-operative global functioning in adult and older patients undergoing cardiac surgery. *J Psychosomat Res* 2006; 60:21-28.

[58]   Ai, AL, Peterson C, Tice T N, et al.: Differential effects of faith-based coping on physical and mental fatigue in adult and older cardiac patients. *Int J Psychiatr Med* 2006; 36(3), 347-361.

[59]   Moser DK, Dracup K: Is anxiety early after myocardial infarction associated with subsequent ischemic and arrhythmic events? *Psychosom Med* 1996; 58(5):395-401.

[60]   Fleet RP, Dupuis G, Martel JP, et al.: Two-year follow-up status of emergency department chest pain patients with panic disorder. *Psychosom Med* 1998; 60(1): 92.

[61]   Lynch P, Galbaraith KM: Panic in the emergency room. *Can J Psychiatr* 2003; 48(6):361-366.

[62]   Eaker ED, Sullivan, LM, Kelly-Hayes M, D'Agostino RB et al.: Tension and Anxiety and the Prediction of the 10-Year Incidence of Coronary Heart Disease, Atrial Fibrillation, and Total Mortality: The Framingham Offspring Study. *Psychosom Med* 2005; 67(5):692-696.

[63]   Paterniti S, Zureik M, Ducimetière P et al: Sustained Anxiety and 4-Year Progression of Carotid Atherosclerosis. *Arterios Thrombo Vasc Biol* 2001;21:136-141.

[64]   Vingerhoets G: Perioperative anxiety and depression in open-heart surgery. *Psychosom Med* 1998; 39:30-7.

[65]   Williams RB: Do benzodiazepines have a role in the prevention or treatment of coronary heart disease and other major disorders? *J Psychiatr Res* 1990; 24 (suppl 2):51-56.

[66]   Haines AP, Imeson JD: Phobic anxiety and ischemic heart disease. *British Med J* 1987; 295:297-299.

[67]   Kawachi I, Colditz GA, Ascherio A, et al.: Prospective study of phobic anxiety and risk of coronary heart disease in men. *Circulation* 1994; 89:1992-1997.

[68]   Kawachi I., Sparrow D, Vokonas PS, Weiss ST: Symptoms of anxiety and risk of coronary heart disease. The Normative Aging Study. *Circulation* 1994; 90:2225-2229.

[69]   Yan L, Liu K, Matthews KA et al.: Psychosocial Factors and Risk of Hypertension: The Coronary Artery Risk Development in Young Adults (CARDIA) Study. *JAMA* 2003; 290:2138-2148.

[70]   Ortega AN, Feldman JM, Canino G, Steinman K, Alegria M: Co-occurrence of mental and physical illness in US Latinos. *Soc Psychiatry and Psychatr Epidemiol* 2006; 41(12):927-934.

[71]   Kubzansky LD, Kawachi I, Weiss ST, Sparrow D: Anxiety and coronary heart disease: A synthesis of epidemiological, psychological, and experimental evidence. *Annals of Behavioral Medicine* 1998; 20:47–58.

[72]   Strike JJ H, Denollet J, Lousberg R, Honig A: Comparing symptoms of depression and anxiety as predictors of cardiac events and increased health care consumption after myocardial infarction. *JAm Coll Cardiol* 2003, 42(10):1801–1807.

[73]   Lynch J, Krause N, Kaplan GA et al.: Work place demands, economic reward, and progression of carotid atherosclerosis. *Circulation* 1997; 96:302-307.

[74]   Theorell T, Tsutsumi A, Hallquist J et al.: Decision latitude, job strain and myocardial infarction: A study of working men in Stockholm. *Am J Public Health* 1998; 88(3):382-388.

[75]   Holmes TH, Rahe RH: The social readjustment rating scale. *J Psychosom Res* 1967; 11(2):213-218.

[76]   Pignalber C, Patti G, Chimenti C et al.: Role of different determinants of psychological distress in acute coronary syndromes. *J Am Coll Cardiol* 1998; 32:613-619.

[77]   Leor J, Poole WK, Kloner RA: Sudden cardiac death triggered by an earthquake. *New England J Med* 1996; 334: 413-419.

[78]   Meisel SR, Kutz I, Dayan KI, et al.: Effects of Iraqui missile war on incidence of acute myocardial infarction and sudden death in Israeli civilians. *Lancet* 1991; 338:660-661.

[79]   Vale SL: Psychological distress and cardiovascular disease. *Postgrad Med J* 2005; 81(957):429-435.

[80]   Fleet RP, Arsenault A, Lespérance F, et al.: Panic disorder in coronary artery disease patients ins associate with reversible myocardial perfusion defects during panic challenge with 35%CO2 [abstract]. *Psychosom Med* 2001, 63:187.

[81]   Tennant C, McLean L: The impact of emotions on coronary heart disease risk. *J Cardiovas Risk* 2001, 8:175-183.

[82]   Schelling G, Kilger E, Roozendaal B, et al.: Stress doses of hydrocortisone, traumatic memories, and symptoms of posttraumatic stress disorder in patients after cardiac surgery: A randomized study. *Biol Psychiatry* 2004; 55:627-633.

[83]   Stoll C, Schelling G, Goetz AE, et al.: Health-related quality of life and posttraumatic stress disorder in patients after cardiac surgery and intensive care treatment. *J Thorac Cardiovas Surg* 2000; 120:505-512.

[84]   Ai AL, Peterson C, Tice TN, Huang BC et al.: The influence of prayer on mental health among cardiac surgery patients: The role of optimism and acute distress symptoms. *J Health Psychol* 2007; 12(4):580-596.

[85]   Williams RB: Do benzodiazepines have a role in the prevention or treatment of coronary heart disease and other major medical disorders? *J Psychiatr Res* 1990; suppl 2, 24:51-56.

[86]   Burg M M., Jain D, Soufer R, et al.: Role of behavioral and psychological factors in mental stress-induced silent left ventricular dysfunction in coronary artery disease. *J Am Coll Cardiology* 1993; 22:440-448.

[87]   Gidron Y, Davidson K, Bata I: The short-term effects of a hostility-reduction intervention in CHD patients. *Health Psychology* 1999; 18:416-420.

[88]   Niaura R, Todaro J, Stroud L, Spiro A, et al.: Hostility, the metabolic syndrome, and incident coronary heart disease. *Health Psychol* 2002; 21(6):588-593.

[89]   J Julkunen, R Salonen, GA Kaplan, MA Chesney, and JT Salonen: Hostility and the progression of carotid atherosclerosis. *Psychosom Med* 1994;56(6): 519-525.

[90]   Matsumoto Y, Uyama O, Shimizu S, Michishita H et al.: Do anger and aggression affect carotid atherosclerosis? *Stroke* 1993 ;24:983-986.

[91]   Gallacher JEJ, Yarnell JWG, Sweetnam PM, Elwood PC et al.: Anger and Incident Heart Disease in the Caerphilly Study. *Psychosom Me*d 1999;61(4): 446-453.

[92]   Kawachi I, Sparrow D, Kubzansky LD, Spiro A et al.: Prospective study of a self-report type A scale and risk of coronary heart disease. *Circulation* 1998; 98:405-412.

[93]   Krantz DS, Olson MB, Francis JL, Phankao C: Anger, hostility, and cardiac symptoms in women with suspected coronary artery disease: The Women's Ischemia Syndrome Evaluation (WISE) Study. *Journal of Women's Health* 2006, 15(10):1214-1223.

[94]   Miller TQ, Smith TW, Turner CW, Guijarro ML et al.: A meta-analytic review of research on hostility and physical health. *Psychol Bull* 1996;119(2):322-348.

[95]   Eaker ED, Sullivan LM, Kelly-Hayes M, D'Agostino RB et al: Anger and hostility predict the development of atrial fibrillation in men in the Framingham Offspring study. *Circulation* 2004;109:1267-1271.

[96]   Chang PP, Ford DE, Meoni LA, Wang NY et al.: Anger in young men and subsequent premature cardiovascular disease: The precursors study. *Arch Intern Med* 2002;162:901-906.

[97]   Williams JE, Paton CC, Siegler IC, Eigenbrodt ML et al.: Anger proneness predicts coronary heart disease risk: Prospective analysis from the atherosclerosis risk in community (ARIC) study. *Circulation.* 2000;101:2034-2039.

[98]   Knox SS, Adelman A, Ellison RC, Arnett DK et al.: Hostility, social support, and carotid artery atherosclerosis in The National Heart, Lung, and Blood Institute Family Heart Study. *Am J Cardiol* 2000; 86(10):1086-1089.

[99]   Chaput LA, Adams SH, Simon JA, Blumenthal RS et al.: Hostility predicts recurrent events among postmenopausal women with coronary heart disease. *Am J Epidemiol* 2002; 156(12):1092-1099.

[100]   Helmers KF, Krantz DS, Howell RH, Klein J et al.: Hostility and myocardial ischemia in coronary artery disease patients: evaluation by gender and ischemic index. *Psychosom Med* 1993; 55(1): 29-36.

[101]   Olson MB, Krantz DS, Kelsey SF, Pepine CJ et al.: Hostility scores are associated with increased risk of cardiovascular events in women undergoing coronary angiography: A report from the NHLBI-sponsored WISE study. *Psychosom Med* 2005; 67: 546-552.

[102]   Williams JE, Nieto FJ, Sanford CP, Couper DJ et al.: The association between trait anger and incident stroke risk: The atherosclerosis risk in communities (ARIC) study. *Stroke* 2002; 33:13-20.

[103]   Suarez EC: Joint Effect of hostility and severity of depressive symptoms on plasma interleukin-6 concentration. *Psychosom Med* 2003;65: 523-527.

[104]   Schulman JK, Stromberg S: On the value of doing nothing: Anger and cardiovascular disease in clinical practice. *Cardiol in Rev* 2007; 15:123-132.

[105]   Denollet J: Type D personality: A potential risk factor refined. *J Psychosom Res* 2000; 49:255-266.

[106]   Denollet J, Brutsaert DL: Personality, disease severity, and the risk of long-term cardiac events in patients with a decreased ejection fraction after myocardial infarction. *Circulation* 1998; 97:167-173.

[107]   Denollet J, Vaes J, Brutsaert DL: Inadequate response to treatment in coronary heart disease: Adverse effects of type D personality and younger age on a 5-year prognosis and quality of life. *Circulation* 2000; 102:630-635.

[108]   Sher L: Type D personality: the heart, stress, and cortisol. *QJM* 2005; 98: 323-329.

[109]   Jarett DB, Lloyd-Jones DM, Garside DB, Wang R et al.: Social avoidance and long-term risk for cardiovascular disease death in healthy men: The Western Electric Study. *Ann Epidemiol* 2007; 17(8):591-596.

[110]   Anda R, Williamson D, Jones D, Macera C et al: Depressed affect, hopelessness, and the risk of ischemic heart disease in a cohort of U.S. adults. *Epidemiol* 1993; 4:285-294.

[111]   Everson SA, Goldberg DE, Kaplan, GA Cohen RD et al.:.Hopelessness and risk of mortality and incidence of myocardial infarction and cancer. *Psychosom Med* 1996;58:113-121.

[112]   Schwarz AM, Schächinger H, Adler RH, Goetz SM: Hopelessness as Associated with decreased heart rate variability during championship chess games. *Psychosom Med* 2003;65: 658-661.

[113]   Stern SL, Dhanda R, Hazuda HP: Hopelessness predicts mortality in older Mexican and European Americans. *Psychosom Med* 2001;63: 344-351.

[114]   Everson SA, Kaplan GA, Goldberg GE, Salonen R et al.: Hopelessness and 4-year progression of carotid atherosclerosis: The Kuopio ischemic heart disease risk factor study. *Arterioscler Thromb Vasc Biol* 1997;17:1490-1495.

[115]   Carney RM, Freedland KE, Miller J et al: Depression as a risk factor for cardiac mortality and morbidity: A review of potential mechanisms. *J Psychosom Res* 2002, 53, 897-902.

[116]   Fraguas R, Iosifescu DV, Bankier B, Perlis R et al.: Major depressive disorder with anger attacks and cardiovascular risk factors. *Int J Psychiatr Me*d 2007; 37(1):99-111.

[117]   DiMatteo MR, Lepper HS, Croghan TW: Depression is a risk factor for noncompliance with medical treatment: Meta-analysis of the effects of anxiety and depression on patient adherence. *Arch Intern Med* 2000; 160:2101-2107.

[118]   Musselman DL, Evans DL, Nemeroff CB: The relationship of depression to cardiovascular disease: Epidemiology, biology, and treatment. *Arch Gen Psych* 1998; 55:580-592.

[119]   Singh RB, Kartik C, Otsuka K, Pella D, Pella J: Brain-heart connection and the risk of heart attack. *Biomed Pharmacother* 2002; 56(2suppl):257s-265s.

[120]   Van der Kooy K, van Hout H, Marjijk H, Marten H et al: Depression and the risk for cardiovascular diseases: systematic review and meta analysis. *Int J Geriatric Psychia* 2007; 22(7):613-626.

[121]   Musselman DL, Tomer A, Manatunga AK, Kinght BT et al.: Exaggerated platelet reactivity in major depression. *Am J Psychiatr* 1996; 153:1313-1317.

[122]   Laghrissi-Thode F, Wagner WE, Pollock BG, Johnson PC et al.: Elevated platelet factor 4 and beta-thromoglobulin plasma levels in depressed patients with ischemic heart disease. *Biol Psychiatr* 1997; 42:290-295

[123]   Study of the effectiveness of additional reductions in cholesterol and homocysteine (SEARCH): Characteristics of a randomized trial among 12,064 myocardial infarction survivors. *Am Heart J* 2007, 154(5):815-823.

[124]   Mischoulon D, Raab MR: The role of folate in depression and dementia. *J Clin Psychiatr* 2007; 68(suppl 10):28-33.

[125]   Roberts SH, Bedson E, Hughes DA, Lloyd KR, et al: Folate Augmentation of treatment- evaluation for depression (FolATED): Protocol of a randomized controlled trial. *BMC Psychiatr* 2007; 7:65.

[126]   Williams A, Girard C, Jui D, Sabina Am et al.: S-Adenolosylmethionine (SAMe) as treatment for depression: A systematic review. *Clin Invest Med* 2005; 28(3):132-139.

[127]   Carney R: Omega-3 acids to improve depression and reduce cardiovascular risk factors.   Accessed   November   27,   2007 htt://clinicaltrials.gov/ct2/show/NCT00116857.

[128]   Anisman H, Merali Z: Cytokines, stress, and depressive illness. *Brain Behav Immun* 2006; 16:513-524.

[129]   Black PH, Garbutt LD: Stress, inflammation and cardiovascular disease. *J Psychosom Res* 2002; 52:1-23.

[130] Miller GE, Blackwell E: Turning up the heat: Inflammation as a mechanism linking chronic stress, depression and heart disease. *Curr Dir Psychol Sci* 2006,15(6):269-272.

[131] Mosovich SA. Boone RT, Reichenber A, Bansilal S, et al: New insights into the link between cardiovascular disease and depression. *Int J Clin Prac* 2007; doi 10.1111:1-10.

[132] Appels A, Bar FW, Bar J, Bruggeman C, De Baets M: Inflammation, depressive symptomatology, and coronary artery disease. *Psychosom Med* 2000; 62:601-605.

[133] Pasic J, Levy WC, Sullivan MD: Cytokines in depression and heart failure. *Psychosom Med* 2003;65:181-193.

[134] Dantzer R, Wollman E, Vitkovic L, Yirmiya R: Cytokines and depression: fortuitous or causative association? *Molec Psychiatr* 1999; 4(4): 328-332.

[135] Libby P, Ridker PM: Novel inflammatory markers of coronary risk: Theory versus practice. *Circulation* 1999;100(11):1148-1150.

[136] Libby P, Theroux P: Pathophysiology of coronary artery disease. *Circulation* 2005;111:3481-3488.

[137] Rauch B, Schiele R, Schneider S, Gohlke H et al: Highly purified omega-3 fatty acids for secondary prevention of sudden cardiac death after myocardial infarction-aims and methods of the OMEGA study. *Cardiovasc Drugs Ther* 2006; 20:365-375.

[138] Capuron L, Miller AH: Cytokines and psychopathology: Lessons from interferon-α. *Biol Psychiatr* 2004, 56(11):819-824.

[139] Danner M, Kasl SV, Abramson JL, Vaccarino V: Association between depression and elevated C-reactive protein. *Psychosom Med* 2003; 65:347-356.

[140] Kop WJ, Gottdiener JS, Tangen CM, Fried LP, et al.: Inflammation and coagulation factors in persons >65 years of age with symptoms of depression but without evidence of myocardial ischemia. *Am J Cardiol* 2002; 89:419-424.

[141] Penninx BWJ, Kritchevsky SB, Yaffe K, Newman AB: Inflammatory markers and depressed mood in older persons: results from the health, aging and body composition study. *Biological Psychiatr* 2003, 54(5):566-572.

[142] Zoririlla EP, Luborsky L, McKay JR, Rosenthal R: The relationship of depression and stressors to immunological assays: A meta-analytic review. *Brain, Behav Immun* 2001; 15:199-226.

[143] Empana JP, Sykes DH, Luc G, Juhan-Vague I, et al.: Contributions of Depressive Mood and Circulating Inflammatory Markers to Coronary Heart Disease in Healthy European Men: The Prospective Epidemiological Study of Myocardial Infarction (PRIME). *Circulation* 2005; 111:2299-2305.

[144] Miller GE, Stetler CA, Carney RM, Freedland KE, et al.: Clinical depression and inflammatory risk markers for coronary heart disease. *Am J Cardiol* 2002; 90:1279-1983.

[145] Shimbo D, Chaplin W, Crossman D, Hass D, et al.: Role of Depression and Inflammation in Incident Coronary Heart Disease Events. *Am J Cardiol* 2005; 96(7):1016-1021.

[146] Vaccarino V, Johnson BD, Sheps DS, Reis SE, et al.: Depression, inflammation, and incident cardiovascular disease in women with suspected coronary ischemia: The

National Heart, Lung, and Blood Institute–sponsored WISE study. *J Am Coll Cardiol* 2007; 50(21):2044-2050.

[147]   Watkins LL, Grossman P, Krishman R, Sherwood A: Anxiety and vagal control of heart rate. *Psychosom Med* 1998; 60:498-502.

[148]   Bjork JM, Dougherty DM, Moeller FG: Symtomatology of depression and anxiety in female 'social drinker'. *Am J Drug Alc Abuse* 1999; 25(1): 173-182.

[149]   Black DW, Zimmerman M, Coryell WH: Cigarette smoking and psychiatric disorder in a community sample. *Ann Clin Psychiatr* 1999; 11(3): 129-136.

[150]   Stoney CM: Plasma homocysteine levels increase in women during psychological stress. *Life Sci* 1999; 64(25):2359-2365.

[151]   Ueland PM, Refsum H: Plasma homocysteine, a risk factor for vascular disease: Plasma levels in health, disease, and drug therapy. *J Lab Clin Med* 1989; 114:473-501.

[152]   Heinz A, Hermann D, Smolka MN, Rieks M, et al.: Effects of acute psychological stress on adhesion molecules, interleukins and sex hormones: implications for coronary heart disease. *Psychopharm* 2003; 165(2):111-117.

[153]   Owen N, Poulton T, Hay FC, Mohamed-Ali V, et al.: Socioeconomic status, C-reactive protein, immune factors, and responses to acute mental stress. *Brain Behav Immun* 2003;17:286-295.

[154]   Bierhaus A, Wolf J, Andrassy M, Rohleder N, et al.: A mechanism converting psychosocial stress into mononuclear cell activation. *Proc Natl Acad Sci US Am* 2003; 100:1920-1925.

[155]   Murray DR, Prabhu SD, Chandrasekar B: Chronic ß-Adrenergic Stimulation Induces Myocardial Proinflammatory Cytokine Expression. *Circulation.* 2000;101:2338-2341.

[156]   Matthews KA, Owens JF, Kuller LH, Sutton-Tyrrell K, et al.: Are Hostility and Anxiety Associated With Carotid Atherosclerosis in Healthy Postmenopausal Women? *Psychosom Med* 1998; 60:633-638.

[157]   Räikkönen K, Matthews KA, Sutton-Tyrrell K, Kuller LH: Trait anger and the metabolic syndrome predict progression of carotid atherosclerosis in healthy middle-aged women. *Psychosom Med* 2004; 66: 903-908.

[158]   Anderson DE, Metter EJ, Hougaku H., Najjar SS: Suppressed anger is associated with increased carotid arterial stiffness in older adults. *Am J Hyperten* 2006; 19(11):1129-1134.

[159]   Suarez EC: Joint effect of hostility and severity of depressive symptoms on plasma interleukin-6 concentration. *Psychosom Med* 2003; 65: 523-527.

[160]   Krantz DS, McCeney MK: Effects of psychological and social factors on organic disease: A critical assessment of research on coronary heart disease. *Ann Rev Psychol* 2002; 53:341-369.

[161]   Rutledge T, Reis SE, Olson M, Owens J, et al.: Psychosocial variables are associated with atherosclerosis risk factors among women with chest Pain: The WISE study. *Psychosom Med* 2001; 63: 282-288.

[162] Fraguas R, Papakostas GI, Mischoulon D, Bottiglieri T, et al.: Anger attacks in major depressive disorder and serum levels of homocysteine. *Biol Psychiatr* 2006; 60(3):270-274.

[163] Peterson C: The future of optimism. *Am Psychol* 2000; 55:44-55.

[164] Ai AL, Peterson C, Bolling SF, Koenig H: Private prayer and the optimism of middle-age and older patients awaiting cardiac surgery. *The Gerontologist* 2002; 42:70-81.

[165] Carver CS, Spencer SM, Scheier MF: Optimism, motivation, and mental health. In N.S. Friedman (Ed), *Encyclopedia of mental health* (Vol.3, pp.41-52). San Diego, CA: Academic Press.

[166] Shen B-J, McCreary CP, Myers HF: Independent and mediated contributions of personality, coping, social support, and depressive symptoms to physical functioning outcome among patients in cardiac rehabilitation. *J Behav Med* 2004; 27(1):39-62.

[167] Bedi G, Brown SL: optimism, coping style and emotional well-being in cardiac patients. *Brit J Health Psychol* 2005; 10:57-70.

[168] Giltany EJ, Geleijnse JM, Zitman FG et al: Dispositional optimism and all-cause and cardiovascular mortality in a prospective cohort of elderly Dutch men and women. *Arch Gen Psychiatry* 2004; 61:1126-1135.

[169] Helgeson VS, Fritz HL: Cognitive adaptation as a predictor of new coronary events after percutaneous tranluminal coronary angioplasty. *Psychosom Med* 1999; 61:488-495.

[170] Pirraglia PA, Peterson JC, Williams-Russo P et al: Depressive symptomatology in coronary artery bypass graft surgery patients. *Ann Thoracic Surg* 1999; 14:668-680.

[171] Sykes DH, Hanley M, Boyle DM et al: Work strain and the post-discharge adjustment of patients following a heart attack. *Psychol Health* 2000; 15:609-623.

[172] van Elderen T, Maes S, Dusseldorp E: Coping with coronary heart disease: A longitudinal study. *J Psychosom Res* 1999; 47:175-183.

[173] Ai AL, Park C, Huang B, Rodgers W, Tice TN: Psychosocial mediation of religious coping: A prospective study of short-term psychological distress after cardiac surgery. *Personal and Soc Psychology Bulletin* 2007; 33(6):867-882.

[174] Lewis SC, Dennis MS, O'Rourke S J, Sharpe, M: Negative attitudes among short-term stroke survivors predict worse long-term survival. *Stroke* 2001; 32:1640-1645.

[175] Sarker U, Sadia A, Whooley MA: Self-efficacy and health status in patients with coronary heart disease: Findings from the heart and soul study. *Psychosom Med* 2007; 69:306-312.

[176] Oxman TE, Hull JG: Social support, depression, and activities of daily living in older heart surgery patients. *J Geron Psychol Sci* 1997; 52b:1-14.

[177] Krause N, Ellis Oxman TE, Hull JG: Social support, depression, and activities of daily living in older heart surgery patients. *J Geron Psychol* Sci 1997; 52B:1-14.

[178] Krause N: Church-based social support and health in old age: Exploring variations by race. *J Gerontol* 2002; 57B:S332-S347.

[179] Powell LH., Shahabi L, Thoresen, CE: Religion and spirituality: Linkages to physical health. *Am Psychol* 2003, 58, 36-52.

[180]   Hughes JW, Sketeh MH, Watkins LL: Social support and religiosity as coping strategies for anxiety in hospitalized cardiac patients. *Ann Behav Med* 2004; 24:179-185.

[181]   Oxman TE, Freeman DH, Manheimer ED: Lack of social participation or religious strength and comfort as risk factors for death after cardiac surgery in the elderly. *Psychosom Med* 1995; 57:5-15.

[182]   Contrada RJ, Goyal TM, Cather C, Rafalson L et al.: Psychosocial factors in outcomes of heart surgery: the impact of religious involvement and depressive symptoms. *Health Psychol* 2004; 23: 227-238.

[183]   Stanek EJ, Oates MB, McGhan WF, Denofrio D, Loh E: Preferences for treatment outcomes in patients with heart failure: Symptoms versus survival. *J Cardiol Fail* 2000; 6(3):225-232.

[184]   Newman S: The psychological perspective: a professional view. *Heart* 2003; 89(Suppl2):ii16-18.

[185]   Screening for depression: recommendations and rationale. U.S. Preventive Services Task Force. *Annals Int Med* 2002; 136(10):760-764.

[186]   Adams K, Corrigan JM, eds: Priority areas for national action: Transforming health care quality. Washington, DC: The National Academic Press, 2003.

[187]   Chung H, Teresi J, Guarnacci P, Meyers BS, Holmes D et al: Depressive symptoms and psychiatric distress in low income Asian and Latino primary care patients: Prevalence and recognition. *Comm Ment Health J* 2003; 39(1):33-46.

[188]   Brown C, Abe-Kim JS, Barrio C: Depression in ethnically diverse women: Implications for treatment in primary care settings. *Prof Psych: Res and Prac* 2003; 34(1): 10-19.

[189]   Gilbody S, Whitty P, Grimshaw J, Thomas R: Educational and organizational interventions to improve the management of depression in primary care. *JAMA* 2003; 289(23):3145-3151.

[190]   Beck AT, Steer RA, Ball R, Ranieri WF: Comparison of Beck Depression Ineventories-IA and –II in Psychiatric Outpatients. *J Personal Assess* 1996; 67(3):588-597.

[191]   Ensel, W. Measuring depression: The CES-D Scale. *Social Support, Life Events and Depression.* N. Lin, A. Dean and W. M. Ensel. New York: Academic Press, 1986.

[192]   Hofer S, Lim L, Guyatt G, Oldridge N: The MacNew heart disease health-related quality of life instrument: A summary. Health and Quality of Life Outcomes 2004. Retrieved October 3, 2007 from http://www.hqlo.com/content/pdf/1477-7525-2-3.pdf

[193]   Hunt SA, Baker DW, Chin MH et al: ACC/AHA guidelines for the evaluation and management of chronic heart failure in the adult: Executive summary: A report of the American College of Cardiology, American Heart Association Task Force on Practice Guidelines. *J Am Coll Cardiol* 2001; 38:2101-2113.

[194]   Berkman LF, Blumenthal J, Burg M et al: Effects of treating depression and low perceived social support on clinical events after myocardial infarction: The Enhancing Recovery in Coronary Heart Disease Patients (ENRICHD) Randomized Trial. *JAMA* 2003; 289:3106-3116.

[195]   Serebruany VL, Suckow RF, Cooper TB et al: Sertraline antidepressant Heart Attack Randomized Trial. Relationship between release of platelet/endothelial biomarkers and plasma levels of sertraline and N-desmehtylsertraline in acute coronary syndrome patients receiving SSRI treatment for depression. *Am J Psychiatr* 2005; 162:1165-1170.

[196]   Shah SU, Iqbal Z, White A, White S: Heart and mind: psychotropic and cardiovascular therapeutics. *Postgrad Med J* 2005; 81(951):33-40.

[197]   Lesperance F, Frasure-Smith N, Koszycki D, Laliberte M-A: Effects of Citalopram and Interpersonal Psychotherapy on Depression in Patients with Coronary Artery Disease. *JAMA* 2007; 297:367-379.

[198]   Fuchs E, Czeh B, Flugge G: Examining novel concepts of the pathophysiology of depression in the chronic psychosocial stress paradigm in tree shrews. *Behav Pharmacol* 2004; 15:315-325.

[199]   Glassman AH, O'Connor CM, Califf RM et al: Sertraline treatment of major depression inpatients with acute MI or unstable angina. *JAMA* 2002; 288:701-709.

[200]   Tuglu C, Kara SH, Caliyurt P, Vardar E, Abay E: Increased serum tumor necrosis factor-alpha levels and treatment response in major depressive disorder. *Psychopharm* 2003; 170:429-433.

[201]   Swenson JR, O'Connor CM, Barton D, Van Zyl LT, et al.: Influence of depression and effect of treatment with sertraline on quality of life after hospitalization for acute coronary syndrome. *Am J Cardiol* 2003;92:1271-1276.

[202]   ENRICHD Investigators: Effects of treating depression and low perceived social support on clinical events after -myocardial infarction: the Enhancing Recovery in Coronary Heart Disease Patients (ENRICHD) Randomized Trial. *JAMA* 2003; 289(23), 3106-16.

[203]   Serebruany VL, Glassman AH, Malinin AI, Nemeroff CB, et al.: Platelet/endothelial biomarkers in depressed patients treated with the selective serotonin reuptake inhibitor sertraline after acute coronary events: The sertraline antidepressant heart attack randomized trial (SADHART) platelet substudy. *Circulation* 2003; 108:939-944.

[204]   Schatzberg AF, Rush AJ, Arnow BA et al: Chronic depression: Medication or psychotherapy is effective when the other is not. *Arch Gen Psychiatry* 2005; 62:513-520.

[205]   ENRICHD Investigators: Enhancing recovery in coronary heart disease (ENRICHD) study intervention: Rationale and design. *Psychosom Med* 2001; 63(5):747-755.

[206]   Van Voorhees BW, Walters AE, Prochaska M, Quinn MT: Reducing health disparities in depressive disorders process of care and outcomes between whites and ethnic minorities: Call for a comprehensive and pragmatic approach. *Med Care Res Rev* 2007; 64(Suppl):157S-194S.

[207]   American Heart Association 2002. *Heart and stroke statistical update*. Dallas, TX: American heart Association.

[208]   Irvine J, Ritvo P: Health risk behavior change and adaptation in cardiac patients. *Clin Psychol Psychother* 1998; 5:86-101.

[209] Katon W, Von Korkoff M, Lin E, Simon G, Walker E, et al: Stepped collaborative care for primary care patients with persistent symptoms of depression: A randomized trial. *Arch Gen Psychiatr* 1999; 56:1109-1115.

[210] Lobo CM, Frijling BD, Hulscher ME, Bernsen RM, et al.: Effect of a comprehensive intervention program targeting general practice staff on quality of life in patients at high cardiovascular risk: a randomized controlled trial. *Qual Life Res* 2004;13:73-80.

INDEX

B

C

D

E

I

N

O

U

V